Audiology Business and Practice Management

Audiology Business and Practice Management

Holly Hosford-Dunn, Ph.D.

Daniel R. Dunn, M.B.A.

Earl R. Harford, Ph.D.

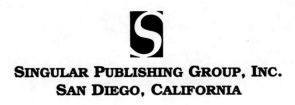

SINGULAR PUBLISHING GROUP, INC.
SAN DIEGO, CALIFORNIA

A Volume in the
Singular Publishing Group
Audiology Series
Series Editor
Jeffrey L. Danhauer, Ph.D.

Singular Publishing Group, Inc.
4284 41st Street
San Diego, California 92105-1197

© 1995 by Singular Publishing Group, Inc.

Typeset in 10/12 Bookman by So Cal Graphics
Printed in the United States of America by McNaughton & Gunn

Library of Congress Cataloging-in-Publication Data
Hosford-Dunn, Holly.
    Audiology Business and Practice Management / by Holly Hosford-Dunn,
Daniel R. Dunn, and Earl Harford.
       p.   cm.
    Includes bibliographical references and index.
    ISBN 1-56593-345-1
    1. Audiology—Practice—Handbooks, manuals, etc. I. Dunn, Daniel R.
II. Harford, Earl R. III. Title.
    [DNLM: 1. Audiology. 2. Private Practice—organization & administration.
WV 270 H825h 1995]
RF291.H67   1995
617.8'0068—dc20
DNLM/DLC
for Library of Congress
                                                    94-24043
                                                     CIP

Contents

Foreword

As audiology moves into the 21st century, one of the most dramatic trends will be the growth of private practitioners. In a very real sense private practice will form the financial foundation for the profession. When we first formed the American Academy of Audiology, in 1988, our initial survey showed that only 25% of members identified themselves as private practitioners. By the year 2000, however, it is estimated that more than 50% of all audiologists will be in private practice. It is widely lamented, however, that audiology training programs are notoriously deficient in preparing students for the private-practice arena. The audiologist who contemplates private practice has been ill-prepared for the vicissitudes of the business world and typically doesn't know where to turn for help.

In this volume authors Holly Hosford-Dunn, Daniel Dunn and Earl Harford confront the problem directly. They begin with an insightful analysis of the broad philosophical currents through which the audiological vessel seeks to steer a successful course, then move into the principles involved in becoming an autonomous provider. The bulk of the book, however, deals with the many very specific issues of day-to-day practice, like marketing, pricing, and reimbursement which confront the private practitioner on a day-to-day basis.

All three authors are eminently qualified for this task. Both Holly and Earl have successfully made the transition from traditional academic audiological environments into private audiological practice. Both know what it is to make a payroll. Both know the bottom line. Their professional expertise is well complemented by the business know-how of Daniel Dunn, an MBA and licensed investment advisor with more than 28 years of experience in computers, staff, business, and financial planning and management. This is virtually the only book of its kind available to audiologists. If you are contemplating private practice you really cannot do without it. If you are in private practice you will find much here that can help you to do a better job. But the most important audience for this book will be those of us in the academic/training program milieu who need to know a lot more about the world of private audiological practice.

James Jerger
Division of Audiology & Speech Pathology
Baylor College of Medicine

Preface

The purpose of this book is to explain sound business and practice management principles and procedures in the independent practice of audiology and relate them to the broader context of patient care. Whenever possible, the text relies on practical examples and eschews theoretical approaches. Much of the discussion is applicable to many audiology settings of varying degrees of autonomy, not just the owner-operated, independent practices that fit the traditional definition of private practice.

From necessity, however, much of the "business" of audiology has been pioneered by dispensing audiologists who have founded and operated their own practices. The text's organizational structure reflects their pioneering efforts. Each chapter covers a specific topic that practitioners will encounter at some point in developing and/or operating practices. Because each chapter is self-contained, the book need not be read cover to cover. However, the chapters are arranged in a loose order that is meant to reflect the sequence in which the topics are encountered in real life. Ideally, the book should serve as a text that is read cover to cover by graduate students or audiologists contemplating a move to independent practice or management careers. It should serve as a reference handbook for audiologists who are managing practices or have their own practices.

Chapter 1 presents the recurring theme that pervades the book: that the foundations of practice autonomy are professional responsibility and management ability. It provides an historical perspective of the evolution of audiology as a profession, looks at where we stand currently, and concludes with recommendations for achieving full autonomy in the coming years.

Chapters 2 and 3 examine internal and external factors that shape the manner in which audiologists practice audiology. These two chapters use personal and societal examples to echo the recurring autonomy theme. Chapter 2 describes five generic audiology practice models that exist in today's market, discussing them in terms of the possibilities for autonomy that they offer practitioners. Chapter 3 looks at how personal attributes and inclinations affect practitioners' career choices in audiology.

Chapter 4 explains how to create a business plan and make it the backbone of a practice. This chapter also serves as the foundation of the book, outlining the general topics that make up the remaining chapters. All readers will benefit from reading Chapter 4 before proceeding to specific topics of interest.

Legal concerns associated with establishing practices are discussed in Chapters 5, 6, and 8. Chapter 5 describes the ways in which audiology practices can legally organize. Arriving at a name, designing a logo, and getting a practice properly registered are addressed in Chapter 6. Chapter 8 and its appendix review the basics of negotiating and writing a lease.

The physical practice is "built" in Chapters 7 through 10. Chapters 7 and 8 focus, respectively, on finding the right place for the practice and securing the location, Chapter 9 goes over office design and equipment needs, and Chapter 10 looks at the computer options available to streamline office function through automation.

Chapter 11 and its appendixes survey the all-important topic of staff planning. This chapter covers recruiting, selection, hiring, orientation, training, and termination procedures. The role of leadership is stressed to audiologists who find themselves in management positions.

A variety of financial issues connect Chapters 12 through 16. Basic accounting and financial management are covered in Chapter 12. Marketing theory is considered at length in Chapter 13, with special emphasis on practical implementation and continuous quality improvement for professional practices. Chapter 14 is really an extension of Chapter 13, but focused entirely on the marketing component of pricing. The financial section concludes with Chapters 15 and 16. Respectively, these two very different chapters address (a) reimbursement issues that audiologists currently face, and (b) new reimbursement issues that we will face as managed competition predominates.

Chapters 17, 18, and 19 are about protecting the audiologist and the practice. Chapter 17 sets out 12 legal guidelines for avoiding legal action, then offers three test cases to illustrate what happens when guidelines are neglected. Chapter 18 informs audiologists and practice owners on steps that are necessary for sound financial planning, including qualified retirement plans for private practices. In a related vein, Chapter 19 discusses methods and considerations for handling the purchase and sale of the independent audiologist's most important financial asset—the practice itself.

The book concludes as it began. Chapter 20 stresses the need for audiologists to learn and develop management skills. The chapter gives a brief history of the development and evolution of management theory. It then examines health care in the 1990s, depicting the opportunities for autonomy that await audiologists who learn about management and the pitfalls that await those who do not expand their training to embrace management concepts, but instead, remain simply as technicians.

Throughout the chapters, a mythical private practice—Cardinal Hearing Services (CHS)—is defined and developed through sample documents, figures, and appendixes. It serves as a convenient and cohesive model for illustrating many of the varied aspects of practice management in self-sustaining, independent audiology settings. Typical management problems crop up periodically as the book progresses and CHS grows. A few of these management problems are described and analyzed in "scenarios." Each scenario includes a series of questions posed to the reader to stimulate thinking about practice management, and suggested answers.

Acknowledgments

A book that takes on as many topics as this one does cannot be written by a few people working in isolation. The final product reflects direct and indirect inputs from many, many people, including people who have taught us, supervised us, worked with us, provided us books and products, and those who have received our services. Although we cannot begin to name them all, we wish to thank all of those people who (perhaps unknowIngly) have contributed to our understanding of how we conduct ourselves as audiology professionals.

Among those who have given their time directly to this project, we would like to give special thanks to the following:

REVIEWERS

Mark Brenzel, Chief Administrator, Northwest Hospital, Tucson, AZ

Donald A. Chaney, CPA and Attorney in private practice, Tucson, AZ

Jim Curran, M.A., Senior Audiologist, Starkey Laboratories

Jeffrey Danhauer, Ph.D., Audiology Editor, Singular Press, San Diego, CA

Alan Desmond, M.A., Owner/Founder, Princeton Audiology, Princeton, WV

Theodore Glattke, Ph.D. Professor, Department of Hearing and Speech Sciences, University of Arizona

Emma Hestand, CPA, Holm & Hestand, Tucson, AZ

Philip L. Hosford, Ed.D., Professor Emeritus, Department of Education, New Mexico State University, Las Cruces, NM

James Jerger, Ph.D., Professor & Head, Division of Audiology and Speech Pathology, Baylor College of Medicine, Houston, TX

Cheryl Runge, M.S., Owner/Founder, Southwest Audiology Institute, Phoenix, AZ

Earl D. Schubert, Ph.D., Professor Emeritus, Hearing Sciences, Stanford University, Stanford, CA

CHAPTER CONTRIBUTORS

Donald A. Chaney, CPA JD

Jack T. Diamond, JD

Terry Griffing

Herbert McCollom, M.A.

Joel Mynders

David Weil, MBA JD

Alexander Woods, MD JD

GENERAL CONTRIBUTIONS, INCLUDING REALLY GOOD IDEAS

Donald Heckerman, Ph.D., Professor of Economics, University of Arizona, Tucson, AZ

Ray Katz, Owner, Katz Hearing Aids, Tucson, AZ

Evey Cherow, M.A., and Mark Kander, MHA, American Speech-Language-Hearing Association, Rockville, MD

Phil Korbas, Owner, MEDI Corp., Benecia, CA

Hector Maese, Owner/Founder, Hector the Hair Stylist, Las Cruces, NM

Kurt Pfaff, M.A., Owner, Hearing Care Specialists, Inc., St. Lous Park MN

From Starkey Labs:

Mike Bastyr
Jim Curran
Randy Drullinger
Larry Greely
Marian Halvorson
Pat Moore
Eric Peterson
Rob Thompson
Dale Thorstad

From Tucson Audiology (past and present):

Maryanne Bellissima, M.S.
Mary K. Gansheimer, M.S.
Barbara Green, LPN
Kresent O. Gurtler, M.A.
Pat Perkins

From Singular Publishing Group, Inc.:

Sadanand Singh
Angie Singh
Marie Linvill
Sandy Doyle
Randy Stevens

Finally, special thanks and appreciation to our families, who were consistently inquisitive and enthusiastic in their support:

Jennifer Fox and Leslie Harford-Fox
Andrew and Daniel Dunn

Appendixes

1

Toward the Era of Autonomous Audiology

OVERVIEW

- Seeds of the Profession
  Our Educational Heritage
  Professional Organization
  The Job Market
  The Hearing Aid

- Historical Summary

- Where Are We Now?

- Where Do We Go From Here?

Autonomous Audiology

"The ascendancy of treatment has made audiology a more balanced hearing health care profession..."

As we approach the 21st century, the profile of audiology differs distinctly from earlier days:

- Growing numbers of audiologists are engaging in independent private practice.
- Our scope of practice continues to expand.
- Our graduate curriculum continues to expand.
- Employment opportunities for audiologists are increasing due to improved techniques and instrumentation for hearing assessment.
- The variety of employment opportunities for audiologists is increasing due to more sophisticated instruments for personal amplification, increased use of cochlear implants, recognition of the equal rights of persons who are hearing-impaired, growing momentum in support of universal hearing screening for infants, and expansion of audiology's role in medical/surgical areas.
- Managed competition in health care is prompting interest in cost-effective services delivered by audiologists and other allied health professionals.
- Audiology comprises research, hearing conservation, diagnosis, treatment, and education. It makes important contributions not only to individuals with hearing and balance problems, but to other disciplines and professions as well (e.g., acoustical engineering, law, neurology, neurosurgery, occupational safety and health, oncology).
- Audiologists are the only professionals uniformly trained and credentialed to provide specialized ser-

vices to the more than 20 million hearing-impaired persons in the United States who have irreversible hearing loss.

The ascendancy of treatment services has made audiology a much more balanced hearing health care profession than at any time in its history. A profile is emerging of audiology as not just a profession that provides assessment for hearing and balance disorders, but as the premier profession for treatment of hearing impairment through personal amplification.

In spite of our unique profile, audiologists currently face formidable threats and daunting tasks as we struggle to gain professional independence in the hearing health care community (cf. Beck, 1994; Clark, 1994; Lovrinic, 1994). Autonomy is the issue as we approach the 21st century. Audiology must become a fully autonomous profession or it will surely shrink into the shadows as a low-profile, ancillary technical vocation.

Audiology at the crossroads

Let us clarify what we mean by the term "autonomous audiology." We will use Webster's (Babcock, 1986) as our source, which states: "living under one's own laws, independent . . . having the right or power of self-government ... being a perfect whole—not forming a part" (p. 148). To take this concept to the next logical step, Webster's helps again with the definition of "independent": "not subordinate . . . not affiliated with or integrated into a larger controlling unit" (p. 1148). The American Speech-Language-Hearing Association uses the following definition in its report on autonomy (American Speech-Language-Hearing Association [ASHA], 1986):

> An autonomous profession is one in which the practitioner has the qualifications, responsibility, and authority of the provision of services which fall within its scope of practice. (p. 53)

Some audiologists may criticize the appropriateness of our use of the term "autonomous audiology," claiming it is contradictory. The critics are correct in pointing out that professionals who are employees and professionals who must be supervised lack the fundamental ingredient of autonomy, namely, self-government (ASHA, 1986). We prefer, however, to take a more optimistic view of our profession and recognize that, even though some audiologists do not enjoy professional independence, audiology as a whole is certainly heading in the direction of autonomy. Recalling the broad definition of private practice given in the Preface, it is important to note that autonomous audiology is not synonymous with the traditional, narrow definition of private practice; rather, autonomous audiology defines a distinct profession that is recognized as such by other health practitioners and the government—regardless of setting.

Evidence of the trend toward autonomous audiology is seen in the following chronology:

1. The founding of the Academy of Dispensing Audiologists (ADA) in 1977.
2. ASHA's policy change in 1978, permitting audiologists to engage in the sale of hearing aids.
3. The establishment in 1987 and rapid growth of the American Academy of Audiology (AAA).
4. ASHA's recognition of audiology as a separate profession (ASHA, 1990) with a professional doctorate as the preferred entry point.[1]
5. AAA's position statement on the professional doctorate as the appropriate entry-level degree for the practice of audiology (AAA, 1991).
6. The subsequent creation of professional doctorate programs in audiology (Au.D.) at Baylor and Central Michigan University in 1993 and 1994.

Emergence of ADA and AAA

To achieve autonomy, audiologists must understand more than just audiology. They must also understand the "business" of health care. It is our intent for this handbook to serve as a useful reference for audiologists in training as well as those currently in practice who wish to become better informed about the business and managerial aspects of practicing audiology in America's health care system.

To understand the significance of autonomous audiology and the contents of this handbook, the following section explores some of the historical background and development of audiology.

---

[1]ASHA LC4-92 supported "the concept of doctoral degrees as the entry level academic credentials for the practice of audiology" (ASHA, 1993, p. 34). LC44-93 supported "the professional doctorate as the entry-level credential for the practice of audiology" (ASHA, 1994, p. 31).

In 1994, ASHA's Council on Professional Standards in Speech-Language Pathology and Audiology (Standards Council [SC]) developed an action plan with the following components: (a) use of *Doctor of Audiology* as the preferred title for the professional doctorate in audiology, (b) change degree requirement for the CCC in Audiology from a Master's degree to the professional doctorate, (c) develop standards for a professional doctorate curriculum, (d) have revised standards ready for peer review by 1/1/1994, and implement them in 2002 (Cherow & Thompson, 1994).

Four Factors that Shaped the Course of Audiology

- *Educational Environment and Curricula*
- *Professional and Learned Societies*
- *Employment Opportunities*
- *Relationship to the Hearing Aid*

SEEDS OF THE PROFESSION

Virtually from its inception and throughout its evolution, the course of audiology has been influenced and shaped by four major factors: (1) the educational environment and curriculum of audiologists, (2) the major professional and learned societies that encompass audiologists, (3) the jobs to which audiologists migrated, and (4) audiology's relationship to the hearing aid. The events, circumstances, and relationships that transpired in these four areas had a profound effect on the development of audiology's autonomy and professional independence. Let us briefly examine each of these areas.

Our Educational Heritage

Our profession was conceived in the armed forces rehabilitation programs during World War II (WW II) by a corps of technical and educational personnel. Many of these people were recruited from university departments of speech pathology, psychology, and education of the deaf. For a period of 3 to 4 years, these pioneers served the needs of hearing-impaired military personnel, testing hearing, select-

Audiology emerged from WW II rehabilitation efforts, but was defined in academia

ing hearing aids, and providing auditory training and lip-reading lessons. After the war, several of these individuals returned to their universities and introduced courses on hearing loss and aural rehabilitation. Events and decisions during this crucial period set the course for audiology to the present day.

Audiology was actually *formed* in academia, although the idea for a discipline[2] came out of the brief experiences of those few people who served hearing-impaired military personnel during WW II. Most disciplines experience a long history of service delivery before establishing a professional[3] school for training. In effect, they start by meeting a need of a cross section of a population and then move into a formal setting, usually a university, to establish a curriculum to teach the discipline. A case in point is medicine, others include dentistry and optometry. When each of their curricula was developed in professional schools, it was shaped in response to the needs of the public. In contrast, the founders of the audiology curriculum shaped the discipline according to the services they envisioned that people with hearing loss needed, what they themselves needed in their work settings, and what was acceptable in a graduate school curriculum. While the discipline was forming, the actual profession was left to develop in a more haphazard fashion as clinicians recognized and attempted to respond to consumer demand.

What if hearing aid dealers had started audiology?

The imperatives of graduate school academia directed the discipline of audiology toward research and diagnosis, rather than treatment and rehabilitation. If the hearing aid dealers of the 1940s had migrated to academia to establish the discipline of audiology, the resulting curriculum would have been much more clinically oriented, and there would be a single group of professionals dispensing hearing aids today, rather than the present dichotomy of audiologists and hearing aid specialists (dealers).

Preparation for clinical service was of secondary importance

In the late 1940s, our "founding fathers" realized they had to gain the acceptance and respect of their peers in the academic community. To do so, they had to manipulate the mission of audiology away from its service-oriented, rehabilitation roots, toward a research and diagnostically oriented academic discipline. Doctoral degrees were awarded to students with the intent of developing a cadre of teacher/inves-

---

[2]*Discipline* is defined as a branch of knowledge or teaching.

[3]A *profession* is defined as an occupation or vocation requiring training in the liberal arts or the sciences and advanced study in a specialized field (Morris, 1973).

tigators and researchers, who had two primary missions: (a) to teach and study hearing and its disorders and (b) to develop new audiology degree programs. Secondarily, the purpose was to develop, but not necessarily provide, new methods for testing and evaluation and, finally, to rehabilitate those with hearing losses.

In masters' degree programs, testing was emphasized over treatment. The quantitative nature of testing blended well with the research orientation of graduate programs. Unlike testing, traditional aural rehabilitation methods did not emphasize systematic observation and implementation, and therefore failed to develop the necessary research base required to become a strong force in graduate studies. It is natural, then, that the area of tests and measurements received the greatest attention in both the curricula and practica of audiologists' education and training. Over time, the quality and utility of aural rehabilitation courses (lipreading and auditory training) declined.

In this milieu, masters' level preparation of student practitioners to deliver clinical *service* was of ancillary importance, and it still is in many programs. Faculty guided masters' curricula toward research to make the programs acceptable in graduate school environments. The very presence of university hearing clinics was justified to collect research data by faculty, rather than to provide clinical services. Often, these clinics provided audiology services free of charge or for only token amounts, to entice persons to seek their services.[4]

Another very crippling birth anomaly affected the future course of audiology. Instead of establishing professional schools of audiology at the outset, our forefathers decided to move in with their relatives, the speech correctionists (as they were called in those days). It would have been a monumental task to establish an independent department or professional school of audiology in any university at that time.[5] On the one hand, hardly anyone knew what audiology was, including some of those whom we now credit as our pioneers. On the other hand, it was fairly easy and expedient simply to add a course here and there to those already existing in speech correction. In most university settings, departments changed their names from "Speech Correction" to

---

[4]Only in recent years have some university clinics endeavored to act as profit centers or at least attempted to price their service fees at a break-even point.

[5]To the best of our knowledge, the only exception to this was the audiology degree program at Wayne State University Medical School, developed by John Gaeth, Ph.D., in the 1950s.

"Speech and Hearing Disorders" or the like. Later, the names were changed to "Department of Communicative Disorders," and audiology remained and is still there today in most cases.

In 1994, there were about 115 audiology programs accredited by ASHA (Harford, 1993), awarding about 700 masters' degrees and 25–30 doctorates annually. Most of these programs have 10 or fewer students enrolled, which makes the per capita cost of their education high and the program income low. Contrast these figures with 15 schools of optometry, graduating about 1,100 Doctors of Optometry each year. This situation dilutes the education and training that audiologists receive. It is impossible for all of these audiology degree programs to maintain excellent standards of training and attract the highest quality educators, especially considering the escalating cost of graduate education.

Why the AuD?

Throughout the history of our profession, it has been the rule for students to terminate their education with the master's degree, rather than to complete the doctorate. Thus, in the work-a-day world, most audiologists are not referred to as "doctor." The absence of this title automatically places the audiologist in a subservient role in the health care system.

Professional Organization

Instead of establishing our own professional society following WW II, audiology moved into the American Speech Correction Association, with the agreement that "hearing" would be added to the association's name. The resulting American Speech and Hearing Association (ASHA) also agreed that audiology would be allowed the freedom to determine its own future (Doerfler, 1991). However, the minority position of audiologists and their disparate interests led to inertial forces within the ASHA that did not fully encourage or support the autonomy and growth of audiology.[6]

In the beginning, the speech correctionists and those interested mainly in hearing loss saw themselves with very similar interests, backgrounds, and missions. But, over the decades, the two groups have drifted apart. Audiologists today are primarily health care providers, whereas a large number of speech-language professionals are educators working in school systems and long-term rehabilitation facilities. The disparate nature of the communicative problems and the different responsibilities and roles of audiologists and speech-lan-

---

[6]This is apparent from the length of time it has taken for ASHA to embrace such issues as audiology licensure, hearing dispensing, and the Au.D. as the entry level for our profession.

guage pathologists today make these two distinctly different professional groups. For example, speech-language personnel serve "clients." Audiologists serve "patients." Yet, ASHA's editorial policy calls for the term "client" to be used instead of "patient" in ASHA publications and public relations media, including audiologic information (ASHA, 1993). What other health care profession refers to those they serve and treat as "clients?"

It is important for all audiologists to keep in mind that the language and lexicon we use influences how we think and how we are perceived by others. If we want to be considered health care providers, we must talk and behave as health care providers, not lawyers, insurance salespersons, financial advisors, speech pathologists, and so on, all of whom have clients.

Speech-language professionals serve clients, audiologists serve patients

The Job Market

Even though evaluation and treatment are the hallmarks of a viable health care profession, evaluation received the most emphasis during the formative years of audiology. Why? Because few in the general public were interested in making repeated visits to a clinic for lip-reading lessons to learn to distinguish between homophenous sounds. They did not constitute a captive audience like that previously encountered in military hospitals. "Hearing therapy" was not nearly as popular as the speech therapy provided by our colleagues working in the same clinics. Most individuals with hearing loss demanded a "quick fix" for their communicative problems, usually via hearing aids. Unfortunately, audiologists could recommend but not sell hearing aids. They could not meet public demand by providing the important fitting, dispensing, and servicing of the instruments. Thus, most adults with hearing loss were fitted by hearing aid dealers, and few returned to the audiologists for therapy.

That left the audiologist with the evaluation of hearing as the area in which to develop unique expertise. Many audiologists who initially started in speech therapy transferred to audiology because it seemed more "objective" and "scientific," and appeared to lead to more immediate results. In the same vein, they gravitated toward audiologic testing rather than aural rehabilitation because testing was more objective and felt more scientific than aural rehabilitation. This view was indirectly endorsed by the ASHA's dim view of hearing aid dispensing and the emphasis in the graduate schools on research-based, quantitative education.

Graduates with audiology degrees soon learned that, although there were only a few jobs for aural rehabilitationists, there were lots of jobs for testers. Over the years, scores of audiologists took jobs that involved primarily the testing of hearing. With few exceptions, these were salaried positions working for otolaryngologists, clinics, hospitals, residential institutions, and agencies, nearly all of which were supervised by physicians. By the mid-1970s, the audiology profession included many individuals with master's degrees who were working for physicians. The major role of audiology in the health care system was to obtain audiometric data for otolaryngologists who managed the patients' ear diseases. Much to the detriment of the profession, audiologists were viewed as technicians by patients as well as by physicians.

> **There were lots of jobs for testers**

This situation was not aided by the fact that most audiologists were not trained at a doctoral level. They lacked the credentials and tools to become teacher-investigators, preferring to pursue the service area rather than research. Too often overlooked was the small cadre of research audiologists that was contributing to the understanding of hearing and its disorders. Unfortunately, job opportunities in research and research funds have always been limited.

The Hearing Aid

Audiology simply could not gain its independence as a health care profession if it were composed of a few researchers and teachers and a large majority of master's level audiologists who lacked the freedom to dispense hearing aids and often functioned as supervised test technicians. There had to be a viable treatment component that could sustain itself as a clinical service, offer fruitful research avenues, and enable practitioners to achieve financial security. Such goals could not be realized solely by providing hearing tests. To realize the goals, audiologists needed to treat hearing problems by dispensing hearing aids and providing short-term aural rehabilitation. But, ASHA's Code of Ethics did not recognize the sale of hearing aids by its members as an ethical practice.

> **ASHA would not allow audiologists to sell hearing aids**

In 1977, the Academy of Dispensing Audiologists (ADA) was founded. This event sent a clear signal that audiologists were going to dispense and sell hearing aids. In April of 1978, the U.S. Supreme Court (U.S. v. National Society of Professional Engineers) ruled it illegal for a professional society's canon of ethics to limit competition among its members (Skafte, 1990). Just 2 months later, the ASHA Executive Board recommended a change in the association's Code of Ethics that would permit audiologists to engage in the retail sale of hearing aids (Skafte, 1990). This action had a profound effect on the course of audiology, even though the recommendation did not find its way into ASHA's Code of Ethics until 1992.[7]

By 1979, a trade journal survey reported that about 900 audiologists were involved in the direct dispensing of hearing aids. Some learned fitting and dispensing techniques from manufacturers. Others spent time as students or staff in Veterans Administration or military clinics, but most had to learn on-the-job, by trial and error. By mid-1985, 2,400 audiologists were dispensing hearing aids; and by the early 1990s the number had reached 5,000, or half of all the hearing aid dispensers in America (Skafte, 1990). In 1992, over 65% of the more than 1.6 million hearing aids sold were dispensed by audiologists (Kirkwood, 1992).

Historical Summary

Because of circumstances and decisions made during the formative period of our profession, audiologists assumed a minority position in university settings and within the ASHA. In this position, they were less than effective in defining audiology goals and furthering audiology objectives. As a result, audiologists became stereotyped as ancillary health care professionals, technically trained to support the medical-surgical community under supervised conditions (e.g., concentrating on site-of-lesion testing, which in many instances had the effect of relegating audiology to a supportive role in a physicians' realm).

Audiologists as technicians

Thus, audiology as a profession foundered and failed to develop the characteristics necessary for autonomy: self-governance, financial security, respected entitlement, and public recognition. Audiology chose to prolong its adolescence by staying subsumed in ASHA and Speech Departments, assuming a technicians' role to physicians, and evaluating but not treating hearing problems. As a result, audiology failed to develop a clear professional identity or assume control of its destiny. Audiology waited 30 years before engaging in the dispensing of hearing aids. When audiologists finally started dispensing, that activity encouraged the development of an independent practice mentality. The emergence of an

Audiology falters

[7]Regarding revisions in the 1991 ASHA Code of Ethics, Resnick (1993) comments that "the approval for audiologists to dispense hearing aids was of great concern to the stated ethics of the Association since the 1991 version did not permit hearing aid dispensing as an ethical practice. Because most audiologists today dispense hearing aids, that change was clearly necessary" (p. 32).

Characteristics of Autonomy

- *Self-Governance*
- *Financial Security*
- *Respected Entitlement*
- *Public Recognition*

independent practice component in turn gave audiologists the opportunity to achieve greater financial security and the means and direction to become autonomous professionals.

WHERE ARE WE NOW?

For audiology to move toward autonomy, we must provide services that (a) are valued by society, (b) offer respectable financial compensation, and (c) belong to us and no one else. We borrowed a technique from Robert Turner's (1992) editorial in the *American Journal of Audiology* to evaluate the contribution of audiological services toward achieving this criterion for autonomy. He provides a table, which we modified and expanded to illustrate our position.

In Table 1–1, we estimate the financial, professional, and overall impact of each audiology service. *Financial impact* is determined by compensation and demand. Taken together, compensation and demand reflect the value assigned to the service by consumers. *Demand* is the volume of business for a particular activity. *Compensation* is the reimbursement relative to the cost of providing the service. A high demand for a service can be good or bad, depending on the compensation. A low volume service may have a negligible financial impact, even with good compensation. For example, consider the category "Basic Evaluation-Pediatric" in Table 1–1. There is a good demand for services to infants and children in special settings; however, reimbursement is often minimal and costs are high, resulting in a poor financial net return for services. In other words, society does not assign a very high value to pediatric audiology at present. In contrast, hearing aids have high demand and reasonable reimbursement. Lucille Beck, in her 1994 Presidential address to the American Academy of

Table 1–1. Financial, professional, and overall impact of audiology services.

Service	Financial Impact		Professional Impact		Overall Impact
	Demand	Compensation	Recognition	Independence	
Basic Evaluation Adults	✓	X	Ø	Ø	Ø
Basic Evaluation Pediatric	✓	X	✓	✓	Ø
Special Diagnostics OAE, ENG, ABR, etc.	Ø	X	Ø	X	X
Hearing Aid Dispenser	✓	✓	Ø	✓	✓

✓ Good   Ø Mixed   X Poor

Audiology, acknowledges the "fundamental importance" of the hearing aid to what we do, noting "that hearing aids drive much of the public interest in our profession" (p. 5).

The *professional impact* is determined by recognition and independence. The ASHA (1986) report on professional autonomy observes that the authority to function autonomously is signified when members of a profession:

1. are a point of entry for services that fall within its scope of practice;
2. select the appropriate candidates for those services;
3. determine appropriate diagnostic methodology and suitable approaches to and duration of treatment;
4. effect referrals for services to be provided by other . . . audiologists as well as by members of other professions. (p. 54)

Professional impact is affected by the image we present to the marketplace, which in turn is determined by the business and ethical choices we make as individual practitioners and as a profession. Chapters 13, 14, and 17 dwell on these issues, but Resnick (1993) sums it up nicely:

Audiology has barely been weaned as an independent profession. It is only just now required to fend for itself in the marketplace. While the dust is still settling audiology is looking around to see what other professions are undertaking to protect their professional image. The fork in the road looms ahead. One way leads to the preservation of a profession; the other leads elsewhere. There may be problems to face on each road. (p. 95)

Recognition means that the audiologist is viewed as the most competent and qualified provider of the services. As Turner stresses, it is difficult to argue that audiology is an autonomous profession when audiologists provide services that are also provided by groups who lack the licensing and credentialing of professionals. A case in point is electronystagmography (ENG), which is administered frequently by technicians. But licensing and credentialing do not guarantee societal recognition: it is not unusual for the female audiologist in the ENT office to be perceived by the patient as "the girl who tested my hearing."[8] Beck (1994) stresses that audiologists must be recognized as limited licensed practitioners *and* identified as qualified providers in any health care reform measures that are passed on state or national levels.

Independence is the right to provide direct care without supervision. Again, ENG and certain other special diagnostic procedures, such as intraoperative monitoring, otoacoustic emissions, and ABR in newborn intensive care units are usually considered to be under the direct supervision of a physician, even when performed by an audiologist. Hearing aid dispensing, however, provides the audiologist the opportunity to differentiate hearing loss from ear disease (Beck, 1994) and to assume control of treatment and follow-up. Even though the audiologist is not the sole provider of hearing aids, this activity clearly establishes an opportunity for independent patient management.

Autonomy requires self-governance

As Turner (1992) concludes, and we heartily underscore, "Remember, that which promotes autonomy will also strengthen clinical programs, regardless of the institutional environment" (p. 2).

In spite of self-induced handicaps, audiology is well on the road to professional autonomy

There is no doubt that the field of audiology is making important progress toward gaining its independence and professional autonomy. The mechanism (AAA) is in place for our self-governance. The precedent has been set and the winds are shifting toward establishing our own unmistakable identity (Au.D.). As a result of our relationship with the hearing aid, the entire profession is gaining greater financial security. These "positioning" steps are changing the public's perceived value of audiology services. It is simply a matter of time before audiologists will be the profession of choice in the mind of the public for obtaining hearing aids and man-

---

[8]This is an autonomy issue, not a gender issue. In the office of one of the authors, patients not infrequently refer to the male audiologist as the "boy who tested my hearing."

aged care for permanent hearing loss. But, there is much work ahead if we are to accomplish the goal of becoming a recognized, independent health care profession.

WHERE DO WE GO FROM HERE?

Now, the profession needs to understand that *it takes more than offering services to achieve autonomy.* If that is what it takes, audiology would have been an autonomous profession years ago. The profession must recognize that the *manner* in which services are marketed and provided plays a major role in realizing its goals. At the same time, it must (a) become self-governing, (b) greatly expand the professional training curriculum, (c) require a doctorate to practice, and (d) emphasize continual upgrading of skills and knowledge through continuing education.

Gaining professional autonomy is not something that happens overnight. Unlike the postadolescent moving into his or her own apartment in one day, gaining professional independence and autonomy is a gradual and dynamic process. Practicing audiology in the 1990s demands insights and skills not expected or recognized by our forefathers. Surely, by the time we reach the year 2000, audiologists must be in step with all of the first-string players in the health care system. Remember, many of those who control our degree programs, our certification criteria, standards and requirements, and who often serve as our spokespersons in the bureaucracies of Washington have not historically perceived themselves as members of the health care system. Hence, we cannot expect them to understand audiology's need to secure itself as an autonomous provider of hearing services. Audiologists must take charge of their own destiny as practitioners and not be guided and misled by those who fail to understand our goals. Consequently, audiologists must become educated and sensitized to political issues. They must be politically active at the local and national levels to shape legislation that is favorable to our profession.

At the same time, it is critical that the training of audiologists for the future, and the continuing education of those in the present, include subjects that have not previously been required for ASHA certification.[9] Autonomous service delivery includes more than the technical skills imparted by our gradu-

Autonomy requires expanded professional training

---

[9]The Report on Private Practice (ASHA, 1991) states that: "Private practitioners, as well as individuals who serve as administrators of educational and health care facilities, have additional education and continuing education needs. These include financial planning and management, personnel management, legal issues and taxes, and marketing" (p. 1).

ate programs. True, audiologists must consistently demonstrate professional knowledge and competence, but the responsibilities of independent practice dictate that audiologists' training must be expanded to include information on ethical and business practices, legal and regulatory environments, market analysis, and quality improvement (assurance).

Global market factors

Why is this? The manner in which services are marketed and provided is gaining importance as we gather momentum toward achieving our autonomy. This is because there are global factors operating that affect our profession and our attempts to achieve autonomy. We must recognize the marketplace factors that are brought to bear on the services of *all* professions. More than ever, services are being scrutinized in terms of quality, cost, and perceived value. They are compared to similar services offered by other professions. Eventually, services of a profession are either embraced and enhanced, or they are discarded or absorbed by other professions.

In the 1990s, the most evident global factors affecting audiology service delivery are health care cost containment, consumer protection, competitive services by other professions, and profound changes in business management (cf., Boyett & Conn, 1992). Each of these factors is a form of market-based quality control: only services that are demonstrably effective, perceived to be widely beneficial, and provided in the most competent and cost-effective manner will survive. Efforts by our professional organizations recognize the threats and opportunities these factors pose to our profession (cf. AAA, 1993). Today's audiologists must demonstrate professional knowledge and competence consistently, but that is not enough. They must perform at this level while:

■ containing costs,
■ justifying fees,
■ maintaining profitability,
■ observing ethical practices and national standards of care,
■ protecting patients and staff,
■ monitoring government and business environments, and
■ maintaining a high level of care.

In short, autonomy comes with maturation and the shouldering of responsibility by those in our profession, as manifest by the broad training and entry-level positioning envisioned for the professional doctorate in audiology.

Finally, there remains one essential characteristic that must be inculcated and internalized by every audiologist to ensure our future as an autonomous profession. That is the integration of the concepts of "caring" and "profession." The way in which we view ourselves as audiologists—and our opinions of the new demands and opportunities presented in the 1990s—may be better understood if the word "calling" is substituted for "profession" or "work." A "calling" is an old-fashioned descriptor of a career, connoting a high level of personal commitment, perhaps greater than we typically associate with today's professions. Thus, a "calling" is a "summons" or a "claim" on one's time or life—a call to duty (*American Heritage Dictionary of the English Language*, Morris, 1973). Although business, management, regulations, and marketing are essential elements of how we do our work, it is altogether more satisfying if these elements are viewed as integral parts of the knowledge base that enables us to perform our *calling as audiologists* to provide the highest quality care for our patients.

Audiology as a calling

REFERENCES

American Academy of Audiology. (1991). Position statement: The American Academy of Audiology and the professional doctorate (Au.D.). *Audiology Today, 3*(4), 10–12.

American Academy of Audiology. (1993, April 29). *Hearing care services and health care reform. Report prepared for the President's task force on national health reform* (pp. 1–14). Houston: American Academy of Audiology.

American Speech-Language-Hearing Association. (1986). The autonomy of speech-language pathology and audiology. Report of the ad hoc committee on professional autonomy. *Asha, 28*(5), 53–57.

American Speech-Language-Hearing Association. (1990). Legislative council report (LC 7-89). *Asha 32*(3), 18.

American Speech-Language-Hearing Association. (1991). Report on private practice. *Asha, 33*(Suppl. 6), 1–4.

American Speech-Language-Hearing Association. (1993). Legislative council report (LC 4-92). *Asha, 35*(3), 34.

American Speech-Language-Hearing Association. (1994). Legislative council report (LC 44-93). *Asha, 36*(3), 31.

American Speech-Language-Hearing Association. (1993). *The language used to describe individuals with disabilities*. Resolution No. RA-35, agenda No. F-1.1, approved by the ASHA Executive Board on August, 12, 1993, pp. 1–8.

Babcock, P. G. (Ed.). (1986). *Webster's third new international dictionary of the English language* (unabridged). Springfield MA: Merriam-Webster.

Beck, L. B. (1994). 1994 Presidential address. Healthcare and audiology: Qualified quality providers. *Audiology Today, 6*(4), 4–6.

Boyett, J. H., & Conn, H. P. (1992). *Workplace 2000*. New York: Plume Printing.

Cherow, E., & Thompson, M. (1994). Standards council plan of action for LC 44-93. *Audiology Update, 13*(2), 6.

Clark, J. G. (1994). Letters to the editor. *Audiology Today, 6*(4), 8.

Doerfler, L. (1991). Remembering how it all began. *Audiology CO-Op Newsletter, 3*(3), 2.

Harford, E. (1993). Impact of the hearing aid on the evolution of audiology. *American Auditory Society Bulletin, 18*(2), 7-108.

Kirkwood, D. H. (1992). U.S. hearing aid sales. *Hearing Journal, 45*, 12.

Lovrinic, J. (1994, July). Looking forward while looking backward. *American Journal of Audiology*, pp. 5–6.

Morris, W. (Ed.) (1973). *The American heritage dictionary of the English language.* New York: Houghton Mifflin.

Resnick, D. M. (1993). *Professional ethics for audiologists and speech-language pathologists.* San Diego, CA: Singular Publishing Group.

Skafte, M. D. (1990). Fifty years of hearing health care. Part 2. *Hearing Instruments, 41*(9), pp. 8–127.

Turner, R. (1992). Editorial. *American Journal of Audiology, 1*(3), 2.

Service Delivery Models: Practice Choices and Practice Constraints

This chapter describes external factors that affect how audiologists practice, if they choose to practice with some degree of autonomy. A few universal factors that affect audiologists' practice choices (and success) are described briefly.

The rest of the chapter surveys five different models of practice delivery that exist in today's hearing health care environment: (I) hospital-based, (II) clinic-affiliated, (III) physician-affiliated, (IV) hearing aid dispensing office, and (V) stand-alone audiology practice. All five models fall under our broad umbrella of "private" practice (as discussed later in the chapter), but they differ from each other in organizational structure, financial risk, referral base, and the degree of control the audiologist exercises over the practice. The models are analyzed according to the advantages and disadvantages that audiologists may encounter in each scenario.

UNIVERSAL FACTORS

Universal factors warrant discussion because they are so obvious that they are occasionally overlooked or considered inconsequential by audiologists, often with dire consequences. They are mundane, but formidable factors that deserve attention when defining a practice.

Latches and Barriers

In most states, one may not practice audiology or dispense hearing aids without obtaining professional licenses. In states without licensure or registration, there are many professional

External Factors Affect How We Practice

- *Licensing and Education Requirements*
- *Competitive Barriers*
- *Community Need*
- *Community Support*

and financial constraints on audiologists if they do not obtain clinical certification by the American Speech-Language-Hearing Association. One should apply for and obtain all pertinent certification and licenses *before* committing to a practice arrangement. Setting such "latches" in advance is good risk management, saves time, and avoids surprises. When entering into a practice arrangement with other professionals, be sure that they, too, have "set their latches."

"Latches" are associated with consumer protection

As opposed to latches, which are usually associated with consumer protection motives, barriers are typically associated with competitive protectionism. This is not always negative. For example, there are audiology practices that provide such excellent service that they discourage competitors from entering a service area. Business analysis in other fields shows, however, that competitors will continue to take the risk of penetrating a market as long as economic profit exists. The result is higher quality service with competitive pricing.

"Barriers" are associated with competitive protectionism

Negative competitive protectionism does exist. An example is when physicians and insurers enter into managed care covenants that exclude nonphysician providers. This is an obvious barrier to autonomous audiology practice. In such arrangements, audiology services may be discounted or even offered at a loss by the otolaryngologist to obtain more desirable surgical cases. In this example, low reimbursement for audiology services reduces the quality of hearing health care in three ways:

1. Services are limited within the "protected" environment.
2. Low-end salaries paid to audiologists in that environment do not attract or keep highly experienced or competent clinicians.
3. Independent competitors cannot survive outside the barrier because economic profit has been destroyed.

Community Need

Needs differ dramatically and obviously according to the setting. In wealthy retirement enclaves, hearing aid dispensing addresses a greater need than otoacoustic emission screening. Other examples are: (a) mining towns, which have a greater need for hearing conservation programs than resort towns; (b) rural areas, which require itinerant practitioners rather than office services; and (c) deaf communities, in which audiologists with signing ability are needed more than those with electrophysiology expertise.

Community Support

Community need and community support are not synonymous. Needed services may encounter either support or resistance due to *educational, regulatory,* or *economic factors.* The following examples illustrate only a few ways in which these factors act on the provision of our professional services.

Educational Factors

An auditory electrophysiology clinic will not be supported in a community, regardless of need, if physicians are not educated about or are biased against Auditory Brainstem Response (ABR) testing. In one case, an audiologist started a stand-alone practice after working in a successful, specialized practice that contracted with hospitals and clinics to perform intra-operative monitoring and diagnostic ABR. After purchasing expensive portable equipment, relocating to an urban area with no competing services, and emulating the former practice in every way, the audiologist found no market. The local physicians had neither education nor interest in electrophysiologic services, despite an obvious need. Faced with financial disaster, the audiologist left the profession and went to work for the ABR equipment manufacturer.

This true example illustrates the necessity of doing a comprehensive analysis of the target market. As a corollary, this example also underscores the importance of carefully selecting target markets and diversifying practices. Here, the practice had only one target market, physicians. There was only one "product," a technical service that had to be ordered by the physicians, who were not well versed in the product. Recalling the admonishment in Chapter 1 that autonomy cannot be achieved by offering diagnostic testing services alone, it is likely that setting up a practice to provide diagnostic services solely for physicians is tenuous, regardless of the services offered.

Regulatory Factors

Meeting needs costs money, so all needs are not met in every community. For needs that are obvious and unmet, government sometimes steps in to solve the dilemmas.

A case in point is industrial hearing conservation. The need to address noise-induced hearing loss existed long before enactment of the Hearing Conservation Amendment (Occupational Safety and Health Administration, 1983) forced industries to develop and support hearing conservation programs. Even today, compliance with the Amendment varies from state to state, depending on enforcement and penalties. Ironically, an audiology practice's success in the hearing conservation arena may depend more on how state regulations are written and implemented than on how much need exists in the community.

Economic Factors

Hearing aids were needed, but not easily afforded, by miners with occupational noise-induced hearing loss. This clear need was not supported in communities with large mining populations until negotiations by the United Mine Workers made hearing aids a covered benefit. Not surprisingly, hearing aid dispensing businesses subsequently proliferated in these locations. The aftermath prompted a need for audiologists and physicians in the communities to perform compensatory examinations on claimants. This need, in turn, was supported by insurers.

A less convoluted example of the effects of economic factors is that digital and programmable hearing aids are more apt to receive support in communities with high socioeconomic levels than in economically depressed areas, even though the need for such devices might be greater in the latter in some cases (e.g., mining communities).

SERVICE DELIVERY MODELS

Service Delivery Models

- Hospital-Affiliated Practice
- Clinic-Affiliated Practice
- Physician-Affiliated Practice
- Hearing Aid Office
- Independent Audiology Practice

For purposes of discussion, we have broadly defined five general types of practices and just as generally called them all "private" practices. This is not done to prompt argument or confusion, but to simplify the discussion so that some useful and general observations can be made.

The first observation is that *all practices that are not part of government or not-for-profit institutions are "private."* "Private" audiology practice occurs in settings where licensed and/or credentialed audiologists provide services that are reimbursed by patients or the patients' health care plans.

The second observation is that "private" practices differ along many dimensions: size, status, position in the health care delivery system, scope of services, administrative duties, and financial security. But primarily, *"private" practices differ in the type and degree of autonomy available to the practitioner.*

The third observation is that the five *practice models* are *not distinct, but overlap to form a continuum.* They are popular categories, probably because they are associated with visual cliches: from the institutional version of hospital-based practices to the store-front vision of hearing aid dispenser's offices. Reality can be quite different: the hospital "clinic" may be a part-time audiologist who works in a cubby hole, while the hearing aid dispensary may be part of a large clinic.

With these observations in mind, and with the knowledge that practitioners will see ways in which their individual situations differ from the models, we will discuss the advantages and disadvantages of the five service delivery models.

Model I: Hospital-Affiliated Practices

In this model, audiologists either contract or are employed to perform audiology services. In either case, the audiology clinic has a supervisor who is an administrator (e.g., business manager, physician director, or both). The clinic can be part of a hospital organization, or it can be one of many clinics that are closely or loosely affiliated with the hospital.

The size of the clinic can vary from one part-time audiologist to a large number of audiologists, often working at multiple sites, under an audiology director with many administrative duties. The case load is made up of inpatients and outpatients, with the relative composition dependent on the type of hospital (e.g., pediatric, rehabilitation, general). The hospital may supply all referrals or only a few. Regarding referrals, the audiologists may be expected to provide only services for scheduled patients in a busy clinic, or they may be expected to increase referrals through marketing to justify their positions.

Test equipment usually is owned by the hospital. The audiologist or clinic director often selects new equipment within a budget set by the administrator and may be responsible for equipment maintenance and calibration.

Scheduling and patient intake are performed by hospital employees in most cases, but scheduling is controlled either by the audiologist or the administration. Patient records are often centrally located. They are maintained in accordance with external credentialing requirements, which also dictate clinic policies for patient care (e.g., infection control, quality improvement).

Typically, fees are set by the director, the business manager, or the two together. Audiologists working on contract may specify their fees for service as part of the contract negotiations. Billing is done by the hospital. Audiologists who contract their services are paid either by the hour or as a percentage of the revenue they generate. In the latter case, the percentage can be based on gross revenues or profit.

Patient management varies widely by setting, depending on the number and types of patients (e.g., pediatric) and types of procedures (e.g., hearing aid fitting, balance assessment). It also depends on who controls scheduling.

Advantages

Hospital settings often have broad and interesting case loads that provide excellent training for audiologists. This is especially true if the audiologists work closely with physicians, as in resident training hospitals. These settings also give audiologists opportunities to learn clinic management skills. This on-the-job training in hospitals is one of the few instances where audiologists get a chance to observe or participate in management.

For salaried employees, the financial advantages of hospital-affiliated practices are fairly standard: a steady income and good benefits, assuming the position is secure. For audiologists working on contract, one of the main advantages of hospital-affiliated practice is the low financial risk because they do not assume overhead expenses. Space, equipment, furnishings, support personnel, scheduling, medical records, and billing are provided by the hospital. If the hospital has a good billing department, third party reimbursement will be better than that allotted to an independent audiologist. Patients' hospitalization plans are usually more comprehensive than their major medical plans. They will cover hospital charges that would not be covered if submitted independently by the audiologist.[1]

Disadvantages

Audiologists often lack autonomy in hospital-based settings. In many cases, they have little control over scheduling, test protocols, equipment, billing, fees, or patient management. In "on-call clinics," they may sit idly for long periods and then be deluged with patients at other times.

Clinic directors may be expected to assume major responsibilities for clinic management, but lack the autonomy to make needed changes in a timely fashion. Often, they must keep their clinics "in the black" without the benefit of a budget or knowledge of changes in assigned overhead expenses. Administrative demands take away from direct patient contact, which is viewed by some audiologists as a disadvantage.

The biggest disadvantage for audiologists on contract is the potential loss of the contract if the clinic is profitable. If the audiologist has marketed and built up the clinic to the point that it is a revenue maker, the hospital is likely to covet all of the revenues. When that happens, there is a good chance the hospital will act to recapture the clinic's revenues by not renewing the audiologist's contract and creating an hourly or salaried audiology position in the clinic. In that case, the position may still be available on contract, but at a lower level of reimbursement.

Model II: Clinic-Affiliated Practices

This model is really a variation of the hospital-affiliated practice, but housed in a stand-alone, out-patient care clinic that is itself composed of numerous smaller specialty clinics such as otolaryngology and audiology. Compared to hospitals, most clinics are small, but they can be very large (e.g., The Cleveland Clinic, Mayo Clinic) and occasionally very specialized (e.g., The House Ear Institute, Shea Clinic).

For the most part, audiology clinics function the same as in the hospital-affiliated model, except that there are no inpatients, there are fewer levels of management, and there are fewer protocols dictated by external accreditation. *In general, the advantages and disadvantages of this model are the same as the hospital-based model.*

---

[1]For example, the hospital can bill Medicare for inpatient audiology services performed by an audiologist who is an employee or has a contract with the hospital. An audiologist cannot bill Medicare for the same services performed on inpatients in a hospital.

Model III: Physician-Affiliated Practices

As external credentialing requirements diminish, individuality flourishes, producing a plethora of possible arrangements in this service delivery model. The ASHA Omnibus survey showed 23.9% of all audiologists working in this arrangement (Cherow & Thompson, 1992). The variety ranges from audiologists who are part-time, hourly employees to audiologists who have partnerships with physicians. In between, and probably most common, are audiologists who work full-time on salary and/or commission or in some kind of contractual or fee-splitting arrangement.[2] In almost all cases, the physician affiliate is an otologist or otolaryngologist, although it is possible and desirable that audiologists may become associated with primary care physicians in the future.

Obviously, the degree of autonomy the audiologist has is dependent on the setting. In the least autonomous arrangements, "management" consists of the medical staff and the office manager. The physicians own the equipment, set the fees, and control billing. They provide most of the referrals and often dictate what tests are to be performed. As in other settings, however, audiologists may solicit referrals from other sources to "pay their way." This last is in quotes because it is unlikely in this situation that audiologists' earned revenues will cover only their own expenses (including salary). Rather, audiologists' revenues are typically adequate to support the audiology practice *and* contribute to the physicians' profitability. In return, the physicians provide the equivalent of room and board to the audiology practice.

In the most autonomous version of the physician-affiliated model, the audiologist and physician work as a team, sharing space, patients, and sometimes equipment costs. The audiologist sets fees and may or may not bill separately, depending on third-party reimbursement in the demographic area. The audiologist exercises a good deal of control over patient management, especially regarding hearing aid treatment.

Advantages

Many audiologists associate with physicians to minimize the financial investment required, guarantee referrals, and ensure third party reimbursement for diagnostic services.

---

[2]Depending on why it is done and how it is done, fee-splitting is not always ethically or legally defensible.

If the physician or physicians are good and prolific ear surgeons, the audiologists have the advantage of exposure to a wide variety of ear disorders and their audiologic manifestations. The association can also mean better patient care in some instances. If the physicians have good management skills, have a high respect for audiologists and their skills, and set financial rewards that are commensurate with those skills, then such positions have advantages. Otherwise, it is unclear what long-term personal or financial advantages the audiologists glean from these arrangements.

Disadvantages

Whenever there are as many unpoliced contingencies on a position as stated above, the disadvantages will likely outweigh the advantages in the long run. The physician controls the audiologist, professionally and financially, in all but the most advantageous situations. Even in the latter, the audiologist at best is perceived as "second fiddle." This is a problem for our entire profession which is not improved by audiologists operating as support staff in physicians' offices.

Audiologists who contract with or work on commission for physicians face the same unpleasant scenario described for hospital-affiliated audiologists. As they expand the practice and boost revenues, their professional stock may not grow correspondingly. At some point, the audiologist is often perceived to be "making too much" and is either let go or asked to take a reduced compensation package.

Model IV: Hearing Aid Dispensing Offices

Since ASHA reversed its ethical stand on hearing aid dispensing by audiologists in 1978, audiologists have progressively assumed 65% of the hearing aid fitting market (Kirkwood, 1992). What used to be unheard of—audiologists working for hearing aid dispensers, or vice versa, or audiologists buying hearing aid businesses—is becoming increasingly common. Some audiologists are electing to be primarily sellers of hearing aids rather than practicing as audiologists who offer hearing aids as one of their service "products."

The dispensing office model assumes that the audiologist purchases or takes over a traditional hearing aid dispensing office. Traditionally, service delivery is nonmedical and product oriented. Emphasis is on promotional types of marketing, and staff may be paid on a commission. Scheduling is emphasized less and walk-ins are not discouraged. Sales are to repeat patients, referrals from old patients, and new patients attracted by promotional activities.

Advantages

If the office is well run, the audiologist/owner inherits an established patient base and referral system. In contrast to the previously discussed models, the hearing aid dispensing office offers the practitioner an opportunity to use a "personal touch" when working with patients. Owning the office, the audiologist has complete autonomy and control of the dispensing process, as long as patients remain satisfied and income exceeds expenses. If the office is successful, it is an asset that the audiologist may choose to sell at some future time.

Disadvantages

There is a self-imposed limitation of services that is very difficult to escape. The marketed product is hearing aids, not audiology. Established patients are not used to paying for hearing tests and are not likely to get used to it now. New patients are not referred by physicians, which eliminates most third party reimbursement. There are no guaranteed referrals, and income may be seasonal. Attracting physician referrals can be difficult because of the murky professional identity assumed by audiologists who "cross the line" into hearing aid dispensers' territory.[3]

Model V: Independent Practices

In this final service delivery model, audiologists work for themselves, exercising as much autonomy as market forces will allow. They must obtain referrals by devising marketing strategies. To the extent that the strategies are successful, they can tailor their referral base to suit their professional preferences. Independent audiologists have many and diverse management responsibilities. These include most of the things covered in the rest of this book, such as purchasing and maintaining equipment, developing scheduling policies, setting fees, establishing billing and collection procedures, assigning work schedules, and recruiting personnel.

---

[3]For further discussion of public professional perceptions in this regard, see comments in Chapter 17 by Dr. Alexander Woods.

Independent practices can be large, but the majority are quite small, as businesses go. They can take the form of widespread, part-time contracts, with the audiologists traveling from site to site, or they can be situated in individual offices, often near medical campuses, but sometimes in franchised locations (e.g., department stores, optical offices). In many cases, they may adjoin an otolaryngologist's office. In that case, independent audiologists are distinguished from Model III because they:

- bill independently for most patients,
- do not share staff (with minor exceptions),
- do not depend on the physician for the majority of their referrals, and
- do not have any fee, lease, or other agreements with the physician that enable either side to control the expenses and profits of the other.

Advantages

This service delivery model gives audiologists the most flexibility and independence. Their autonomy gives audiologists high visibility as recognized professionals in their community. This in turn can foster strong clinician-patient relationships in which patients view the audiologist as they view their doctor. This is gratifying to the clinician because patients are more likely to show compliance with recommendations and follow-up.

In contrast to Models I, II, and III, independent audiologists can become successful without fear that success will cost them their position. In contrast to Model IV, they can expand their diagnostic services as the market allows without confusing or angering their patients. Finally, successful independent practices are assets that can be sold to the right buyers for a profit.

Disadvantages

It is expensive to start or purchase an independent practice. Initial start-up costs must be recovered as soon as possible to minimize risk. Leases are signed that commit the audiologist for several years. The result of so much risk is that audiologists usually work very hard in the early years or fail in the process.

Unlike Models I, II, and III, there are no guaranteed referrals. Referral sources fluctuate, and seasonal trends affect the monthly patient census. Agencies, schools, and other contracting sources may lose funding, switch to a competitor, or bring the contract in-house. The audiologist has to regularly monitor these and other measures of practice success and use them to forecast the future.

Third party reimbursement is more difficult for independent practitioners, because few insurers recognize our services as autonomous. A final disadvantage is that complete autonomy brings full liability. No hospital or clinic entity stands between the audiologist and a malpractice or general liability lawsuit. Likewise, there is no large bank account or cash reserve to cover slow periods or unanticipated expenses.

SUMMARY

External factors affect the way in which audiologists practice. Some of the major factors are: (a) local licensing and education requirements, (b) competitive barriers, (c) community need, and (d) community support.

The "private" practice of audiology occurs in settings where licensed and/or credentialed audiologists provide services that are reimbursed by patients or the patients' insurers. The service delivery models are quite variable in terms of setting and professional autonomy. Five overlapping models are described and discussed in terms of autonomous advantages and disadvantages: (I) Hospital-affiliated, (II) Clinic-affiliated, (III) Physician-affiliated, (IV) Hearing aid dispensing office, and (V) Independent practice.

REFERENCES

Cherow, E., & Thompson, M. (Eds.) (1992). Audiologists respond to 1992 ASHA omnibus survey. *Audiology Update, 11*(1), 14–17.

Kirkwood, D. H. (1992). U.S. hearing aid sales. *Hearing Journal, 45,* 12.

Occupational Safety and Health Administration. (1983, March 8). Occupational noise exposure: Hearing conservation amendment; final rule. *Federal Register, 46,* 9738–9785.

3

Personal Considerations Associated with Autonomous Practice

There are probably as many ways to manage audiology practices as there are individuals directing them. Our codes of ethics, scopes of practice, external credentialing, and market demands dictate general structures of viable audiology practices, but these leave a good deal of room for the expression of personal preferences in the conduct of autonomous practices. This chapter will address some of the personal considerations associated with defining a practice.

Think Long and Hard About:

- **Level of Commitment**
- **Degree of Expertise**
- **Expectations**
- **Self-Image**
- **Attitudes and Biases**
- **Long Term Goals**

An honest self-appraisal is an important first step

The first step for audiologists considering autonomous practice is to think long and hard about their level of commitment, degree of expertise, personal and professional expectations, self-image, attitudes and biases, and long-term goals. Personal acknowledgment of these considerations allows individual practitioners to realistically define the types of practice in which they can function comfortably and successfully enhance personal satisfaction while making a positive professional contribution.

COMMITMENT LEVEL

In general, the more autonomous the position, the higher the level of commitment required by the person who fills the position. Independent practice typically carries more risk and obligation than is required in hospital- or physician-based practices. The latter, in turn, may be less secure than employment in schools or other government agencies. When examining the autonomy continuum, it is wise to remind oneself that autonomous practice is a big step and ask "Am I sure I want to do this?" Likewise, when examining the opposite end of the continuum, it is wise to remind oneself that the proverbial "spinning of dials" often prompts the question "How much longer can I stand to do this?"

Finding (or changing) one's place on the autonomy continuum is aided by graduate education, continuing education, reading, and experience. Whenever possible, students should take advantage of as broad a variety of internships and externships as their graduate programs provide. The Report on Private Practice (American Speech-Language-Hearing Association [ASHA], 1991b) "encourage(s) University programs to include practicum in private practice settings . . . [and] encourages(s) private practitioners to accept students for clinical practicum" (p. 1). By carefully assessing the varied training situations, students can develop impressions that will guide them in selecting a broad Clinical Fellowship experience, pursuing a research or clinical doctoral program, or seeking employment in a hearing aid dispensing office.

Continuing education courses through AAA, ADA, and ASHA are available and being developed on all aspects of audiology practice. ASHA's Task Force on Audiology recommended that "ASHA should foster the attitude toward, and attainment of, professional autonomy in the course of training and in varied work settings where professionals practice. The growing movement of professions to private practice underlies the significance of this strategy" (ASHA, 1988, p. 43). Numerous, excellent articles are available enumerating the requirements and demands of independent practice in audiology (cf. Feldman, 1988).

The following commitments are identified by the current authors and others (cf. ASHA, 1991a) as requisites of independent practitioners. These points and others are examined by Curran (1986) in Appendix 3-A. Briefly, audiologists must be willing to:

Drive, determination, and hard work are important attributes

- enthusiastically respect the profession
- assess and take risks
- supervise and administer personnel and programs
- promote themselves and the profession
- work more hours, at least for a few years
- go without income for period(s) of time

DEGREE OF EXPERIENCE

Autonomous practice requires a high level of expertise in the profession. The audiologist must be adept, adaptable, and appreciative of the theoretical underpinnings that moor the clinical tests. Audiologists do not emerge from school with these attributes fully developed. Their development requires repeated practice and exposure to unforeseen work situations and to patients with unusual histories, symptoms, results, or affect.

The demand for experience is growing as the scope of practice expands: the Task Force on Clinical Standards identified 23 procedures in the range of services offered by audiologists (ASHA, 1993). These are enumerated in Table 3–1. Many of these procedures are broadly defined, requiring years of training and experience (e.g., hearing aid assessment, balance system assessment). It is no surprise that the profession and its governing bodies have endorsed a clinical doctoral degree as the entry-level academic credential for the practice of audiology.

It is also not surprising that audiologists in full-time independent practice in 1992 reported that they had previously worked an average of 7.6 years in the field before taking on the responsibility of independent practice (Cherow & Thompson, 1992). But the number of years of experience is not enough in itself. There is a good deal of truth to the observation that a person who has worked 10 years has either 10 years of experience or just 1 year of experience 10 times.

The Committee on Private Practice (ASHA, 1991a) poses the following questions to prospective independent practitioners:

■ Do you have the necessary experience?
■ Do you have an established reputation?
■ Are you a good clinician?
■ Are you willing to learn what you don't know?

A good "business head" helps tremendously

We would add to this list "Are you a business person?" Either through training or experience or preferably both, the autonomous practitioner must be able to run a business in which the professional services are rendered. *It is important to stress that this expertise is required not only of those in independent practice. Clinic directors and their staffs must also be conversant in business management, if they hope to maintain their clinics and their quality of customer service.*

Continuing education fills gaps

Courses in business, accounting, and law are available through community colleges and business schools. Information, training, and counseling regarding small business are available through the Small Business Association's "incubator program" and SCORE program.

Table 3–1. Audiology preferred practice patterns.

1. Hearing screening
2. Speech screening
3. Language screening
4. Follow-up procedures
5. Consultation
6. Prevention
7. Counseling
8. Aural rehabilitation assessment
9. Aural rehabilitation
10. Product dispensing
11. Product repair/modification
12. Basic audiologic assessment
13. Pediatric audiologic assessment
14. Comprehensive audiologic assessment
15. Electrodiagnostic test procedures
16. Auditory evoked potential assessment
17. Neurophysiologic intraoperative monitoring
18. Balance system assessment
19. Hearing aid assessment
20. Assistive listening system/device selection
21. Sensory aids assessment
22. Hearing aid fitting/orientation
23. Occupational hearing conservation

PERSONAL REQUIREMENTS AND EXPECTATIONS

Audiologists who plan to work autonomously must be highly motivated, energetic, and robustly healthy. They should have strong self-images, manage stress effectively, know how to handle unstructured time, and have a network or support system on which to rely. If their network involves family members, they need to ensure that the family is supportive and also willing to bear the risks. Likewise, practitioners must clearly identify and maintain their family responsibilities. It is also helpful if they like to network rather than operate as mavericks.

**Greater
independence**

What are the expectations of those who decide to work autonomously? It is reasonable to ask why anyone would wish to practice autonomously in view of the personal and education demands, and the risks. After all, over two thirds of all human service businesses fail within the first 5 years, and job security is rapidly becoming a thing of the past as hospitals reorganize to contain costs. Probably the only really good answer is: "I like what I do and want to do it in the best possible manner." This desire for professional autonomy, or what Peters (Peters & Waterman, 1982) calls the search for excellence, drives people to perform beyond expectation, often with significant personal sacrifice. Audiologists are not an exception, although our field has not always encouraged such excellence when it was associated with entrepreneurial endeavor.

Financial gain

Entrepreneurial enterprise in other fields is associated with financial reward, albeit often deferred. Increased financial gain is an important expectation of audiologists who endeavor to succeed in autonomous practice, either in the clinic or in independent practice. Although it cannot be the foremost goal (as that must always be patient care), financial reward certainly is an important motivating factor. This is appropriate because Americans typically associate financial reward with a strong work ethic, increased responsibility, and high motivation. The amount of financial remuneration varies widely from one practice setting to another. Audiologists must determine their individual financial goals and tailor their professional endeavors accordingly.

Personal autonomy

In addition to professional autonomy and financial gain, a third expectation is personal autonomy. There is the freedom to accommodate work hours to one's lifestyle, bring the baby to work, and schedule vacations. It is doubtful that successful audiologists avail themselves fully of these opportunities, but there is something to knowing that the possibilities exist!

ATTITUDES AND BIASES

The following are individual and institutional perspectives that affect audiology negatively. We refer to them collectively as "chips on our shoulders" and expect that they will drop off as our profession matures.

Chip #1: "Private" Practice Stigma

Vestiges remain of a prejudicial attitude toward "private" practice, especially in some academic settings. Basically, the attitude reflects the damaging myth that commerce and audiology are ethically incompatible. It is not surprising that this attitude is encountered occasionally—after all, audiologists have dispensed hearing aids "ethically" only since the late 1970s. Paradoxically, clinic directors rarely encounter this prejudice, although they often perform tasks similar to independent practitioners (e.g., fee setting, product pricing, promotion).

As private practice increases, the old stigmas fade

The prejudicial attitude toward independent practice should disappear as audiologists achieve a more universal agreement on the appropriate means of marketing, recommending, and fitting amplification; as an expanded scope of practice gains universal acceptance (e.g., cerumen management); as audiologists settle into a defined niche in the health care system; and as graduate curricula adopt practice management courses for audiologists. Nevertheless, audiologists considering autonomous practice must disabuse themselves of this attitude's influence. It can have a devastating and insidious effect on the practice if it results in the practitioner being uncomfortable discussing charges and billing procedures with patients or referrals. Audiologists cannot maintain good self-images if they are worried that others in the profession will view their practice choice in this biased manner. It is doubtful whether audiologists can attract referrals, especially from professionals, if they carry this chip on their shoulders.

Chip #2: The Specialist Mentality

Another "chip" has to do with attitudes toward certain patient groups. Especially in today's competitive climate, it is difficult to practice autonomously while simultaneously restricting services. This is not to say that one should not develop specialty expertise (e.g., pediatric audiology). On the contrary, the creation of a specialized practice is an important means of distinguishing oneself and obtaining referrals by demonstrating "excellence." However, in general practices audiologists must be prepared to effectively handle cases outside their preferred specialty areas. Audiologists who view themselves solely as specialists are usually best utilized in large clinics or educational settings. The autonomous audiologist, on the other hand, is typically a practitioner who is comfortable and competent with all age groups and all procedures for which there is a demand in the community and is willing to meet those demands.

Chip #3: We Don't Do Windows

A third "chip" is the "I don't do windows" attitude, in which audiologists choose not to perform certain functions (e.g., discussion of billing, answering the phone) on the basis that they are not "audiology." The alternative is to hire nonaudiologists to perform these tasks. But in today's work place, nonproducing employees are an expensive anachronism (cf., Boyett & Conn, 1991). Only those who are "close to the product"—in this case hearing care—can expect to keep positions. It is important that we not allow our hard-earned professionalism to blind us to the importance of the more mundane aspects of service delivery. For example, discussing billing is part of being an audiologist if such discussion improves service delivery.

Chip #4: Taking Things Personally

Not every patient or customer encounter goes as planned by the audiologist: patients dispute charges or refuse to comply with recommendations; customers demand services or contractual agreements that strain professional bounds or capabilities. Some audiologists take these actions personally. They respond to the patients or customers in an emotional and occasionally adversarial manner.

An extreme version of this fourth chip is the audiologist who always assigns blame (elsewhere) when problems or miscommunications arise, rather than assuming responsibility for correcting the situations. The more autonomous the position, the more necessary it becomes to handle unpleasant situations objectively and dispassionately. Audiologists who cannot or will not assume responsibility for defusing abusive encounters are more appropriately placed in other settings.

PROFESSIONAL AVERSIONS AND AFFINITIES

It is as important to know what you do not want to do as it is to know what you want to do. The previous section pointed out that independent practitioners are more likely to be generalists than specialists, but this does not mean one must do every procedure under the scope of practice to succeed.

Indeed, it is difficult to imagine providing a high quality of service if one dislikes performing it. As an example, if you really do not wish to work with children, then consider locating in a retirement community. Conversely, skip retirement communities if you strongly favor diagnostic over hearing aid services.

Professional likes and dislikes extend to such basic decisions as practice size and time allocation. The yardstick of success is not measured in units of patient visits, employees, or office expansions, but rather in units of financial stability, personal satisfaction, and quality of service. All three are as possible in small practices as in large ones, but the professional's time is allocated differently. For audiologists who prefer direct patient care and like to control as many aspects of the care as possible, a small practice may be most satisfactory. For others who prefer to manage people and administer service delivery, a larger practice is better.

Evaluate strengths and weaknesses—capitalize on the strengths

Not all audiologists share the same patient care ethic. Independent practice provides the best forum for audiologists who want to assume full responsibility for all aspects of their patients' care. Less autonomous positions limit the clinicians' direct responsibility. The ASHA Committee on Private Practice notes that "In private practice there is a direct contract between the clinician and the client . . . . In nonprivate practice situations there is a third person or agency contracting with the clients and the clinician" (ASHA, 1982, p. 19).

LONG-TERM GOALS

Not surprisingly, many audiologists discover an increasing desire for personal and professional autonomy as they gain experience and confidence in the workplace. Long-term goals need to reflect this growth process, providing avenues for upward mobility and allowing time for continuing education, networking, and fulfillment of community responsibilities. It is important to gain perspective on one's work by periodically defining the relationship of the audiology practice to one's "life" goals. Such examination prevents job burn-out and allows one to continue practicing audiology as a calling.

Self-appraisal is an ongoing process

SUMMARY

Our field is maturing and broadening in scope, providing increasing opportunities for autonomy in clinic and independent practice settings. Choosing your point of comfort on the "autonomy continuum" requires a careful inventory of your commitment level, expertise, personal attributes, personal expectations, attitudes and biases, and long-term goals.

REFERENCES

American Speech-Language-Hearing Association. (1988). Report of the Task Force on Audiology II. *Asha, 30*(1), 41–45.

American Speech-Language-Hearing Association. (1982). Questions and answers on private practice. *Asha, 24*(11), 19–20.

American Speech-Language-Hearing Association. (1991a). Considerations for establishing a private practice in audiology and/or speech-language pathology. *Asha, 44*(Suppl. 3), 10–21.

American Speech-Language-Hearing Association. (1991b). Report on private practice. *Asha, 33*(Suppl. 6,), 1–4.

American Speech-Language-Hearing Association (1993). Preferred practice patterns for the professions of speech-language pathology and audiology. *Asha, 35*(Suppl. 3), 1–102.

Boyett, J. H., & Conn, H. P. (1992). *Workplace 2000.* New York: Plume.

Cherow, E., & Thompson, M. (1992). Audiologists respond to 1992 ASHA omnibus survey. *Audiology Update, 11*(1), 14–17.

Curran, J. R. (1986). The ten commandments of hearing aid dispensing. *Seminars in Hearing, 7*(2), 219–228. New York: Thieme.

Feldman, A. S. (1988). Some observations about us and private practice. *Asha, 30*(1), 29.

Peters, T. J., & Waterman, R. H., Jr. (1982). *In search of excellence.* New York: Warner.

APPENDIX 3-A

The Ten Commandments of Hearing Aid Dispensing[1]

James R. Curran, M.S.

The "Ten Commandments of Hearing Aid Dispensing" first appeared nearly 10 years ago, and although events and the passage of time have changed the conditions of dispensing somewhat, their essential message is as up-to-date and pertinent for the audiologist engaged in an autonomous dispensing practice as when they were first published a decade ago.

1. THOU SHALT BE TIRELESS IN THE PROMOTION OF THY PRACTICE

Does it appear strange that this "commandment" is listed first? It is not only the first, but perhaps the most important of the commandments.

For an audiologist immersed in the day-to-day routine of diagnostic clinical activities either as a student, instructor, or as an employee in an agency or medical setting, the shift in emphasis that must occur when one begins dispensing hearing aids in private practice sometimes comes as a wrench. Suddenly, a matter in which the individual placed little importance begins to assume gigantic proportions.

The nature of hearing aid dispensing can be summed up in one sense by understanding that it has been, since its inception, a product in search of a consumer. The hearing aid has been resisted historically because it represents to many hearing impaired persons a form of social stigma. With the exception of glasses, it is not fashionably acceptable to wear devices that advertise a disability, especially one that has come, for some, to be associated with senility and deterioration of the faculties. Therefore, the biggest challenge to the early dispenser was to develop methods for attracting customers. Potential customers did not, on the average, walk into offices voluntarily; in addition, the instruments of the early days were big, clumsy, inefficient, and underpowered. Continuing to today, dispensers have engaged in as many forms of advertising and promotion as they have been able to devise, in order to motivate hearing impaired persons to try their products.

If one of the primary objects of private practice is to dispense hearing aids to those who are candidates for amplification as part of a total rehabilitation program, then it becomes imperative that the audiologist also learn how to obtain a steady source of clients. Not only must the techniques for obtaining referrals be learned and practiced, they must be practiced with a diligence that borders on fanaticism. Promotion of the audiologist's services

---

[1]Reprinted from "The Ten Commandments of Hearing Aid Dispensing" by James R. Curran. *Seminars in Hearing,* 7(2), 219–228, with permission. Copyright 1986 Thieme, Inc.

must assume a level of importance perhaps greater than that of any other activity in the office, especially in the first few years, or the practice may fail. There is nothing more tragic than the picture of a superbly trained clinician sitting in a lonely office waiting for the telephone to ring, wasting his or her training, and losing self-esteem because he or she will not or cannot engage in promotional activities. Another way of looking at it is to realize that when a hearing aid office is sold, the most valuable asset of the business is not the furnishings or location, but rather its list of active users. There is constant subtle, often unrecognized competition between dispensers for clients who either are wearing amplification or who are willing to.

Sometimes it is not in the nature of the clinician to believe that he or she has the necessary skills to engage in successful public relations. It takes a willingness to overcome natural reticence in order to "blow one's horn." Sometimes the nature of the task is not understood. Public relations is nothing more than steady attention to the minutia of promotion and publicity, including meetings, mailings, bulletins, sales visits, letters, telephone calls, advertisements, and notices. It is never missing an opportunity to let people know you are in practice. It is never letting a day go by without making some sort of contact with a prospective customer or referral source. It is not without reason that the small businessman will join as many social and civic organizations as possible. It is with this purpose and intent that the doctor, lawyer, or other professional becomes active in social, charitable, and professional organizations. The talks one gives to various consumer organizations, the in-service training one is able to provide, visits to referral sources,

agencies, and institutions are all part of a master plan to make one's service known and understood.

There is a difference between conducting these familiar activities within and without the private practice setting. In private practice, they become critical to success, not just another necessary professional duty. As such, they must be elevated to a very high level of importance in the audiologist's mind. They may be boring, they may be tedious to execute, they may be frightening, and they may be unexciting; they are also imperative. In my experience, it is this single factor, the willingness to promote one's services persistently and tirelessly that often constitutes the difference between being successful and remaining marginal.

The foregoing is not meant to diminish the importance of providing the highest quality professional care. However, you cannot dispense a hearing aid and use your skills and training to provide the rehabilitative services required unless someone who needs your help is sitting across the table from you. Engross yourself in this reality, and all other things being equal, your practice will be a success. Ignore it, and you may soon be unself-employed.

2. THOU SHALT HEED GRAVELY THE MESSAGE OF THE BOTTOM LINE

The bottom line will tell you what equipment and furnishings you may purchase for your practice, how much you may pay yourself, whether you may hire additional help, whether your practice is improving or is on the downswing, and whether you can expand or not. It will also become, if studied with diligence and care, your touchstone for success, and prevent you from getting into financial difficulty. A well-thumbed set of financial statements, often referred to during the week, or even daily, eventually becomes an indispensable internalized reference point for making decisions.

I do not subscribe to the point of view that the audiologist cannot become a good businessman, but I do feel that audiologists have not had the opportunity to be exposed to businesslike thinking. They have had neither mentors nor models. Therefore, they do not have the feel for conducting a practice on a businesslike basis. It is not difficult eventually to learn the basics of what appears to be the arcane world of financial statements, but it is difficult to realize finally how vitally important they are. They must motivate your decision-making and guide your business way of life. It is somewhat similar to learning masking; the theory is not too difficult to understand with a little work, but putting it into practice is an altogether different story. Only after restudying the principles and after encounters with live patients does the process become an automatic part of the audiologist's clinical armamentarium. In both cases, much more than theoretical understanding is necessary; daily practice is required before the person owns the procedures.

This all implies that a certain amount of discipline must be brought to bear on business decisions as dictated by the financial health of the business. The purchase of a brand new dual-channel digital audiometer may have to be postponed, and instead one must get along with the clunky but serviceable 15-year-old channel and a half for another year or two, because the purchase of a new audiometer cannot be justified. Not enough revenue is being generated to

pay the bills; therefore, the owner must raise prices or search out alternative ways to obtain new business. Unpaid accounts must be placed for collection. A branch office becomes unprofitable and, despite the business it is generating, must be closed and employees let go to halt the drain on reserves. Third party payments are held up by political or other decisions beyond the clinician's control; consequently, the planned combination seminar or vacation one was planning during the winter months must be cancelled. Any number of similar decisions may be adversely affected by the state of the bottom line.

Making appropriate decisions based on the financial state of the business is necessary in order to protect the business. They are inevitably difficult to make, but to ignore or dismiss the story that the balance sheet tells will surely imperil the practice. Sometimes this is a painful lesson for the clinician to learn. He or she mistakenly believes that in the end, one's professional experience and skills are the primary ingredients for success and will be all that are required to overcome obstacles. Lip service is paid to the importance of taking business management principles seriously, but when the time comes, either they have not been learned or they are not acted on. The woods are filled with brilliant, professionally competent entrepreneurs who acted similarly, and eventually watched their dreams go up in smoke.

3. THOU SHALT BE WILLING TO LEARN AND USE FINE MOTOR SKILLS

It is one of my beliefs that all of the methods that have been proposed for the selection of hearing aids are, to a greater or lesser extent, rather unreliable. They are crude in their ability to predict which specific set of electroacoustic parameters or which specific hearing aid will provide the most benefit. They only provide approximations of the desired result, and often cannot be repeated. As a result, almost all instruments require some form of post-fitting adjustments to be satisfactory. Desired changes in performance can be affected subsequently either by adjusting trimmers or switches (electrical) or by altering the shape and dimensions of the coupling system (acoustical). The latter necessitates learning modification techniques that entail the development and use of fine motor skills.

It is astounding how often I hear statements like this from some audiologists: "I make the recommendation for amplification and let the dispenser (or technician) do the earmold, venting, modifications, etc." This point of view is probably permissible for the nondispenser to hold, but it should have no place in the thinking of the dispensing audiologist. It is incomprehensible to me that a dispensing audiologist would want to turn over to someone else the modifications, repairs, and other maneuvers that accompany the fitting process. Not only are modifications important for providing fit and comfort or for dealing with feedback problems, they can be used to enhance speech recognition in given instances. Motor skills can only be learned by doing, by repetition, and the beneficial outcomes that occur when modifications and minor repairs are properly effected cannot be fully appreciated unless the dispenser is directly involved in the process.

Perhaps some of the reluctance to perform modifications reflects an attitude that such work is less significant than site of lesion testing, less impor-

tant than being able to read research critically, or less professionally acceptable than conducting research, and therefore is not important enough to be a part of the preparation audiologists receive. Could this be the reason why so many audiologists are emerging from training programs without these skills and without an appreciation of their value? If so, I would point out that other health professionals undergo training in and rely strongly on using fine motor skills in the conduct of their professional practice, including medical doctors, dentists, and those in the optical field. I would rather dislike to have a denture fitted by a dentist who was not highly skilled in the mundane arts of filing, bending, cutting, and adjusting.

I feel there may be other reasons for reluctance to modify, however. Unless clinicians have had, somewhere in their background, training or experience, some success in developing physical dexterity through sports and manual or industrial arts training, they may feel quite inadequate about their ability to perform the required maneuvers. Having never experienced success in activities requiring mastery of physical skills, they harbor some doubt or anxiety about their ability to be adept enough, and feel clumsy and awkward. I am reinforced in this view, because when I conduct modification seminars, I always see a small number of clinicians, both male and female, who despite insistent exhortation and ample opportunity, hold back and refuse to avail themselves of the opportunity to learn how it feels to work on an earmold or an in-the-ear hearing aid. At the same time, many of their peers cannot wait to get started and are enthusiastic about learning this aspect of the art of dispensing.

The fact is that most persons learning a new skill will feel, to a greater or lesser extent, some anxiety and fear that they will not perform well. It is uncomfortable in the beginning, but with practice, everyone improves. The joy and feeling of competence that one experiences when these important maneuvers are mastered is difficult to describe. Patients who have never had good listening experiences or whose instruments have been poorly fitted can be taken care of with the simplest of techniques, easily and quickly. Clinicians discover that they have answers for serious problems literally "at their fingertips," and hearing aid dispensing suddenly becomes less difficult and unpredictable than it initially seemed to be.

4. THOU SHALT DEVELOP BROAD SHOULDERS

The buck stops at your desk. When a user returns to your office for the sixth or seventh time with vague complaints, appears to be impossible to satisfy, and not only your patience but your options for correcting the complaint appear to be close to exhaustion, then is the time to tell yourself that there really are no problems connected with hearing aid fitting that you are unable to handle. This idea, the willingness to do whatever it takes to resolve difficult fitting problems whenever they occur, is one of the fundamental attitudes that one must hold to be successful in dispensing. You cannot walk out the back door when problems walk in the front. There was a time when the dispenser relied heavily on handholding and counseling, to pacify the irate customer, asking the user to be patient, using soothing words to

resolve problems for which there were simply no other solutions. Today, there are so many options for altering performance, so many alternative methods for providing appropriate amplification, that it is usually no longer necessary to resort to this. This is not to say that counseling is not critical to the fitting process, but rather that it should not be utilized as the sole method for solving fitting problems.

Your self-esteem as a dispenser should grow as you internalize this altitude. It will require that you invest yourself in learning as much as possible about the technology and methods that are used to ensure satisfaction. Feelings of competency and self: sufficiency result as problem-solving skills and understanding improve. However, one must walk a fine line between that of being responsible and that of being a "caretaker." Caretakers get affirmation and feelings of self-worth by pleasing others. There are a high number of caretakers in the health professions; unconsciously defining one's self worth according to whether the patient is happy with his amplification (and by extension, with you) can lead to feelings of disillusionment, depression, and burnout. There is a point beyond which the professionally responsible clinician should not venture in the attempt to resolve customer problems. On the one hand, it is important to roll up one's sleeves whenever the problem presents itself and to not shirk responsibility; on the other hand, it is important to maintain a sense of detachment toward the customer and know when one's feelings of self-worth might be getting entangled in the process. When the latter occurs, it is best to remove yourself from the fitting by acknowledging that there is little more that you can do to improve things. Sometimes, this might entail a refund, or not accepting a person as a customer, or simply being firm that all that can be done by you, has been. Before one can do these things with equanimity, one must have assured one's self, however, that indeed, the most probable avenues have been explored.

5. THOU SHALT BELIEVE DEVOUTLY IN THE EFFICACY OF AMPLIFICATION

When one enters into dispensing, one is entering into a highly active, dynamic, synergistic environment. Competition hones and whets the level of services that are offered, results in ever-improving products and accessories, and is constantly producing provocative ideas and interesting challenges. This is not the setting for a person who has but a half hearted commitment to the idea of the value of amplification as the prime, operative determinant in the auditory rehabilitation of the hearing-impaired individual. Without this focused dedication, the clinician may never experience the continuing satisfaction: of providing consistently effective fittings. It is permissible to wonder if one will be successful, to worry about the future of the business, to question the correctness of a fitting, but it is not permissible to doubt that hearing aids are the single most significant factor in the rehabilitative process.

The lack of commitment I am speaking about may take more than one form. It is evident in a clinician's thinking when before the fitting, he or she dwells more on the problems and difficulties that the patient is going to have. It is revealed when it is emphasized to the patient that if the hearing aids do not work, they can be returned to the manufacturer at no charge. It manifests itself whenever the audiologist refrains from being aggressive in recommending amplification to a reluctant patient when it is clearly evident that the patient has communicative difficulties, will benefit from amplification, and is an ideal candidate for hearing aids. It stops the dispenser from strongly recommending two hearing aids instead of one, when it is patently obvious that the individual not only needs but is a perfect candidate for binaural amplification. It makes it difficult for the audiologist to charge properly for rehabilitative devices, as if the clinician had doubts about the instruments' (and his or her) essential benefit and worth. It shows when the private practitioner markets the practice with emphasis on auditory training, speech-reading, industrial hearing testing, and diagnostic testing, with amplification occupying a less prominent position in the structure of services.

If you wonder where you stand on the commitment spectrum with reference to hearing aids, perhaps the answers to the following questions will be revealing:

1. Does the person have a hearing loss?
2. If so, is he or she a candidate for amplification?
3. Similarly, will he or she benefit from amplification?
4. If so, is there anyone more qualified than you to do the fitting?
5. If you do the fitting, do you want the fitting to fail?
6. If you do the fitting, do you want it to be successful?
7. If you do the fitting, are there hearing aids capable of delivering the amplification you think is required?

8. Do you think hearing aids are overpriced?

9. Do you deserve a good income? Even if it is based on the sale of hearing aids?

10. If the fitting fails, or is only partially successful, should you get paid for your time, effort and judgment?

11. If the fitting is successful, how much value should be placed on your assistance in restoring or improving the individual's communicative effectiveness?

12. If hearing aids were not available, would you still be able to provide to the patient the same effective level of rehabilitative services?

13. Are you proud to be a hearing aid dispenser?

14. Do you feel at ease in discussing fees and costs?

The questions may help you find and address areas in your thinking that need thoughtful analysis.

6. THOU SHALT KISS THE 8-HOUR DAY GOODBYE

There are two speeds in private practice: top speed and faster. There never is enough time, it seems, to get all the work done in a normal working day. Especially when beginning the practice, the new dispenser usually functions as part-time secretary, bookkeeper, repair technician, and marketing specialist while conducting a full-time audiological and dispensing practice. Most clinicians find that the end of the working day runs into or past the dinner hour, and neither weekends nor holidays are inviolable. Visits to referral sources must be sandwiched in between appoint-

ments, attendance at conventions and conferences must be limited, telephone calls and letters are done on the run, visits to nursing homes and hospital beds entail skipping lunch. The pressure usually lets up a little as the practice expands, and new help is hired in the office, but the demands on the owner's time never appear to slacken, because new responsibilities appear to replace those delegated to other employees. Most dispensers, however, would not have it any other way. The payoff in lieu of the leisurely work day is the freedom to run the practice as one feels it should be, the right to make professional and business decisions without fear of second-guessing, no limitation on income growth, and the self-satisfaction of building a business and seeing it succeed. The milieu of heightened productivity is addictive, and in comparison to the slow pace of institutions and agencies, healthy and mitigative.

7. THOU SHALT GET BY WITH AS LITTLE AS POSSIBLE IN THE BEGINNING

When clinicians ask me for advice on starting an autonomous dispensing practice, I tell them what I think the most important factors are, but one point especially disconcerts them. I strongly recommend that they start their practice with a minimum of outlay for furnishings, equipment, and rent. I suggest that they forego their desire to have attractive new furniture and desk, opt for a small, easily paid for office space, and postpone ordering any but the most basic audiometric and similar equipment. This rubs some audiologists the wrong way, because part of the dream of private practice is to possess the best in equipment and have a great-looking office in a correct location. Audiologists will borrow incredible amounts of money to get started, with little or no assurance that they will generate enough income to pay it back. When I see this happen, I conclude that the clinician has a skewed sense of values and may indeed be heading for disappointment.

The new dispensing audiologist learns that one can do good audiometry in a quiet environment without the benefit of a prefabricated room, if need be. A well-trained audiologist recognizes when room noise levels may be interfering with results and adjusts for it. A single channel (or channel and a half) audiometer will do perfectly well for hearing aid fitting in the beginning, at least until enough revenue is generated to pay for a more elaborate audiometer. A reconditioned older impedance unit will be perfectly serviceable for the first year or two; neither your patients nor your diagnostic conclusions will suffer from the fact that it is not new.

Fixed, recurring expenses such as rent, electricity, and heat must be critically evaluated to make certain the new business does not have too big a nut to crack. I know of very few practices that were started from scratch and were immediately profitable unless close attention was paid to keeping overhead low. You will be grateful for the fact that you were prudent enough to ensure that your ongoing monthly expenses were kept small. Usually, the new practice does not generate income in the beginning at a level that will allow a high debt service.

Fight the temptation to spend on furniture, a big desk, and plush office. One reflects professionalism by being neat, competent, and industrious; the quality of office furnishings does not define the quality of services. Rather, be conservative and use the funds you would have spent on decor and equipment to handle cash-flow emergencies or slumps that inevitably occur the first few years.

If the preceding seems to err on the side of excessive caution, check it out with any audiologist in private practice. Better yet, ask one who has some used office furniture and equipment for sale.

8. THOU SHALT TREAT THY COMPETITORS WITH RESPECT

Starting a new practice is exciting. Besides the fun of being one's own boss, the prospect of being able to increase one's income significantly is very heady. At the same time, it is frightening, because the success of the business rests squarely on one's shoulders. After years of academic training or working for someone else, the audiologist makes the decision to enter into private practice and business. Unless one has had prior experience, business is a whole new world, and not a particularly well understood one. Additionally, the product that the audiologist is dispensing is not particularly well understood, either. Fitting hearing aids well requires the development of a high degree of art and judgment to compensate for the lack of predictability that accompanies the fitting process. Art and judgment are attributes that take time to acquire, and most new dispensers are relatively deficient in them.

Combine these conditions and one has the ingredients for a large dose of insecurity. Being insecure and doubtful about one's knowledge and skills or one's ability to be successful is normal, but it is such an uncomfortable feeling that it may be dealt with by repression or denial. These feelings will not go away if not faced up to and dealt with and can reappear without warning. One of the common ways for a person to hide insecurity from others (and oneself) is to blame others for things that go wrong, or to act in a hostile, arrogant way toward them.

As a result, in their anxiety to be successful, some dispensing audiologists do foolish and detrimental things. They speak negatively to their customers about the dispenser who sold them their previous aids. Probably the worst thing, any salesman can do is knock competition to the potential customer. They isolate themselves from state or national organizations that represent dispensers and work politically to weaken them instead of using them as resources to further their own competence in dispensing, or they badger and threaten manufacturers to stop supplying products to competitors, usually on flimsy grounds. They blame the manufacturer or the manufacturer's representative for their failed fittings, suggesting that the product is at fault. This is understandable, and one of the risks the manufacturer takes, but the rage, hostility, and contempt that sometimes accompanies the complaint is out of proportion to the alleged offense and makes it difficult for the manufacturer to want to help out the dispenser when a favor is needed. In short, their attitude seems to be that their beliefs and practices represent the only truth, and everyone else's are fraudulent or inferior.

When I first started dispensing, I received a wonderful and welcome piece of advice from a veteran dealer whom I had previously mistrusted. He said, "Welcome to the world of hearing aid sales. I will be fitting some of your customers over the years and you will be fitting some of mine. That's the way it's always been and the way it always will be. That should not stop us from being friends as well as competitors, because we have more in common than we have differences." As time passed, I realized the truth of his words and have never regretted following his advice. Competitive nonaudiologist dispensers as a group actually welcome the autonomous freestanding dispensing audiologist to the business. What they dislike is the audiological dispensing facility that is tax-supported, for they feel the latter has an unfair advantage and is supported by their tax dollars. However, most feel that audiologists upgrade hearing aid dispensing when they enter into it. They understand very well the nature of fair competition and are comfortable with it.

With respect to manufacturers, I can say without hesitation that they are nearly always willing to extend themselves for those dispensers who try to resolve problems in a courteous and reasonable way. If the company is in the wrong and will not own up to its mistake, the dispenser should exercise his or her option to take business elsewhere. However, no amount of screaming or verbal abuse by the dispenser will persuade the company that the dispenser is entitled to any extra consideration or care, whether warranted by the facts or not. In this small industry of ours, it is wise to remember that what goes around, comes around, and sometime in the future the dispenser may be in the position of having to ask the manufacturer for assistance. Needless to say, it is always much easier if one has not burned one's bridges behind.

9. THOU SHALT ADOPT A FLEXIBLE HEARING AID EVALUATION PROTOCOL

Just as mature adults have the right to question the proscriptions and regulations they were subjected to as children, so too do dispensing audiologists have the right to change their mind about the hearing aid evaluation procedures they learned. There are far too many conditions that are encountered that are not covered by the rules. For example, you may be called to a nursing home to test and fit hearing aids to a bedridden, retarded, cerebral palsied individual who is unable to participate in the testing. There are no written procedures for this type of case, and if for example, establishing uncomfortable listening level for speech is one of your key measurements, there will be no fitting, unless you are able to change your criteria and approach.

Usually the procedure we first learn assumes the most validity in our minds, and changing that point of view or procedure can make one feel like a heretic or apostate. However, familiarity is not reason enough to eschew change when it becomes necessary, nor is it reason enough to judge critically the work of others that does not follow orthodox guidelines. Twenty years ago the mention of the master hearing aid elicited frowns and murmurs of disapproval; some of the most enlightening research of the past 5 years has been performed and continues to be performed using the master hearing aid. The estimation of gain and saturation sound pressure level (SSPL) 90 from pure-tone thresholds fails to take into account individual differences, yet the concept in one form or another comprises the basis for the selection of performance parameters for most custom in-the-ear hearing aids. Recently, it has become fashionable to find fault with comparative evaluations of hearing aids using speech recognition tests; yet large numbers of clinicians perform some type of speech testing to estimate the ultimate effectiveness of the fitting. There is a ground swell of interest in probe microphone measurements; nevertheless, it is not well understood that they only measure distribution of energy at the tympanic membrane and tell nothing about the individual's perception of the speech signal.

It does not take a genius to recognize that all measurement procedures are lacking. Yet each has its adherents, and each when properly used in the hands of a dispenser who feels comfortable with it is capable of providing adequate amplification for a given patient. Nevertheless, it is not wise to adhere rigidly to one method, so that when a new procedure arises, which will inevitably happen, it cannot be easily accommodated to and incorporated into the practice.

10. THOU SHALT BE FRIENDS WITH THY CUSTOMERS

It can be tempting to adopt a modern, detached way with patients, to follow the dispassionate model of the busy medical specialist. However, here is a tip: Your friendly competitor down the street who always has the coffee pot on and takes a minute or two to catch up with the lives of his patients and tells corny jokes is stealing your income away. Given the choice of two equally competent dispensers, one of whom is more personal and "homey" in his or her delivery of services than the other, which of the two do you think the average elderly patient will want to return to? There are no courses you can take that will help you to prepare for this reality. You must realize the importance of this yourself and do whatever is needed to make your office a pleasant, relaxed, and comfortable environment. You must learn to conduct your business with a personal touch, and encourage your employees to do likewise.

Remember, that you are no different from the patients you serve, except perhaps in age. Remember, too, that senior citizens have lived full lives and have had dreams, sorrows, and joys similar to yours. Remember that they have experienced far more than you and have gained wisdom and serenity in the process. Realize that they certainly prize your professional judg-

ment and skill, but that they also value the comfort and familiarity of friendships. As one becomes older, and as friends and companions begin to die, one begins to appreciate even more the chance to be sociable.

You will read and hear about the pitfalls of getting too close to your patients, about the need to be objective in your relationship with them. You will find some customers who will abuse your friendship; some will become overly dependent, and return to your office weekly with problems or excuses to talk to you because they are lonely, and this will impinge on your precious time. You will learn to deal with these problems in good time. If you are not prepared to accept these minor inconveniences, then you may not be prepared to start dispensing on your own.

Starkey Laboratories,
Eden Prairie, Minnesota

The Business Plan

Business Plans
The benefit from a business plan comes from the time and effort the audiologist puts into writing it

Business plans are working documents that provide guidance and direction to practices as they start out, expand, add new services, obtain financing, make management decisions, and maintain control. A good business plan is a concise but very comprehensive document that defines the core attributes of the practice. An effective business plan *is* the business; so much effort needs to go into its formulation, writing, and updating.

This chapter briefly describes the main topics addressed in business plans, but does not attempt a comprehensive text on *how* to write a plan. Most of the topics receive fuller treatment in later chapters, and a sample business plan is provided in Appendix 4-A. There are entire books dedicated to the topic of writing business plans and they are recommended reading for anyone contemplating opening an autonomous audiology practice.[1]

BUILDING BLOCKS

A business plan needs to reflect the unique characteristics of the individual audiology practice. As tempting as it may be to hire an outside consultant to write it, a large measure of the benefit that a business plan provides comes from the time

---

[1]Books on business plans are available in the business sections of public libraries and bookstores. In particular, see the series by Oasis Press entitled "Starting and Operating a Business in [state of interest]," published for each of the 50 states. The Small Business Administration (SBA) has 15 to 20 page guides to business plans. Contact the Small Business Development Centers (SBDC) at (800) 633-6450 to find out about local seminars on market research and business planning. Software packages are also available to help build and tailor business plans.

and effort the owner/founder puts into creating the plan. In this way the plan reflects the practitioner's vision of the practice. Although there is no set content, to be of maximum value to its authors and others who have a legitimate interest in the practice, every plan should contain the elements itemized in Table 4–1. Each of the items in Table 4–1 is described briefly in this chapter and illustrated in Appendix 4-A. More detailed explanations are found in later chapters.

Executive Summary

This summary appears at the front of the plan but it is written last, based on elements of the developed plan. It is meant to provide a quick overview for executives (e.g., administrators, bank loan officers) who must make important decisions about the practice after reviewing elements of the plan. The Executive Summary is no more than two pages. It covers:

A quick overview

- Current status: When the practice began or is expected to begin;
- A description of products and services;
- Target markets;
- Unique practice strengths (e.g., experience, location, equipment, or products);
- Short- and long-term practice plans;
- Financial projections;
- Money needs, if financing is sought.

Business Concept

The business concept documents the founder's vision of the practice. It must convey the founder's view of why the practice will survive and even flourish in the marketplace. In

The vision

Table 4–1. Elements of a business plan.

Executive summary

Business concept

Market analysis

Marketing Plan

Operation and organization plan

Financial analysis

Risk analysis

Overall schedule

general business this is referred to as the *unique selling proposition* (Whitmyer, Rasberry, & Phillips, 1989).

This section describes the practice's products and services and details the factors that make the practice unique. The market niche or target market is defined along with an assessment of the market potential. That assessment comes from a market analysis.

Market Analysis

Go or no go?

The market analysis (also called a market survey) serves to validate or invalidate the business concept. Before money and time are committed to opening or expanding a practice, the market's characteristics deserve a hard look. Who are the customers? Who is the competition? What is the potential of the market today and in the future? For a complete discussion of marketing, refer to Chapter 13.

Numerous sources for gathering market information are available. Obtaining this information involves research from *primary* and *secondary* sources. Primary data are collected directly, for example, by conducting surveys and interviewing competitors or the public to establish acceptance of a new practice in a community. Secondary data generally are obtained from public sources. Census data provide valuable demographic information, the Chamber of Commerce may have performed research on spending patterns in the targeted market, and the Small Business Administration (SBA) may have information of local interest to the practice.

The *scope of the market* is the first characteristic determined in the analysis. Scope defines geographic attributes of potential target markets. For most practices the scope is localized to a community or, in larger communities, to specific areas within the community. This topic is covered in Chapter 7.

The next step in Market Analysis is to characterize competitors according to their market share, growth rate and potential, strengths and weaknesses, and receptivity to another practice entering the market. For small unincorporated competitors, this analysis relies mainly on primary research and guesswork. Even guesswork estimates are valuable because trying to answer specific questions forces the new practice to look at the marketplace. Information on all corporations is available from Dun and Bradstreet[2] sur-

---

[2]Contact Dun and Bradstreet Information Services at: Customer Service Center, 899 Eaton Avenue, Bethlehem, PA 18025-9922. Telephone: (800) 999-3867; FAX: (215) 882-7400.

veys in many states. If hospitals or public universities are competitors in the market area, information is also available from secondary sources.

Assessing *market potential* is the final step in the market analysis section. Factors to consider include: (a) state of the economy today and as it is forecast in the near- (12 months) and long-term, (b) seasonality of the market, (c) status of audiology and hearing aid technology (e.g., Is it stable or are new break throughs predicted?[3]), and (d) legal or political factors that may influence the market (e.g., are there future plans to change licensing or dispensing requirements?).

Armed with the market and customer characteristics, an evaluation of the competition, and an assessment of market potential, the writer of the business plan is ready to write a marketing plan.

Marketing Plan

The Marketing Plan
- *Revenue Forecast*
  - *Revenue Sources*
  - *Sales Estimates*
- *Services and Products*
- *Fees*
- *Product Positioning*
- *Quality*

The *marketing plan* forecasts revenues, defines how services and products will be provided, determines their pricing, describes promotional strategies, and depicts how the practice intends to stand behind its products and services.

---

[3]Cochlear implant and cochlear nucleus implants are an example of scientific and technological breakthroughs that will affect the profession. Another recent example is the development and clinical implementation of otoacoustic emissions testing.

Traditionally called sales forecasts, the *revenue forecast* identifies sources of practice revenue by product and service and then constructs *market sales estimates*. Market sales are the estimated sales to a specified customer base in a specified geographical area within a specified period (Leza & Placencia, 1988). For a beginning practice, the forecast should be projected out monthly for the first year and yearly for the next 2 years. An example of a monthly forecast for hearing aid sales in shown in Appendix 4-A (see Figure 4–A.1). The important thing to remember is that this analysis is *not* meant to determine how much the practice is going to make, but what number of services and products will realistically be provided in the specified time frame. For instance, the example in Appendix 4-A forecasts hearing aid sales for a new practice in the first year. Because the average sale price of hearing aids in that practice is not known, the ordinate simply shows the number of instruments that could be dispensed if things go as planned. The sale price affixed to the product will be determined subsequently, taking into account cost of sales and other costs of the practice (costs are discussed in the financial section of the business plan). At that point, an actual revenue forecast can be completed.

The marketing plan next describes what *services and products* the practice will provide and how it will provide them. Some services (e.g., diagnostic testing) can be provided only by licensed or certified audiologists and may therefore cost more than other services and products that do not carry this requirement (e.g., hearing screening, minor hearing aid repairs, basic hearing aid orientations). Cost of services, quality of services, time management, and revenues are integrally entwined in decisions of service delivery, for example, using licensed hearing aid dispensers or audiology aides will lessen costs but increase supervision time. There is also the potential for decreased quality (perceived or real) and subsequent revenue declines when services are provided by nonaudiologists.

The *fee schedule* simply states what the charges will be for the services and products described above. Fee setting is a complex topic that is addressed in Chapter 11. Two basic rules must be observed when doing this portion of the business plan. The first rule is that fees have to be consistent with the market: a practice is likely to fail if it sets fees that are well above (or below) the prevailing rates established by insurance providers. Indeed, a practice that does choose to set rates much higher needs assurance from its market analysis that the target market will value its services at those rates. The second rule is that revenues must cover costs: A practice will certainly fail if expenses outrun income. Services must pay for themselves, product pricing must cover wholesale costs, and both must also cover overhead and profit requirements.

Once services and products are identified, analyzed by market demand and form of delivery, and priced, the marketing plan proceeds to describe how those services and products will be positioned. This requires extensive planning and preparation, as discussed in Chapter 13. The business plan briefly describes how the practice plans to contact target markets, what features of the practice will be promoted, and what media will be used to reach the markets. For example, the practice may use pamphlets and newsletters to identify itself to physicians in the community and yellow pages and local newspapers to identify itself to patients.

Lastly, the practice must articulate its *position on quality and service* and communicate that position clearly to its employees as well as its clients and suppliers. The practice must have a constancy of purpose for products and service that focuses on innovation and constant improvement in delivery of the products and services to the final customer (Walton, 1986).

Operation and Organization Plan

The operation and organizational plan is complex and comprehensive. It states the *legal form* of the practice. It defines the location, describes the *facilities*.[4] This section analyzes current and projected capabilities of the practice and sets out a corresponding *organizational structure*. That structure addresses personnel requirements, growth plans, training requirements and the use of professionals from outside the practice. Figure 4–A.2 in the Appendix 4–A of this chapter is an example of a simple organizational structure. For further information, refer to Chapter 11.

Financial Analysis

The financial plan answers many questions for the practice and those outside the practice who may be approached regarding financing. The financial section identifies sources of funding, how much money is needed, when the funding is required, and for what purposes it will be used. Tools that

Money—how much, when, and for what purpose?

---

[4]For complete discussions of the italicized items, refer to Chapters 5, 7, and 8.

help the practice demonstrate these requirements are a *proforma profit and loss statement* for the next 5 years, a *cash flow analysis* for the next 3 years, and a chart that calculates the *break-even point for the practice.* This is a difficult section for many audiologists who are new to the business world. Most financial institutions have their own versions of these forms, which can be helpful guides when constructing these calculations and graphs.

Risk Evaluation

Practices will face an array of risks that run the gamut from rising costs, threats from competition, shifts in key technologies, to economic changes in patient care models. The plan provides a view of the risks facing the practice and how the practice plans to address or mitigate the impact of these risks.

All practices will face tax, legal, and insurance risks as part of doing business. Hiring outside experts to address legal, accounting, and insurance matters will help reduce exposures in these areas.

Overall Schedule

The plan closes with an overall schedule that documents when *major milestones* are projected. This schedule allows the owner/founder and other interested parties to monitor general progress of the business as it relates to the plan. The schedule can be in an outline format that shows projected dates for starting and completing the business concept, marketing analysis, marketing plan, operation and organization plan, the financial plan, and risks. Under each of the headings are subheadings such as revenue forecast, products and services, pricing, advertising, and product/service warranties for the Marketing Plan. As the plan is implemented, the outline is used to note the dates that sub-headings are completed, along with comments concerning the milestone.

To supplement the outline or as an alternative, key elements of the plan can be charted on a time line. The entire plan can be shown on a special time line known as a Gantt chart which illustrates target and actual dates. Gantt charts are commonly used in production scheduling (Stoner & Wankel, 1986). They can be done by hand or through various software packages available for PC systems. Figure 4–A.3 in this chapter's appendix is an example of a Gantt chart for an audiology practice.

Major milestones

Gantt charts

SUMMARY

A good business plan helps a new practice get off on the right foot. As a working document that is periodically reviewed and updated, it is useful when the practice needs to expand or obtain financing. It is also an important means of maintaining focus on the true mission of the enterprise.

The plan should identify the unique *business concept* of the practice. It defines the products or services, the unique selling point, and the target market and its potential to the business.

The plan reviews *market research* which summarizes the scope of the market, analyzes competitors' positions, and market potential. A *marketing plan* is then proposed. The marketing plan presents revenue forecasts based on the products and services that will be offered. It submits a schedule of fees and product charges, summarizes strategies to promote and support those products and services, and sets forth a statement on quality of service.

The *organization and operation* section summarizes the legal form of the practice, its location, facilities, and organization structure. The *financial plan* presents standard financial analyses to identify when, how much, and for what purpose funding is needed. *Risk analysis* addresses strategies to deal with potential internal and external threats to the success of the enterprise. The business plan concludes with an *overall schedule* of projected milestones for the business (e.g., opening day, hiring first staff, break even point).

Each section of a good business plan warrants a great deal of forethought and research as it is conceived and composed. It is important to be realistic and perhaps somewhat conservative, rather than overly optimistic. The issues inherent in a good plan receive further discussion in later chapters.

REFERENCES

Leza, R. L., & Placencia, J. F. (1988). *Develop your business plan.* Grants Pass, OR: Oasis Press.

Stoner, J., & Wankel, C. (1986). *Management.* Englewood Cliffs, NJ: Prentice-Hall.

Walton, M. (1986). *The Deming management method.* New York: Perigee Books.

Whitmyer, C., Rasberry, S., & Phillips, M. (1989). *Running a one person business.* Berkeley, CA: Ten Speed Press.

APPENDIX 4-A

Sample Business Plan for a Dispensing Audiology Practice

CARDINAL HEARING SERVICES (CHS)

Audiology and Hearing Dispensing

A NEW PROFESSIONAL PRACTICE IN HEARING HEALTH CARE

Dr. A, Ph.D.

President

January 19--

Credit Line Request of $30,000.00

CARDINAL HEARING SERVICES

TABLE OF CONTENTS

EXECUTIVE SUMMARY

Cardinal Hearing Services (CHS) is a private practice that will offer comprehensive audiology and hearing aid services to people of all ages in the greater Central City area. CHS is a subchapter-S Corporation founded by Dr. A, an audiologist and hearing aid dispenser with many years of experience in a variety of practice settings.

CHS will begin offering services on January 2, 19--. It will be located in the Physicians Medical Building, Suite 100, adjacent to Central City Hospital. The practice will offer diagnostic audiometry, pediatric hearing evaluations, special tests for auditory and balance disorders, and hearing aid fitting, including programmable instrumentation.

CHS will begin operation with Dr. A performing all audiology services, assisted by an audiology aide, Mr. B. Mr. B is an licensed practical nurse with an undergraduate degree in Speech and Hearing. Mr. B plans to take the [state] hearing aid examination in May 19--. Although services will be available to everyone, CHS's target markets will be senior citizens, high-risk infants and toddlers, and industrial sites requiring hearing conservation programs.

CHS is in a strong position to perform well because the Central City area is currently underserved by audiologists. CHS's position is further strengthened by several factors: Dr. A's background and credentials, CHS's location on the only medical campus in Central City, the large and growing size of its target markets, and recent and continuing technological advances in hearing health care.

CHS will apply for a line of credit of $30,000 to fund unanticipated expenses and eventual expansion, if needed. Start-up costs will be funded from Dr. A's personal savings. The break-even point is predicted to occur after 9 months (January 19--). The practice is expected to grow to the point that a staff audiologist will be hired at the end of the second year. A second office is planned in 5 years, on the assumption that Central City continues to grow and a second hospital or medical plaza is constructed.

BUSINESS CONCEPT

Cardinal Hearing Services (CHS) is an independent private practice that will provide complete diagnostic audiology services and hearing aid dispensing to patients of all ages in the Central City area. The goals of CHS are to provide the highest quality hearing services to Central City residents in a cost-effective manner while maintaining an atmosphere that is professional and friendly. CHS is outstanding for several reasons:

1. Its founder, Dr. A, possesses exceptional training in audiology, management, and business practice, stemming from many years of experience in a variety of audiology service settings, including academic institutions, Veterans Administration hospitals, private hospitals, and hearing aid dispensing practices;

2. Staffing will be in "teams" of professionally trained individuals: every service encounter (e.g., telephone call, walk-in, or scheduled appointment) is with a certified audiologist, clinical fellow in audiology, audiology aide, or some combination of these staff;

3. Patient referrals by primary care physicians will account for at least 60% of all services provided, based on the location of the practice and the marketing plan;

4. Sophisticated test equipment (e.g., auditory brainstem response, computerized programmable amplification) and office equipment (e.g., computer networking, billing by modem) will allow comprehensive and accurate service delivery that is more cost-effective than is available from local competitors.

5. Services will be maintained at "cutting edge" because all staff will be required to stay technically current by participating in continuing education that is formal (e.g., conferences) and informal (e.g., on the job training, reading journal articles, discussions with manufacturers and other professionals).

MARKET ANALYSIS

Scope

The market scope encompasses greater Central City, with a population of approximately 100,000 according to census reports. Major market segments within that population are: (1) retirees, (2) infants and young children, and (3) industrial workers. Central City is primarily a retirement community, due to its temperate climate. The Chamber of Commerce estimates that 30,000 of the residents are retired to Central City from other locations, and that 40% of nonessential services (e.g., restaurants, theater) are purchased by these residents. In addition, these residents have a higher utilization of the hospital than the rest of the population. Most retirees have purchased homes in development enclaves clustered within a 3 mile radius of the community hospital. With our office located in the medical building adjacent to the hospital, CHS expects to provide services to 35% of this target market within the next five years. Published figures suggest that 35–50% of persons over 65 years of age have hearing losses that warrant amplification.

Central City has the only tertiary intensive care nursery (ICN) in the eastern portion of this state and there are few services available in outlying areas. Central City Hospital oversees the care and follow-up of over 80% of sick infants born in a 100-mile radius. CHS plans to contract within the next year with the hospital to perform hearing screening on all ICN babies and outpatient follow-up on those who fail the screening (published research estimates the latter to range from 6–10% of infants in the ICN). CHS's location adjacent to the hospital in the Physicians Medical Building will make such an arrangement convenient for patients and staff.

Over the years, Central City's low cost of labor, liberal business tax incentives and lenient environmental policies have attracted several small industrial plants. However, the shift to a service-oriented retirement community coupled with stricter enforcement of OSHA guidelines have placed an increasing burden on these factories to protect their workers. Hearing conservation programs are being established in some plants. CHS plans to capture 50% of this market in the next 5 years.

Competition

Central City is currently underserved by audiologists and other health professionals, undoubtedly because of its remote location and low cost of labor. According to hearing industry statistics and discussions with hearing aid manufacturers, over half of the hearing aids dispensed in this area are coming from sales-oriented hearing aid franchises that do not employee audiologists and maintain only satellite offices in Central City. There are two audiologists in private practice. One works in a local ENT office and performs on-call audiology. The physician refers patients who need hearing aids to one of the franchises. The other audiologist operates a solo practice in the downtown area. It has been static for many years, but does receive referrals from the only other ENT physician in the community. Little diagnostic audiology is performed, and the owner has not stayed up to date on current amplification technology.

Central City Hospital is private but also functions as the county hospital. New state regulations will require hearing screening in tertiary ICNs within the next year. The hospital has no funds budgeted for test equipment, nor does it have any employees trained to operate hearing test equipment or interpret results. A survey of hospital administrators and local pediatricians indicates a strong interest in contracting with CHS for ICN screening and follow-up.

The state university is located in Central City. It has a large Communications Disorders graduate program that is accredited for SLP but not for audiology. The University program has an active clinic that provides services primarily to low income groups within the community and to the schools. CHS views the university program and clinic as an auxiliary support service rather than a competitor. Informal surveys of the faculty and students by the founder of CHS showed that they are dedicated to service delivery and enthusiastic about the type of practice CHS proposes to bring to Central City.

There are two large industrial audiology businesses with mobile equipment that are headquartered in the adjacent state. According to telephone interviews CHS conducted with their owners, neither company considers it cost-effective to add Central City industries to their "routes" because of the small number of employees (<50 per site). However, they are interested in contractual arrangements with CHS to perform on-site screening and hearing conservation training.

Market Potential

According to the most recent census information, Central City is growing more rapidly than cities its size in other parts of the country, and its proportion of retirees is higher and growing more rapidly. The average income of Central City residents is lower than average, but the average income of the retiree market is higher than average. Zoning is favorable for the development of more retirement enclaves. Another professional medical building is slated to break ground near the hospital in 2 years. As already mentioned, state and federal laws are prompting implementation of hearing services at the hospital and at industrial sites. Industry is not expected to grow in this area, and may decrease as regulations raise the cost of doing business. But even this may be favorable to CHS, because our efforts to be cost-effective through the use of computerized technology will in turn reduce the overall cost to the industries of implementing hearing conservation programs.

Recent breakthroughs in computer, test equipment, and hearing aid technology are favorable for CHS. Faster CPUs and printers, video and sound cards, and better modem and fax technology will improve handling of patient data and patient training, while reducing staff time associated with indirect patient care. Equipment to test otoacoustic emissions promises faster, less expensive, infant hearing testing. If deep insertion and programmable hearing aids are fitted properly, these products will expand the market of hearing aid users by increasing the acceptance of the product by consumers and by offering more appropriate fittings. At present, CHS's competitors have not incorporated these technologies into their practices.

All of the above suggests that there is very good market potential in Central City for a high quality, comprehensive audiology and hearing aid dispensing practice. It also suggests that the market can accommodate more than one such practice. CHS expects to prevail because: (1) it will enter the market first, (2) it will maintain a high quality of services and professional relations, and (3) it will expand as the market grows.

MARKETING PLAN

Revenue Forecast

Hearing aid sales will constitute the majority of practice revenues for CHS, because of the large retiree target market and because of growth in the hearing aid industry. According to Hearing Industry Association annual sales statistics, the hearing aid industry in the United States has grown at an average annual rate of 5.6% for the last 4 years on record. CHS expects to grow at that rate or better over the next 3 years.

Hearing aid sales will also be important to boost cash flow in the first year of the business, as revenues from diagnostic services slowly build with increasing physician referrals. The monthly sales forecast in Figure 4-A.1 assumes an average of five hearing aid sales per month for the first quarter, rising thereafter by an average of two aids per month for the rest of the year. Many of the retirees return north in the warm summer months, and the sales forecast reflects this seasonal trend. Second- and third-year revenue forecasts from hearing aid sales predict slower growth in the second year, reaching a ceiling of 20 aids per month in the third year. Although not shown, it is predicted that this ceiling will rise by 5 aids per month around the fifth year, due to repeat fittings or updated fittings for established patients.

Diagnostic revenues are expected to constitute about 10% of total revenues in the first year of the practice, but the percentage will steadily increase in the second and third years as the number and type of physician referrals increase, the ICN hearing screening and follow-up program is implemented, and a second audiologist comes on board. Our long-term goal is to reach a position where 30% of gross profits are generated from diagnostic services.

Revenues from industrial hearing conservation programs will account for 1% of total revenues in the first year, rising to a maximum of 5% over the next 2 years.

Service and Product Delivery

CHS will offer diagnostic hearing testing (e.g., audiometry, acoustic immittance) for all age groups, including pediatric. Services will be provided by a certified audiologist or by a clinical audiology fellow under direct supervision. Pediatric audiology will be performed with a certified audiologist and test assistant who is either a clinical fellow or an audiology aide. Cerumen removal, when it is necessary, will be performed by trained staff.

Special testing for auditory (ABR, otoacoustic immittance) and balance (ENG) disorders will be performed by a certified audiologist or by a clinical audiology fellow under direct supervision.

Hearing aid consultations, orientations, and checks (in sound field or by probe microphone) will be performed in a team approach in which the certified audiologist and clinical fellow or audiology aide work together with each patient. Electroacoustic analyses, hearing aid cleaning, and minor modifications and repairs will be performed by any of the staff, based on availability.

Fees

The following fee schedule [at this point in the business plan a fee schedule would be inserted] was determined by:

1. surveying all audiology providers in the area,
2. procuring "usual and customary" values and reimbursement profiles from third party payers (e.g., Medicare, Blue Cross/Blue Shield),
3. requesting recommended sale prices from hearing aid manufacturers,
4. estimating fixed and variable costs of the practice,
5. including a 5% profit margin and a 5% return on investment.

Marketing

Marketing will begin with an announcement of the practice in the local newspaper, followed by a mailing to local health professionals inviting them to an Open House. A marketing package will be sent to local primary care physicians, containing a cover letter of introduction, practice brochures, appointment cards, maps, and brief biographies of staff members.

The long-term marketing of the practice will focus on the primary care physicians, with a goal of increasing diagnostic services to 30% of total revenues. Typed reports will be sent to physicians within 24 hours of seeing a referred patient. A physicians' "News Update" will be compiled and mailed quarterly, detailing new developments in auditory/ vestibular research and hearing aid technology, and explaining reimbursement and insurance issues regarding hearing care. Physicians and their staff will be provided with calibrated hearing screening equipment. The staff will be trained in its use and the equipment will be checked and maintained periodically. CHS management will meet annually with each physician to answer questions, provide information, and ensure that the quality of CHS services is satisfactory.

In addition, CHS will work closely with hospital administrators to provide hearing screenings in the ICN and at pediatric follow-ups. CHS will provide hearing screenings or lectures for hospital health fairs and in conjunction with other hospital promotions to the public.

In the first year of the practice, costs will be covered mainly by hearing aids sales. This will require short-term advertising directed to the public. Brief announcements of new hearing developments will be placed as advertisements in the local newspaper. There will be two direct mailings to targeted markets.

Long-term direct marketing will consist of an annual newsletter and an annual telephone call to all patients to insure that they are satisfied with CHS services and inform them of any changes in the field or our practice. In addition, CHS will host an annual holiday "drop in" party in December to which all patients are invited.

Service and Product Support

All diagnostic services will be performed in a comprehensive fashion, documented, and dealt with in an ethical manner. Full disclosure of procedures, fees, and nonrefundable service fees associated with product dispensing will be provided in all instances. Written descriptions of CHS's insurance billing procedures will be given to patients. Products will be dispensed with a written, signed contract, with a 30-day trial period, and with a written warranty guarantee of at least 12 months. Patients will be notified within 30 days of their warranty expiration.

In all cases, patients will be treated with respect and their needs will be given first priority by staff members. In cases of misunderstandings or product defects, every effort will be made by all staff to obtain satisfaction for the patient.

OPERATION AND ORGANIZATION PLAN

CHS is organized as a sub-chapter S corporation in [state]. It is located in the Medical Arts Building of the Central City Hospital, Suite 100. Facilities consist of 1000 square feet, divided into a waiting room, office/reception area, hearing testing room, two consultation rooms, hearing aid modification lab, storage area, and bathroom. A kitchen area is shared with an adjacent suite. Suite 100 is on the first floor and access is direct from the dedicated parking area.

CHS will begin operation with one audiologist, Dr. A, and one audiology aide, Mr. B (see diagram of the Organization Structure in Figure 4-A.2). Mr. B is an LPN with an undergraduate degree in speech and hearing. Dr. A will perform all testing and hearing aid consultations and checks, as well as hospital and physician marketing. Mr. B will assist with patient care and perform scheduling and back office duties. Outside professional services will be provided by a banker, accountant, attorney, equipment service technician, and computer technician. *[Note: In most cases, these important people should already have been identified and interviewed prior to writing the business plan. List their names, addresses, and associations here.]*

Another audiologist or clinical audiology fellow is expected to be added to the staff to assist both Dr. A and Mr. B at the end of year two. The current facilities can be fully staffed by two full-time audiologists and one full-time audiology aide. If further expansions are required (e.g., another hospital is built in Central City or target markets appear in another part of town), CHS anticipates the need to staff another office with an audiologist and audiology aide.

FINANCIAL ANALYSIS

Financing of $40,000–50,000 will come initially from Dr. A's savings. This will cover projected start-up costs of $30,000, 6 months of salary for Dr. A and Mr. B, and 6 months of rent. This should be sufficient, according to the attached pro-forma profit and loss statement and cash flow analysis *[Note: Typically, these charts would be included at this point in the business plan. For examples based on data in this business plan, see Figures 12–5 and 12–6 in Chapter 12.]* Based on these analyses, the practice should break even at the end of the first year (discounting the large depreciation expense taken in the first year). Equipment costs should be recovered by the end of year three. To deal with unanticipated expenses effectively and provide for expansion to a second office, CHS will seek a 1-year, renewable credit line of $30,000 with an interest rate tied to prime.

Risks

The major risks to this enterprise are:

1. Dr. A's health,
2. a malpractice award against CHS and Dr. A due to negligence,
3. increased competition from audiologists or otolaryngologists,
4. sudden and severe downturn to the economy.

CHS has evaluated these risks and taken the following precautions or stances: (1) Dr. A's health is good and CHS has taken out disability and life insurance policies for her; (2) Dr. A and Mr. B are credentialed, competent, and caring, which goes a long way toward warding off negligence suits, however CHS has taken adequate malpractice insurance to cover their business actions in the office, while driving, and in the hospital; (3) if competition increases to the point that profit disappears, the weaker practices will fail first. CHS realistically does not view itself as a weak practice and therefore believes it will survive if survival is possible. This belief is strengthened by the fact that CHS has not targeted ENT referrals as a primary source of revenues; (4) sudden and inexorable downturns in the economy cannot be anticipated and sometimes cannot be survived. CHS plans to retain 50% of profits in savings to ward off such disasters to the extent possible.

OVERALL SCHEDULE

A schedule of important business milestones, predicted and achieved, is depicted in Figure 4–A.3. As shown by the figure, CHS has completed its business plan, identified and leased a site for the practice, hired an audiology aide (Mr. B), and established working relations with an accountant, attorney, insurance agent, and several hearing aid manufacturers.

The next major milestones are to acquire a line of credit, move into the site, design a yellow page advertisement, get business forms printed, and commence working on April 1, 1995.

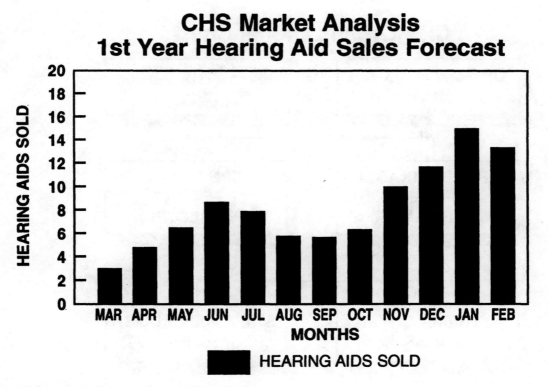

Figure 4–A.1. Sample monthly sales forecast.

CHS Organizational Chart

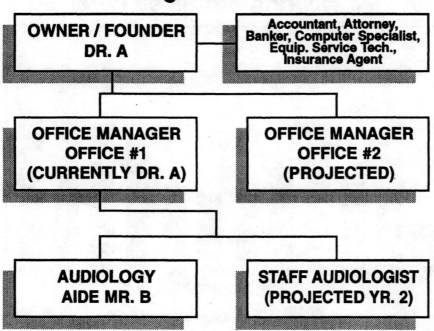

Figure 4–A.2. Sample organizational structure.

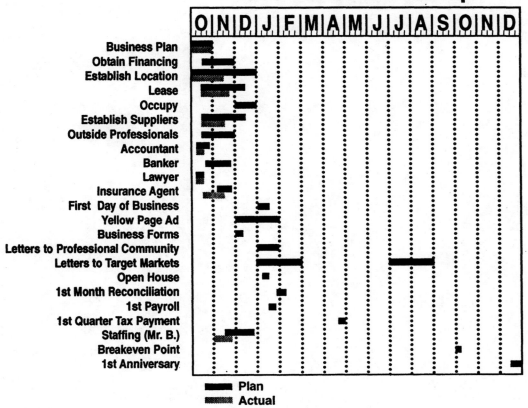

Figure 4–A.3. Sample Gantt Chart.

5

Legal Business Entities

Organizational Forms

- **Sole Proprietorships**
- **Partnerships**
- **Corporations**
- **S Corporations**
- **Limited Liability Companies**

This chapter is intended for audiologists who are considering setting up their own practices or going into practice with one or more individuals. The *choice* of practice model is not at issue here. As discussed in Chapter 3, practices can be set up with a hospital, clinic, physician, or hearing aid business, or as an independent office. Rather, the issues in this chapter are *how audiologists are paid, taxed, and made liable.* If audiologists function as independent contractors and/or collect fees directly (e.g., fee for service, third party reimbursement) or indirectly (e.g., percentage of billings, capitation), they are functioning as businesses and must report their business incomes to the government. In that event, they must decide what business form their practice is to take and initiate the steps required to establish it.

The three basic types of business organizations are proprietorships, partnerships, and corporations. In this chapter, we discuss five versions of these business forms: sole proprietorships, partnerships (general or limited), corporations (C-type), S corporations, and a new hybrid called Limited Liability Companies. A summary of the key characteristics of each business form is provided in Appendix 5-A.

This chapter is *not* intended as a definitive guide to setting up a business entity. Indeed, entire books written by business experts are devoted to this topic. Rather, this chapter attempts to familiarize audiologists with the legal forms of businesses and the basic legal obligations associated with those organizations. Audiologists contemplating private practice should consult with their attorneys and accountants before deciding which form of business to adopt for

Use an attorney to select the best organizational form

their practices. In general, audiologists should select the form of organization that allows them to function in the least costly manner in the long run while limiting taxation and liability exposures as much as possible.

SOLE PROPRIETORSHIP

This is a business owned by one individual. It does not exist apart from the proprietor. The owner is the sole proprietor and the business is the sole proprietorship. No one else can own any part of a proprietorship but the single owner[1].

A sole proprietorship is the oldest, simplest, most common, and least-expensive-to-initiate form of business organization. It does not exist apart from its owner, who can begin the business with no formality beyond obtaining required licenses and permits. As pointed out by Metzger (Metzger, Mallor, Bannes, Bowers, & Phillips, 1989), a person may have a sole proprietorship without intending to create one: "Few people consider the business-form decision. They merely begin their businesses. By default then, a person going into business by herself automatically creates a sole proprietorship when she fails to choose another business form" (p. 760).

Sole proprietorship is most common, simplest, and de facto business form

In 1990, sole proprietorships constituted 72.4% of all businesses filing United States tax returns (United States Department of Commerce, 1992). At present, no statistics are available on the percentage of audiology practices that are sole proprietorships or other forms of business.

Sole proprietorships typically are small, because they are owned by single individuals. If the owner uses a trade name for the business, it must be registered as a fictitious business name[2] with the city, county, or other governmental agency, along with the owner's name. The business is then designated as "doing business as" (dba) whatever trade name was registered.

The owner must also obtain relevant business licenses, sales tax licenses, and enroll to pay state and federal unemployment insurance and Worker's Compensation insurance[3]. The business may have employees, but they are actually employees of the owner. If there are no employees, the owner

---

[1]Except in community property states, where a spouse is a co-owner.

[2]For further information on fictitious business names, see Chapter 6.

[3]For information and samples of forms referred to in this chapter, refer to General Appendix I at the end of the book.

can report business income using his or her social security number. However, in most cases, owners apply to the IRS for an Employer Identification Number (EIN) for reporting and paying payroll withholding and social security taxes. They are assigned a payroll tax number by the state as well.

All of the income of a sole proprietorship belongs to the proprietor, who reports business profits as personal income for tax purposes and is subject to self-employment tax. In other words, no formal tax return is submitted in the business's name (Meiners, Ringleb, & Edward, 1988). Instead, the owner files a federal Schedule C (Form 1040), "Profit or (Loss) from Business or Profession," in addition to the regular Form 1040, "U.S. Individual Income Tax Return" (Whitmyer, Rasberry, & Phillips, 1989).

The owner has practically complete freedom to make business decisions with minimum legal restrictions. If the owner decides to cease doing business, he or she simply discontinues the proprietorship. Similarly, if the owner dies, the business dies too.

Risks Associated with Sole Proprietorships

Sole proprietorships are risky for the owner because they are simply an extension of the owner. Thus, the proprietor is personally liable for all financial obligations "including debts on contracts signed only in the name of the business" (Metzger et al., 1989, p. 760). If the assets of the business are not sufficient to cover creditors' claims, the owner must be prepared to cover those claims from his or her personal assets, even to the point of declaring bankruptcy.

Even in favorable situations, it is more difficult to raise capital in a sole proprietorship than in other business forms, because lending institutions are less likely to lend to individuals than to companies. In many cases, alternatives for raising capital are limited to the owner's own resources (or resourcefulness). Keeping the business solvent may be the biggest risk associated with sole proprietorships.

A sole proprietor assumes all risk

The risks to the owner extend beyond unlimited financial liability. Because the business is not a legal entity, it cannot be sued or sue. In legal actions, the owner is sued personally by creditors of the business, and the owner can be sued personally for acts of employees of the business. In the event of a legal suit where the business operates under a trade name, the suit would be addressed for example to "Anne Hall, dba Cardinal Hearing Services, Inc." If the business is damaged, the owner must sue the perpetrators personally.

A final risk is that associated with self-employment. Not only must sole proprietors pay self-employment tax, but their nonemployee status usually makes them ineligible for fringe benefits such as health plans. However, if the sole proprietor and his or her spouse are not covered by another health plan, up to 25% of health insurance premiums for the sole proprietor may be allowed as a deduction before adjusted gross income. In some cases, under new IRS rules, a sole proprietor may obtain a full deduction for medical plan costs if his or her spouse is an employee of the business (Chaney, 1991a).[4] The sole proprietor *is* eligible for a pension contribution,[5] if the business shows a profit.

PARTNERSHIPS

This is a business that has more than one owner, with each owner designated as a "partner." In theory, there can be an unlimited number of owners in a partnership. The idea of a partnership is to pool financial resources, skills, and talents to augment financial strength, improve day-to-day operations, increase profits, and combine the managerial skills and judgments of the partners. According to 1990 federal tax returns, 8.75% of businesses in the United States businesses are partnerships.

As in sole proprietorships, owners of partnerships must have the required business and tax licenses and tax identification numbers and partnerships can be created with no other legal formalities. Partnerships exist whenever two or more people agree, orally or in writing, to conduct a business venture for profit, or if they simply arrange their affairs as if they were partners. Because the agreement may be either expressed or implied, a partnership situation may exist even without the participants knowing or desiring it.

> Partnerships are legal arrangements based on expressed or implied agreements

Although they may be constructed informally, partnerships have definite legal status, and there is a great deal of legal formality associated with their operations. For historical reasons, which are summarized in the next section, the legal bases for addressing partnerships vary, depending on circumstances and location.

---

[4]Be sure to check current laws and IRS positions before setting up an employee health benefit program, as the laws and IRS positions change (as they did in 1994).

[5]Refer to Chapter 18 for more information on personal and business financial planning.

There are two basic types of partnerships: general and limited. General partnerships are most common in professional associations such as law firms, physician and dental groups, or audiology practices. In a general partnership each partner contributes money, property, labor, or skills. Each partner shares control of business operations, and each shares in the profits (or losses) of the business.

Limited partnerships are a special version of general partnerships in which there are two different *types* of owners. One type of owner is like the owner in a general partnership, contributing efforts and perhaps capital to running the business. The other type of owner contributes capital and shares profits, but does not participate in the operation of the business. In short, the second type of owner views the business as a financial investment. Unlike the operating partners who possess unlimited liability, partners who only invest have liability that is limited to the extent of their financial investment. Limited partnerships basically are tax shelter ventures[6] that are not likely to apply in professional organizations. For this reason, nothing more will be said about limited partnerships.

Historical Review of Partnership Law

Partnerships are an ancient form of business, dating back to Babylonian times. As Metzger et al. (1989) point out "The definition of a partnership in the sixth-century Justinian Code of the Roman Empire does not differ materially from that in our laws today" (p. 761).

Partnerships in the United States originally were treated according to English common law. By common law, partnerships were viewed like sole proprietorships with multiple owners. The business was an extension of the owners and not a separate legal entity. Multiple owners had unlimited liability, and law suits were brought by or against owners, rather than the business. In modern legal terms, this view of partnerships is know as the "aggregate theory."

Partnerships were the most important form of business in the United States for much of the 1800s. Undoubtedly, many prob-

---

[6]A Revised Uniform Limited Partnership Act (RULPA), passed in 1976 and amended in 1985, governs limited partnerships in most states. A limited partnership cannot be created informally. It requires filing of a certificate of limited partnership with the state. The attraction of limited partnerships as tax shelters was diminished by the Tax Reform Act of 1986, which limits tax deductions for partnership losses only to offset income from other passive investments.

lems arose at common law over the activities of these "nonentities." As a result, much of partnership law was codified into statutory law with the passage of the Uniform Partnership Act (UPA) in 1914.[7] This law has been adopted in the District of Columbia and in every state but Georgia and Louisiana.

The UPA expresses an "entity theory" which recognizes partnerships as legal entities in some circumstances. For example, partnerships are required by UPA to keep financial records of the business, even though federal income taxes are paid on the partners' individual tax returns and not by the business. Partnerships may own property and may be allowed, in some circumstances, to continue after the death of a partner.

The UPA also views partnerships according to the aggregate theory. Partnerships still cannot be sued or sue; they have no life apart from their owners; they are not employers of partners and therefore do not provide unemployment benefits to partners who leave the business.

Partnerships are legal entities in some cases but not in others

Creating and Running General Partnerships

To avoid disputes and ensure success of the enterprise, future partners need to work with an attorney to write a contract known as "articles of partnership." This contract must include the partnership trade name, which is registered with state authorities just as in a sole proprietorship. The contract should specify the location, purpose, and duration of the partnership. It should also spell out the financial and management contributions of the individual partners, method and amount of compensation to partners, accounting methods, dissolution procedures, and arbitration methods. Appendix 5-B is an example of a basic partnership agreement for an audiology/hearing aid dispensing practice.

Write a partnership agreement

For the most part, partners can specify their arrangements with each other as they see fit. A few general rules apply, however, unless the articles of partnership state differently. All partners are general managers of the partnerships and have equal say in the management of the business. Most decisions are made on a majority vote. Partners share ownership and profits equally, regardless of their contributions. Partners (even "silent" ones) have unlimited lia-

---

[7]The UPA is far too comprehensive to receive even a cursory review in this chapter, but it is very important to the operations of partnerships. A copy of the UPA (approximately 10 book pages in length) can be obtained at a nominal cost by writing to the National Conference of Commissioners of Uniform State Laws, 676 N. St. Clair Street, #1700, Chicago, IL 60611, or by calling (312) 915-0195.

bility for the debts of the business and are liable for the actions and decisions of other partners in the business.

Most importantly—and unalterably under the law—partners owe a "fiduciary duty" to the business and the other partners. Fiduciary duty means that partners must act in good faith for the good of the partnership, demonstrating trust, confidence, honesty, and loyalty. For example, partners cannot put their own interests before that of the business in financial transactions. This conflict of interest is known legally as "self-dealing." Partners may not disclose confidential matters of the business. They must devote full time to the business and not compete with it without consent. Partners must demonstrate reasonable care and skill in performing their assigned duties and must fully disclose all information about the business to their partners.

In terms of taxation, partnerships are almost invisible entities and, like sole proprietorships, are taxed on net income. Partners may allocate income and loss as they wish to different partners at different times in the tax year. All partners are nonemployees and therefore all income to each partner is subject to self-employment taxation. Partners are eligible for pension contributions, but nonemployment status prevents tax deductions for fringe benefits such as health insurance, just as in a sole-proprietorship. The only requirement of the partnership is that a "K-1" notice must be filed annually with the IRS, indicating the revenue distributed to the partners (Whitmyer, Rasberry, & Phillips, 1989).

Terminating General Partnerships

Two legal terms apply to termination of partnerships. "Dissolution" occurs whenever a partnership's ownership changes, or if events make the partnership unlawful. "Winding up" occurs when the assets of the partnership are liquidated.

If an owner dies, retires, resigns due to violations of the partnership agreement, or withdraws from the business for any reason (e.g., incapacity, bankruptcy), the partnership may not engage in any new business and must be dissolved. Dissolution does not always mean stopping the enterprise. For example, one partner may sell his or her business interest to another person. The old partnership is automatically dissolved by this action, but a new partnership can be formed with the purchaser and the remaining partners. In this event, the original partners retain unlimited liability for acts of the former partnership, and the new partner assumes some of the liability as well.

If the enterprise stops as the result of dissolution, "winding up" procedures start. In a winding up, the value of the business is established and creditors of the partnership are paid first. Loans to the partnership by the partners are paid next, and finally, remaining profits are distributed to the owners.

Advantages and Disadvantages of Partnerships

Partnerships offer an opportunity for audiologists and other hearing health professionals to work together in a mutually beneficial way that promotes creativity and team work. They are easy to start, and they may be more financially robust than sole proprietorships. To some extent, they are recognized as legal entities. Partnerships benefit from the combined strengths of the partners' training, management skills, and judgment. The partners' fiduciary duties dictate that they will give their personal attention to the business.

Partners have unlimited liability for the acts of the other partners. If one partner does not exercise good judgment, that partner can cause not only the loss of the partnership's assets, but the loss of the other partners' personal assets (Active Corps of Executives, 1993). Partnerships may be slow to respond to crises and opportunities because decisions must be based on agreement of the partners. Unless there is a well thought-out contractual agreement, internal disputes and divided authority can become significant problems in partnerships.

Partners have unlimited liability

A tax advantage of general partnerships is that special allocations are allowed so that income distributions do not have to be equal to all partners. A potential tax *dis*advantage is that all net income in a general partnership is subject to payroll taxes.

CORPORATIONS

Corporations are the creation of corporate law over the last two centuries. Corporations are classified as "for profit," "not for profit," and "government-owned." For profit corporations are further classified as "closely held" or "publicly held" corporations. The classification depends on size (close corporations usually have fewer than 50 shareholders) and whether stock can be purchased by the public. Subchapter S corporations are smaller (not more than 35 shareholders), special, closely held corporations that are taxed like partnerships. This chapter will concern itself only with for profit, closely held corporations, devoting a special section to S Corporations.

In contrast to sole proprietorships and partnerships, corporations are recognized by law as separate entities for liability and tax purposes. A corporation is legally a "person" whose life is independent of that of its owners. As a "person," the corporation has constitutional rights such as freedom of speech, protection against unreasonable search and seizure, and the right to sue and be sued. Because the corporation is an entity that can be sued, the individual owners avoid unlimited liability against their personal assets *except in cases of their own personal negligence*[8] (Chaney, 1994b). This is the main reason for small businesses to incorporate. However, the owners of small corporations are rarely shielded from business creditors, because financial institutions and other businesses (in audiologists' cases, hearing aid manufacturers, property managers, lending institutions) almost always require that the business owners co-sign personally for the business.

Corporations are separate entities

The owners of a corporation are called shareholders or stockholders. Ownership is freely transferable through the sale of stock. In forming a corporation, the owner(s) transfers money and sometimes property to the corporation and receives capital stock in exchange. Profits are distributed to shareholders in the form of dividends. Shareholders need not work in the business, and employees of the business need not be shareholders. Shareholders who work in the business are employees of the corporation and receive compensation in the form of salary as well as dividends.

As a very simplified example, an audiologist who owns a private practice employing two people decides to incorporate for liability reasons. After incorporation, the business appears no different than before, except that all assets (e.g., equipment, furniture and fixtures, bank accounts) now belong to the corporation and the owner has been issued a stock certificate. The audiologist/owner is the sole shareholder and becomes an employee of the corporation. The corporation pays salaries to all three employees (including the owner) and withholds federal, state, social security, and Medicare taxes. If the business is profitable, the corporation may pay the profits to the owner as a dividend. Subsequently, the owner and the corporation file separate, annual tax returns. In the event that one of the nonshareholder employees has an automobile accident while on company business, the corporation,

---

[8]An owner/employee or employee cannot avoid liability by claiming that in committing negligence he or she was acting as an employee of the corporation.

and not the owner, is primarily liable. By contrast, if the owner is found personally negligent in a malpractice suit, the owner and the corporation are both liable.

A practice owned and operated by several audiologists will probably want to incorporate (or form a Limited Liability Company, as discussed in a later section), but not put very large assets like a building into the corporation. This is mainly for liability and asset protection. For example, a group of audiologists may practice together in a building or office that is owned by one of the audiologists (Dr. A). If they incorporate and one of the other shareholders (Mr. B) later performs an act of negligence, the corporation and Mr. B can be sued. If Dr. A was not involved in the negligent act, she cannot be sued, and the building is protected from the lawsuit as a personal asset. On the other hand, if Dr. A had sold the building to the corporation, it would be an exposed asset in any lawsuit brought against the corporation.

Creating and Running a Corporation

Corporations are incorporated in individual states according to statutes. A business may incorporate in only one state, but this does not prohibit it from doing business in other states. State statutes vary greatly in terms of their leniency toward corporate management. The audiologist(s) should always discuss incorporation thoroughly with an attorney who is knowledgeable about their particular state's statutes.

The basic requirements for incorporation are that an application, a filing fee, and the corporation's notarized *articles of incorporation* must be filed with the state. The state must also be notified of the fiscal year-end of the corporation. The articles of incorporation include the name, address, statutory agent (the person on whom any future lawsuit against the corporation would be served), and purpose of the corporation. The articles also give the names and addresses of the principals and describe the class of stock and its par value. Figure 5–1 is an example of articles of incorporation for a small practice.

File articles of incorporation with the state

In most states the existence of the corporation begins when the Secretary of State stamps the articles of incorporation "Filed," although some states still issue a certificate of incorporation as proof of a corporation's existence. An accepted copy of the Articles of Incorporation must be sent for publication (e.g., in the county in which the corporation is doing business). The state automatically issues a corporate charter recognizing the existence of the corporation as a legal entity.

Articles of Incorporation
of
Cardinal Hearing Services, Incorporated

This is notice to everyone of the following:

That we, the undersigned, have associated ourselves for the purpose of forming a corporation for profit under the laws of the State of _____, and for that purpose to hereby adopt the following Articles of Incorporation:

ARTICLE I

The name of the corporation is Cardinal Hearing Services, Incorporated.

ARTICLE II

The purpose for which this corporation is organized is the transaction of any and all lawful business for which the corporation may be incorporated under the laws of the State of _____. The corporation initially intends to conduct audiology and hearing aid dispensing business.

ARTICLE III

The corporation shall have the authority to issue one thousand (1,000) shares of common stock (no par).

(NOTE: Keep in mind the issuance of shares of stock is the issuance of a security and therefore subject to securities law).

ARTICLE IV

The name and address of the initial statutory agent of the corporation is: Mr. C., Attorney at Law, 1 North Street, Central City, State.

ARTICLE V

The known place of business of the corporation shall be Physicians Medical Building, Suite 100, 1 Medical Drive, Central City, State.

ARTICLE VI

The initial Board of Directors shall consist of two Directors. The names and addresses of the persons who shall serve as Directors until the first annual meeting of shareholders, or until their successors are duly elected and qualified are: Dr. and Mr. A., 1 South Street, Central City, State.

ARTICLE VII

The incorporators of the incorporation are: Dr. and Mr. A., 1 South Street, City, State.
(NOTE: Home addresses must be shown for incorporators and directors).
DATE: January 1, 19--

_____
Dr. A, Incorporator

_____
Mr. A, Incorporator

Figure 5-1. Articles of Incorporation. This example is for Cardinal Hearing Services, Inc., a small practice in a community property state that is owned by Dr. A and her spouse (Adapted from *Overview of Closely Held Business Law in Arizona* by D. Chaney, pp. 24–25, 1994b. Copyright 1994 State Bar of Arizona, reprinted with permission).

Once the corporation exists, the shareholders are expected to hold an organizational meeting to enact the corporation's by-laws, issue the stock, and elect a board of directors. Figure 5–2 is an example of the organizational minutes and by-laws of a small corporation. The organizational minutes (which can be in a form similar to a Shareholder Agreement) need to be completed, stock certificates issued,[9] an accounting system established, and various applications for identification numbers made.

Although these steps may seem like unnecessary formalities in companies with one or two owners, they are a good means of forcing the owners to think through management decisions in advance, thus avoiding future problems. For protection of shareholders in liability lawsuits and tax audits, minutes of annual shareholders meetings should be maintained. A "minutes book" should also document "equipment purchases, shareholder compensation arrangements, corporation to shareholder or shareholder to corporation lending, advertising strategies, financial arrangements" (Hoops & Sliwoski, 1988, p. 42).

In many states, a closely held corporation may be managed by the shareholders as if it were a sole proprietorship or partnership, rather than by a board of directors elected by the shareholders. This has obvious advantages for small businesses, especially when there are only one or two shareholders. Many state statutes allow a corporation to "make an election" to be a close corporation, usually by stating the election in the articles of incorporation or organizational minutes. Whether managed by a board of directors or by shareholders, the fiduciary duty of the managers to the corporation is essentially the same as that expected of general partners in a partnership.In close corporations, the management issues addressed in the shareholders agreement are very similar to those in a partnership agreement (see Appendix 5-B).

Closely held corporations can be managed like sole proprietorship or partnership

Terminating a Corporation

As in a partnership, termination involves dissolution and winding up. The corporation stops doing any new business upon dissolution. Dissolution occurs by one or more of the following: (a) the shareholders vote to dissolve, (b) the life-span stated in the articles of incorporation expires, (c) a leg-

---

[9]Blank form stock certificates are available through office supply stores that sell legal items.

ORGANIZATIONAL MINUTES AND BY-LAWS
OF CARDINAL HEARING SERVICES, INC.

Following acceptance of Articles of Incorporation of Cardinal Hearing services, Inc., a meeting of the sole incorporators, shareholders, directors, and officers was held. The meeting was conducted by such individuals, Dr. A and Mr. A who acknowledged the corporation became effective on January 1, 19--.

At the meeting, the following business was transacted and the following agreements made on behalf of the corporation.

Ninety-three (93) shares of common stock were issued to the Mr. and Mrs. A family Trust dated October 1, 19--. It was agreed for tax purposes an S Election would be made and timely filed with the Internal Revenue Service.

It was unanimously resolved and agreed that Dr. A would act as president of the corporation and make all management decisions and Mr. A would hold the offices of Secretary and Treasurer. Both individuals agree to act as directors.

It was agreed a corporation checking account would be opened and initial funding would be payment for the stock. It was agreed the CPA firm operated by Ms. D would be hired to keep corporate books and prepare governmental reporting forms such as S Corporation tax returns. It was acknowledged annual operations of the business would be confirmed by accurate information on tax returns as well as Corporation Commission reporting.

It was acknowledged that as the sole manager of the corporation the president, Dr. A, would make arrangements for an appropriate business lease location. For convenience purposes, the shareholders, directors, and officers waive notice of any corporate meetings whatsoever and acknowledge corporate decisions shall be made by Dr. A.

It was agreed the above shall serve as Minutes of the organizational meeting as well as the By-laws of the corporation.

Effective Date: January 1, 19-- (date of incorporation)

_____

Dr. A, Shareholder, Director, President, Manager

_____

Mr. A, Shareholder, Director, Secretary, Treasurer

Figure 5–2. Organizational Minutes and By-laws. This example is for the same small company whose Articles of Incorporation are shown in Figure 5–1.[12] (Adapted from *Overview of Closely Held Business Law* in Arizona by D. Chaney, p. 26, 1994b. Copyright 1994 State Bar of Arizona, reprinted with permission).

---

[12]State laws differ as to the requirements for organizational meetings, by-laws, and minimum formal requirements for the formation of corporations. The example in Figure 5–2 is not meant to serve as a template for individuals setting up corporations. When establishing a company, always work with an attorney who is well versed in corporate and tax law in the state in which the practice will be incorporated.

islative act in the state of incorporation, (d) court decree in the state of incorporation, or (e) corporate bankruptcy.

Following dissolution, the corporation's management or a court-appointed trustee see to completion of the business's affairs. The corporate assets are then liquidated to pay off creditors, and remaining profits are distributed to the shareholders.

Advantages and Disadvantages of Corporations

The Small Business Administration (ACE, 1993) summarizes the advantages of a corporation as:

1. The life of the business is perpetual.
2. The stockholders have limited liability.
3. Transfer of ownership is easy (sales of stock).
4. Management is generally more efficient.
5. It is adaptable to both small and large business. . . .

Disadvantages . . . are:

1. It is subject to special taxation.
2. It is more difficult and expensive to organize than other forms of ownership.
3. The corporate charter restricts the types of business activities in which the corporation may engage.
4. It is subject to many State and Federal controls. (p. 16)

An additional advantage of *regular* corporations is that health and disability premiums are tax deductible to the corporation.

One disadvantage not acknowledged in this list is the "piercing of the corporate veil," which has significant implications for audiologists in private practice (Hoops & Sliwoski, 1988). The phrase describes situations in which parties may legally sue the stockholders as well as the corporation, thus piercing the liability protection supposedly associated with incorporation. As Hoops and Sliwoski point out, there are three conditions where this applies:

1. Some states prohibit or limit shareholder protection for professional practice corporations.
2. If the corporation is grossly undercapitalized, the corporate entity may be deemed a sham.
3. If an individual owns most of the shares and runs the corporation as a personal business (e.g., no separate bank account, business conducted in the owner's personal name), then *shareholder domination exists*, and the corporation is the *alter ego* of the shareholder.

In such cases, the corporation may be dismissed as a legal entity, because it appears to exist solely to shield the owner from liability.

S Corporations

An advantage of corporations is limited liability of share-holders, but a major disadvantage is the double taxation on regular corporations. A corporation pays federal income taxes on its income and shareholders pay federal income taxes on the income they receive from the corporation. In addition, serious corporate and personal "double taxation" can occur on sale of assets when the business is sold. *Limited liability is maintained and double taxation is avoided by choosing the S Corporation election and complying with IRS requirements.*

Also known as "small business corporations," S Corporations are close corporations that may consist of no more than 35 shareholders. The S Corporation is a legal entity like any other corporations, but is taxed like a partnership.

IRS Election as an S Corporation

The S Election (Form 2553, "Election by a Small Business Corporation") should be sent to the IRS after the articles of incorporation have been filed with the state (i.e., after the official date of incorporation). However, *the S Election must be made and received by the IRS within 75 days of the date of incorporation.* The S Election should be sent by certified or registered mail with return receipt requested.

Like individuals, sole proprietorships, and general partnerships, the fiscal year of an S Corporation is from January 1 to December 31. Although S Corporations do not pay taxes, they are required to file state and federal information tax returns by March 15 each year.

Special Tax Attributes of S Corporations

Shareholders in an S Corporation pay taxes on business earnings as though they were in a partnership, thereby avoiding the double taxation of regular corporations. These earnings are allowed to "flow through" to the shareholders, who report them on their individual federal income tax returns for that year.

Although the owners report the income and pay taxes on it, they need not take the income in the year it is reported. The money may stay in the corporation and be taken in the form of dividends in subsequent years. As simple as an S Corporation seems, there are key concepts that must be understood to properly distribute earnings.

Reasonable Compensation

The IRS requires that a "reasonable amount" of compensation to S corporation shareholder employees must be subject to payroll tax (FICA wages). In other words, an audiologist who owns an S corporation cannot avoid paying FICA withholding and take all profit as dividends.

Chaney (1994b) points out a possible payroll tax savings in an S Corporation. In cases where the corporation's net income is derived from employees as well as the owner's efforts, the courts have held that net income derived from nonowner employees is not to be ignored. In these cases, the owner may be justified in taking a portion of net income not subject to payroll tax. Careful records would be necessary to document each employee's contribution to overall production of the business. The audiologist should consult with an accountant or tax attorney before deciding how to distribute net income.

In the case of an audiology practice, the potential payroll advantage seems most applicable in practices employing one or more nonowner audiologists or hearing aid dispensers and in which there is no qualified retirement plan.

Retirement Contributions

For shareholders who elect to take some of the business's net income as distributions not subject to payroll tax, the lower FICA wages means less Social Security credit *and* a lower contribution to a qualified retirement plan (i.e., pension or profit sharing plan). The potential payroll tax savings described in the previous section may be smaller or offset by tax savings a shareholder may realize by fully contributing to a qualified retirement plan. In contrast to sole proprietorships and partnerships, shareholder employees of S Corporations can make pension contributions on all income subject to FICA taxes. However, practitioners with a large number of nonkey employees typically will not be able to afford a pension-type plan.[10]

Tax Events

It is important to remember that shareholders *must* pay taxes on all non-FICA distributions in the year they occur,

---

[10]For further explanation, refer to Chapter 18 on Financial Planning.

whether they take the earnings or not. Failure to recognize this fact can result in serious cash flow problems due to unanticipated "tax events." For example, a new and highly successful practice owner might pay off equipment loans with profits in the first year or two of business without keeping enough cash reserve to pay taxes on the profits.

One Class of Stock

S Corporations have a "one class of stock" requirement. This means that, in the case of multiple shareholders, all distributions not subject to payroll tax must be proportional and made on the same day. Whereas partnerships may specify the allocation of income/loss to different partners, S corporations cannot. For example, if the S Corporation has two 50% shareholders and one takes a $1000 dividend on July 1st, then $1000 *must* be distributed to the other shareholder on the same day, whether he or she wants it or not!

Fewer Fringe Benefits

Unlike regular corporation shareholders, S corporation owners cannot write off health and disability insurance premiums. They are deductible to the corporation, but taxable to the shareholder/employee (Jenkins, 1993).

To Incorporate or Not to Incorporate

After reviewing the list of advantages and disadvantages, the incorporation decision remains unclear. Attorneys favor incorporation for liability protection; other professionals are less supportive. The following quotations provide a good summary of the ambiguity surrounding the incorporation decision. The first quotation, from a CPA and tax attorney, is pro incorporation.

> It would seem any business with multiple owners should incorporate (rather than forming a partnership) if the owners' activities create liability exposure; this would help "insulate" other owners from the negligence of another owner. Further, it would seem any business (no matter whether one or more owners) should incorporate (whether an S election is made or not) if the business has products liability exposure and/or non-owner employees with activities which create liability exposure (such as driving a business vehicle or installing parts or equipment). (Chaney, 1994a, p. 14)

The second quotation, from an academician and CPA, is less enthusiastic about incorporation:

Though the authors would not presume to give definitive final advice about the incorporation decision..., we have observed that clinicians seeking professional services concerning the incorporation decision continue to receive advice slanted in favor of incorporation, often to the financial detriment of their private practice. There is no obvious explanation for this slant. One might speculate that accountants and lawyers do not handle enough business in this area to understand the realities of communication disorders private practice incorporation. (Hoops & Sliwoski, 1988, p. 44)

LIMITED LIABILITY COMPANIES

A Limited Liability Company (LLC) is a new form of business entity. It is treated as a partnership for tax purposes but provides members[11] with the limited liability that corporate shareholders enjoy. LLCs appear to have special benefit for multiperson professional practices, because they provide members with limited liability for acts of malpractice by other members of the company (Research Institute of America, Inc. [RIA], 1992).

Like S Corporations, LLCs avoid corporation double taxation. In addition, LLCs have several advantages over S Corporations:

LLCs have some advantages over S Corporations

Owner Requirements. In contrast to S Corporations, LLC members may be foreign individuals, trusts, corporations, or partnerships.

Distribution of Net Income. LLCs may have different classes of ownership interest, thus avoiding the "one class of stock" restriction of S Corporations. This means that cash distributions may be allocated to different members as the LLC sees fit, rather than having to make all distributions proportional to ownership and at the same time (as required in an S Corporation) (Chaney, 1994b).

No IRS Election. IRS election is not required.

Legal and Tax Requirements for LLC Status

LLCs are entities that are created by state statute. It is likely that the large majority of states, if not all states, will have LLC statutes in place by the time this book is published. An LLC does not exist officially until it has filed Articles of Organization with the state. It is governed by either an operating agreement (written or unwritten, depending on state

---

[11]Owners in an LLC are referred to as members rather than partners.

requirements) or regulations. Operating agreements are similar to partnership agreements, and regulations for LLCs are similar to corporate by-laws (RIA, 1992).

To qualify as an LLC for federal tax purposes, *a business must lack at least two of the following characteristics in the eyes of the IRS:*

■ limited liability
■ continuity of life
■ centralization of management
■ free transferability of interests

For example, a member-managed audiology LLC does not have the corporate characteristic of centralized management. If the audiology LLC operating agreement prohibits transfer of interest to a third party without permission of other partners, it lacks the corporate characteristic of free transferability. Failing these two characteristics allows the company to be federally taxed as an LLC.

State tax treatment of LLCs does not always parallel IRS treatment: "even in states which allow the formation of LLCs or recognize out-of-state LLCs, the tax treatment of an LLC as a partnership for state tax purposes is not assured" (RIA, 1992, p. 9).

LLCs have risks and uncertainties

Currently, there are risks and uncertainties associated with operating as an LLC. As with any new entity, neither state or federal authorities are uniformly familiar with LLC classifications and administration, nor is there a body of judicial interpretation associated with this new entity.

SUMMARY

The basic organizational forms of business are sole proprietorships, partnerships, and corporations. Sole proprietorships are the easiest and least expensive to set up and run, but they carry the most risk to the owner and are difficult to capitalize. Partnerships are easy to establish and offer the advantages of camaraderie, joint effort, and greater financial strength. Partnerships are subject to more legal controls than proprietorships, and owners have full liability for themselves as well as the other partners. Corporations take more time and money to set up and are subject to more legal control and taxes than either proprietorships or partnerships. Corporations offer liability protection to owners, except in cases of malpractice or when the corporate veil is pierced. S Corporations are a means of functioning with corporate liability protection while being taxed like a partnership or sole proprietorship.

A new type of business entity, the Limited Liability Company, is recognized in many states. It combines the tax advantages of a partnership with the limited liability advantages of a corporation. Because this type of organizational form is so new, owners and partners should work closely with tax and legal consultants when setting up and operating LLCs.

It is important to review one's business situation and goals with an accountant and an attorney before deciding what organizational form the business should assume.

REFERENCES

Active Corps of Executives (ACE). (1993). Points to consider in planning and operating a successful business. SCORE: U.S. Small Business Administration, 1–16.

Chaney, D. (1994a). *Closely held business law in Arizona: Business owner guide and attorney/CPA desk reference.* Tucson, AZ: Author.

Chaney, D. (1994b). *Overview of the closely-held business formation process.* Tucson: State Bar of Arizona.

Hoops, H. R., & Sliwoski, L. (1988). The Tax Reform Act of 1986 and the private practice incorporation decision. *Asha, 30*(1), 41–44.

Jenkins, M. D. (1993). *Starting and operating a business in Arizona. A step-by-step guide.* Grants Pass, OR: Oasis Press.

Meiners, R. E., Ringleb, A. H., & Edward, F. L. (1988). *The legal environment of business.* New York: West Publishing.

Metzger, M. B., Mallor, J. P., Barnes, A. J., Bowers, T., & Phillips. M. J. (1989). *Business law and the regulatory environment. Concepts and cases (7th ed.).* Boston: Irvin.

Research Institute of America, Inc. (1992). *Limited liability company (LLC) can be preferred choice of entity.* New York: Author.

United States Department of Commerce. (1992). *Statistical abstracts of the United States* (GPO Stock Number 003-024-08160-1, p. 519). Washington, DC: Government Printing Office.

Whitmyer, C., Rasberry, S., & Phillips, M. (1989). *Running a one-person business.* Berkeley, CA: Ten-Speed Press.

APPENDIX 5-A

Attributes of Five Types of Organizational Forms

Attributes	Sole Proprietorship	General Partnership	Regular Corporation	S Corporation	Limited Liability Company
Simplicity	Simple to establish and operate	Simple, but good to have written partnership agreement	Legal formalities required to establish/operate	Same as regular corporation, but must file election with IRS	Like partnership but must record with the state to get LLC status
Federal tax on profits	Owner taxed at individual rates	Partners taxed at individual rates	Corporation taxed at higher rates	Shareholders taxed at individual rates	Members taxed at individual rates
Double taxation on profit distributions	No	No	Yes	No	No
Deduction of losses by owners	Yes	Yes	No. Corporation must carry losses to offset future profits.	Federal: Yes State: No	Federal: Yes State: ?
Social Security Tax on owner/employee earnings	15.3% of owner's or partner's self-employment earnings up to a wage base limit; 2.9% on earnings above the limit. Half of contributions are deductible on individual income tax.	Same as sole proprietorship	15.3%: Corporation and owner/employee each pay 7.65% up to wage base limit; 1.45% each on wages each on limit.	Same as regular corporation.	Same as sole proprietorship and partnership
Unemployment taxes on owners earnings	No	No	Yes: Federal and State	Same as regular corporation	Federal: No. State: ?
Retirement plans	Keogh Plan (Owner cannot borrow from plan)	Keogh Plan (10% partner cannot borrow from plan)	Pension and profit-sharing, same as Keogh plans but participants can borrow from plan	Same as regular corporation but 5% shareholders cannot borrow from plan	Same as partnership
Owner taxes on medical, disability, and group term life insurance	Not deductible[a]	Not deductible[a]	Deductible by corporation. Not taxable to owner/employee.	Deductible by corporation for 2% shareholders. Not deductible to shareholders[a]	Not deductible[a]
Taxation of Dividends	Fully taxable to owner	Fully taxable to partners	Table to corporation, but 70% not subject to federal income tax	Fully taxable to shareholders	Fully taxable to members

[a]But 25% of owner's medical premium is deductible from adjusted gross income in some circumstances.

APPENDIX 5-B

Sample Partnership Agreement

This Professional General Partnership agreement is between the following two certified audiologists who are licensed as hearing aid dispensers in [State]:
Dr. A, Ph.D.
Mr. B, M.A.

TERM: The effective date of this Professional General Partnership is the date of execution reflected below, and the term of the partnership is indefinite, with the proviso the partnership may be terminated according to the provision of this agreement.

REQUIRED CAPITAL CONTRIBUTIONS: The partners acknowledge and agree no capital contributions whatsoever are required.

CAPITAL ACCOUNT: A separate capital account shall be maintained for each partner. Each capital account shall be increased by any capital contributions of the partners, and by any allocable share of income, gain or profit, and reduced by distributions to partners and any allocable share of any deduction or loss of the partnership. Capital accounts shall be maintained in accordance with provision in this agreement, as well as any tax law requirements.

RESTRICTIVE COVENANT DURING TERM OF THE PARTNERSHIP: During the term of the partnership, no partner shall carry on, directly or indirectly, the practice of audiology or hearing aid dispensing outside this partnership within the state of [State]. *(NOTE: This type provision could be modified to allow any partner to supplement income by working part-time for another hearing health practice, so long as it does not interfere with partnership business, probably with a prohibition against direct solicitation of partnership patients.)*

PARTNERSHIP MANAGEMENT PROVISIONS: Regarding management of partnership affairs, it is agreed partners shall have equal rights and management of partnership affairs. However, it is specifically agreed that any partnership contract, no matter the type, shall not be entered into, if the amount of such contract is in excess of $3,000, without the unanimous approval of both partners. It is specifically agreed this unanimous voting requirement shall apply to each transaction, whether represented by one agreement or more than one agreement; for example, if an office complex is contemplated to be built by the partnership, all related contemplated contracts shall be aggregated as to the building of such complex, and all such contracts shall be subject to he voting requirement above, if in the aggregate, the $3,000 limit is met. It is specifically agreed the following type transactions shall be subject to a unanimous voting requirement of partners, no matter the dollar amount involved: (1) Modification of the partnership agreement, (2) employment arrangement, whether as an employee or contractor, (3) institution or modification of a partnership qualified benefit plan, (4) further equity issuance (further issuance of any partnership interest). It is agreed any other type contract, including but not limited to, a least contract, loan contract, or otherwise, shall be subject to the $3,000 provision above.

It is agreed if a partner experiences a disability as defined below, management of partnership affairs shall be all in the other nondisabled partner. In the event that one partner has full management authority, that partner agrees management decisions shall be made by such partner, through the exercise of reasonable and prudent business decisions. It is agreed management decisions made under this disability provision shall not subject the managing partner to liability from the other partner, or the partnership, so long as such management decisions ere made on a reasonable basis, and without neglect for the interests of the other partner, and the partnership. For this management purpose, disability is defined to mean that a partner is unable for a period of thirty (30) consecutive days or more, to carry on the practice of audiology or hearing aid dispensing, because of any health problem(s) whatsoever, for at least twenty-five (25) hours per week.

The partners acknowledge they shall in good faith, attempt to share practice responsibilities and working hours, approximately 50/50. Further, partners agree to make themselves reasonably available to make management decisions.

PARTNERSHIP TAX ALLOCATIONS: It is agreed each partner shall be entitled to a 50/50 share of income, gain, deduction, loss, and credit, so long as the partners are sharing approximately equally partnership work responsibilities, and distributions, approximately 50/50. In the event that partners are not sharing management work responsibilities approximately 50/50, for example, in the event of a disability, it is agreed partnership tax attributes of income, gain deduction, loss, and credit, shall be allocated to respective capital accounts on a pro rata basis, determined by number of hours (*NOTE: This could be gross collections*) worked by respective partners. It is agreed any required tax allocations shall be made.

PARTNERSHIP DISTRIBUTIONS: No partner shall receive a salary for services rendered, nor shall any partner receive any interest on a capital contribution. Distributions of partnership cash shall be made to partners on a monthly basis on a 50/50 basis during period of time the partners are sharing work responsibilities equally. For periods of time that partners are not sharing partnership management and work responsibilities approximately equally, such as in the event of a disability, partnership distributions shall be made to the respective partners on a monthly basis, on a pro rata basis, according to number of hours worked by each respective partner.

However, no cash distribution to partners shall be made, which will lower the partnership operating cash balance below $3,000.

PARTNERSHIP SPECIFIC EXPENSE LIMITATION PROVISIONS: Regarding business travel, education seminars, library materials, journals and other educational materials, the partners agrees as follows. It is agreed during any partnership tax year, such expenses incurred by each respective partner shall be limited to $3000, paid by the partnership. It is agreed if such expenses incurred by a partner exceed $3000, that such partner shall be required to pay such expenses personally, or reimburse the partnership within sixty (60) days following the end of any partnership tax year, in which the partnership has paid for any partner, more than $3000 of such expenses.

It is agreed business automobile travel shall be calculated at the Internal Revenue Service standard mileage rate. It is agreed business miles shall have the same definition as for tax purposes (business miles would not include commuting mileage from office to home and back). The partners agree to keep adequate records (for tax purposes) and to document business miles, as well as any expenses incurred.

VACATION AND SICK DAY PROVISIONS: Each partner shall be entitled to partnership distributions as calculated above, for each week of vacation, in which case the partners shall be deemed to have worked forty (40) hours, and shall constitute an equal work week for tax allocation and distribution purposes. Each partner shall be entitled to four (4) weeks of vacation per calendar year, provided such vacation shall not unreasonably interfere with the performance of partnership duties. The partners agree to reasonably cooperate to make a determination as to vacation taken by each respective partner, taking into account existing partnership "work load."

The partners, in addition, shall be entitled to five (5) sick days per calendar year.

The partners agree at the end of each calendar year, to reasonably calculate any unused vacation and sick days, and it is agreed a partner shall be entitled to a specific future distribution in an amount based upon a net earning per day calculation as set forth below. It is agreed the calculation shall be made by dividing two hundred fifty (250) (the approximate number of work days per year) into the partnership net income reflected on the partnership return, and the partner having not utilized full vacation and sick days, shall be entitled when such calculation can be reasonably made, to a distribution equal to the "net per day" times that partner's "extra unused vacation and sick days."

PARTNER MISCONDUCT PROVISION: In the event a partner commits professional misconduct as defined below, the other partner shall have the option to purchase all of the partnership interest of the partner committing professional misconduct, on the same terms and conditions as set forth below, in the event of death, but for a total purchase price equal to one-third (1/3) of the purchase price in the event of death. Partner misconduct shall be defined to mean fraud, misappropriation, embezzlement, intentional and material damage to property of the professional partnership, including but not limited to, patient relationships, chronic addiction to alcohol or narcotic drugs, and conduct intentionally and materially detrimental to the best interest of the professional partnership.

MALPRACTICE INSURANCE PROVISIONS: The partners agree the partnership shall pay for and keep in force audiology malpractice insurance in an amount equal to that which is normal and customary in type, features, and limit, for practitioners engaging in the practice of audiology and hearing aid dispensing in the state of [state]. It is acknowledged as of the date of this agreement, such audiology malpractice insurance coverage is at least one million dollars ($1,000,000), and a current three million dollar ($3,000,000) aggregate.

THIRD PARTY PARTNERSHIP INTEREST SALE PROVISIONS: In the event a partner wishes to sell his entire partnership interest (but not less than all) to another nonpartner party who is a licensed audiologist or hearing aid dispenser, the following terms shall be binding upon the partners. It is acknowledged and agreed that a partnership interest may not be transferred to a nonlicensed and noncertified audiologist/hearing aid dispenser.

If the owner/partner receives an offer, whether or not solicited, to purchase all of the partnership interest, and if the partner is willing to accept it, the partner may transfer all (but not less than all) of the partnership interest, only after the selling partner has afforded the other partner the following rights of first refusal. The partner desiring to make the sale and transfer of all of the partnership interest must first notify the other partner in writing of the desire to buy the partnership interest by the proposed transferee of the exact and complete terms of the offer, which must be signed by the proposed transferee/licensed audiologist/hearing aid dispenser. The other partner (nonselling partner) shall have the right to purchase all of the partnership interest on the same terms and conditions of the offer.

It is specifically agreed that the nonselling partner in no event shall be required to pay a purchase price of more than one hundred twenty-five percent (125%) of fifty percent (50%) of the fair market value of the entire practice.

Written notice of the terms and conditions of the proposed third party offer shall be provided by the other partner by hand delivery to the nonselling partner. After receiving notice, the nonselling partner shall have thirty (30) days to exercise the right of refusal, by way of written notice hand delivered to the selling partner; if the nonselling partner does not provide written notice within the thirty (30) day period, the selling partner may sell the entire partnership interest under the terms and conditions of the offer, to the third party.

If any payment agreed to be made by a partner exercising such a right of refusal is not made, the selling partner shall have the right to retain any previous payments made, and either have the entire partnership interest retitled to the selling partner with no additional consideration to the defaulting party, and/or exercise any other breach of contract or other lawful remedy, such remedies to be cumulative. However, it is agreed the purchasing partner shall be allowed no less than a thirty (30) day grace period before default in payment is deemed to have occurred, allowing the selling partner remedies as above.

It is agreed any third party offer must reasonably comply with any legal or tax requirements.

In the event of a sale to a third party, it is agreed the third party shall be required to enter into an agreement exactly the same as this agreement (or as may be modified in writing and signed by the parties in the future). The party receiving the offer agrees to inform the third party (proposed purchaser) immediately of all terms in this agreement, and shall provide a copy of this agreement to the third party at the time the written offer is received.

Additionally, each partner agrees in the event one partner sells an entire partnership interest, whether to the other partner (party to this agreement), or to any allowable third party, the selling partner agrees not to compete directly or indirectly in providing any audiology or hearing aid dispensing related services within a three (3) mile radius of the practice location on the date of sale, for eighteen (18) months following the date of sale, unless the practice is repossessed as above. It is acknowledged indirect solicitation within the restrictive area and time period shall be allowed; see the definition below.

DEATH OF A PARTNER AND LIFE INSURANCE PROVISION: Each partner shall purchase (and pay premiums upon the life of the other partner), substantially identical life insurance policies, at all times during the term of this agreement between the initial two partners in a policy (proceeds) amount of not less than $150,000. The partners agree in the event of the death of one of the two partners, all of the partnership interest of the deceased partner shall be purchased by the other partner as follows: The purchase price shall be 50% of the fair market value of the entire practice. The purchase price up to the amount of insurance proceeds shall be paid with insurance proceeds referenced above. Any remaining purchase price shall be paid to the estate of the deceased's partner (or successor, such as a designated beneficiary), pursuant to the installment payment method set forth below. Any excess proceeds shall be retained by the purchasing partner.

Each partner shall provide the other partner proof of insurance. Each partner shall be the beneficiary and owner of the policy purchased by him on the life of the other partner for purposes of this agreement. Each partner shall provide proof of payment of premiums to the other partner. Upon the death of the first partner to die, the surviving partner shall collect the proceeds on the policy owned by him on the life of the deceased partner for purposes of this agreement, and shall apply as much of the proceeds as may be necessary to purchase the partnership interest of the deceased partner at the price set forth above. It is agreed the unpaid portion of the purchase price shall be paid over a five (5) year period in sixty (60) equal monthly installments, with the principal balance to bear interest at the prime rate. It is agreed there shall be no prepayment penalty. It is agreed the estate or any other beneficiary(ies) entitled to such payments shall have a security interest in the partnership interest being purchased. It is agreed during such "pay off" period, the interest rate charged (prime rate—see definition below) shall fluctuate up or down for each calendar year, according to the prime rate on December 31, with the interest rate for the next twelve (12) month period to be adjusted accordingly with equal monthly payments adjusted according to the remaining principal balance on December 31, based upon the remaining number of monthly payments at the adjusted prime rate.

It is agreed the first of the sixty (60) monthly payments shall be due on the first (1st) day of the seventh (7th month, following death of a partner, with remaining monthly payments due on the first (1st) day of the next fifty-nine (59) months. It is agreed the initial prime rate shall be determined by the prime rate on the fifteenth (15th) day before the first (1st) payment is due. It is further agreed the purchasing partner shall be allowed a thirty (30) day grace period before being in default, but to avoid default, the purchasing partner shall pay in addition to the installment payment due, a late fee of twenty-five dollars ($25) per day.

In the event of default, the payees shall have all cumulative rights under law, but may repossess the partnership interest only if it is transferred to another certified/licensed audiologist/hearing aid dispenser. Any agreed upon purchase price by such a certified/licensed person shall reduce the amount due by the defaulting partner. It is further agreed, the unpaid defaulted balance shall bear interest at the prime rate as calculated above, until paid.

In the event of the simultaneous deaths of both partners, or in the event of the death of the surviving partner within thirty (30) days after the death of the first partner to die, the partners and/or appropriate successors shall retain insurance proceeds and the successors of the partners are directed to act reasonably and quickly to sell the practice in its entirety, and split the proceeds, including any installment payments, 50/50.

The estate plans of the partners shall be consistent with, and not contradict this provision.

DISABILITY OF A PARTNER: The partners agree they shall obtain and pay for personally, disability income insurance on the respective partners, for substantially identical policies, to be enforced at the effective date of this agreement, and to remain in force throughout the term of this agreement. It is acknowledged a copy of both such policies shall accompany this agreement, and shall be incorporated into this agreement. Each partner shall pay personally, such premiums on his own respective disability policy.

Disability for purposes of this agreement, shall mean the inability of a partner to carry on day-to-day partnership affairs, including the usual practice of audiology/hearing aid dispensing, on a routine basis, for a one hundred eighty (180) day consecutive period, for an average of at least twenty-five (25) hours per week.

In the event of such disability of one partner, the other partner shall be required to purchase all of the partnership interest of the disabled partner, at a price equal to fifty percent (50%) of the fair market value of the entire practice, determined as of the date of disability (defined above).

The full purchase price shall be paid on the same terms and conditions as set forth in the death provision above (sixty (60) equal monthly installments, with principal to bear interest at the prime rate, etc.). However, during the sixty (60) month payment period, any required payment shall be reduced or eliminated by the amount of any disability payment received in the prior month, by the disabled partner. In the event the disabled partner dies before having received the entire purchase price, payment of the purchase price shall be made to the Successors of the then-deceased partner.

In the event both partners meet the definition of disability within a thirty (30) day period, the partners agree to cooperate to sell the entire practice on a commercially reasonable basis.

In the event of disability of one partner, resulting in the purchase arrangement under this provision, the disabled partner within ninety (90) days of disability, shall have the right to purchase for the then-existing value, the life insurance policy on the life of the disabled partner, with the proviso that the entire value must be paid in a lump sum within the ninety (90) day period.

In the event of disability and purchase by one partner, the selling partner shall be subject to the same practice restriction as set forth in the third party partnership interest sale provisions.

DEFINITION AND DETERMINATION OF FAIR MARKET VALUE: Fair market value is defined as the price at which the practice would be exchanged between a willing buyer and a willing seller, each having reasonable knowledge of all relevant facts, neither acting under compulsion, with equity to both. The phrase with equity to both means that no unfair advantage to buyer or seller results from the transaction. The fair market value is to include goodwill, which reflects the excess of the purchase price of the business, over the fair market value of the business, tangible assets to be disposed. It is agreed the purchasing party shall assume any outstanding liens against any property being purchased, and that any such assumed obligation shall reduce fair market value.

Fair market value shall be agreed upon by the partners and/or either of their successors, as appropriate, within thirty (30) days of the event causing the need to determine fair market value. If, within the thirty (30) day period, fair market value is not determined by the unanimous agreement of the partners and/or appropriate successors, the determination of fair market value shall be submitted to the American Arbitration Association for a final and binding decision. If for any reason the American Arbitration Association is unwilling and/or unable to make a determination of fair market value, the involved parties shall have the right to pursue the determination of fair market value by way of any other lawful manner of enforcement, including, but not limited to, filing a lawsuit.

Any time period affected by the delay in determination of fair market value, shall be delayed a reasonable period of time, until fair market value has been determined pursuant to this provision, and the affected provisions shall thereafter by enforceable.

DEFINITION OF PRIME RATE: Prime rate is defined as the rate charged by the _____ Bank (or its successor) to its best commercial borrowers, with respect to ninety (90) day borrowings.

ENCUMBRANCE OF A PARTNERSHIP INTEREST: Other than provided under this agreement, a partnership interest shall not be pledged, encumbered or hypothecated, without written permission of all partners, and any appropriate successor, such as a payee under this agreement.

DEFINITION OF DIRECT AND INDIRECT SOLICITATION FOR RESTRICTIVE COVENANT AGREEMENT PROVISIONS: The parties acknowledge this agreement contains various restrictive provisions, such as in the event of the sale of a partnership interest to a third party, which provisions contain phrases such as "direct and indirect solicitation." It is agreed indirect solicitation shall include only advertisements in any phone book or other publication, including but not limited to, a newspaper and magazine, of general circulation. It is agreed any other type of solicitation, such as direct mailing, including zip code type mailings, or direct contact, such as by telephone, shall be included in the definition of direct solicitation.

SPOUSAL PROVISIONS: It is agreed in the event a married partner becomes divorced, that the partnership interest of the spouse shall be assigned pursuant to the property settlement agreement, or order of the court to the spouse/partner. It is further agreed in the event the court determines under law that it is fair and equitable that the nonpartner spouse receive compensation for some or all of such partnership interest, that the divorcing partner shall purchase such partnership interest on the terms and conditions that the parties agree is fair and reasonable, or on the terms and conditions as ordered by the court.

Further, in the event an unmarried partner contemplates marriage, it is agreed before such marriage takes place, if lawful, a prenuptial arrangement shall be entered into by the prospective spouses, stating the partnership interest subject to this agreement, shall be and shall remain subject to the terms and conditions of this agreement, with the nonpartner spouse being required to sign the spousal consent below. Such prenuptial contracts, shall be in conformity with then existing [State] law.

<u>DISSOLUTION AND LIQUIDATION</u>: The partnership shall be dissolved upon the sale of all or substantially all of the property owned by the partnership. If the partnership is dissolved as a matter of law such as by the death of a partner, a new partnership shall be reconstituted immediately by all remaining and any successor partners with such partnership to contain the exact same terms and conditions as this agreement. It is specifically agreed no partner shall voluntarily withdraw from the partnership without unanimous consent of all partners unless such partnership interest is transferred pursuant to this agreement or required by law. If a partner withdraws in violation of this agreement or applicable statutory law, the other partners in the partnership may recover any and all such damages and additional costs including additional tax and accounting and legal fees caused by such. In the event of dissolution of the partnership, unless the partnership is reconstituted as above, distribution of assets and proceeds from liquidation of the partnership assets shall be applied in the order as follows:

[NOTE: The above provision disallows voluntary withdrawal by any partner; that language may be removed and replaced with language which allows a partner to voluntarily withdraw indicating how to calculate amounts due the withdrawing partner or what negative capital account restoration is necessary. Especially in a professional partnership situation voluntary withdraw might be in the best interest of partners who would wish to practice outside of any restrictive area; further, a retirement age applying to all partners could be utilized after which voluntary withdrawal is allowed.]

1. Payment to creditors of the partnership, other than partners in order of priority provided by law;
2. Payment to partners for indebtedness, if any, of the partnership to partners, in proportion to total loans made by them to the partnership;
3. Payment to the partners in accordance and in proportion to capital account balances, with the proviso following distribution, any partner with a negative capital account shall immediately restore such by a cash contribution in an amount to bring the capital account to zero with such cash to be used to pay remaining liabilities and/or distributed to the other partners such as to reduce their capital accounts to zero.

<u>ARBITRATION PROVISIONS</u>: The parties agree in the event there is a dispute arising from this contract, the matter shall be submitted to the American Arbitration Association in [City], [State] and that such controversy shall be determined under their then-existing rules by an arbitrator selected by the American Arbitration Association and that decision which may be in the form of an award of damages against one part and in favor of the other part or otherwise shall be final and binding upon the parties, and a judgment thereon may be entered in the appropriate court of the State of _____. If at the time a dispute arise, the American Arbitration Association is unable or unwilling to make a binding determination, the parties may litigate the matter in any other lawful manner, provided, however, this clause shall not limit either party's right to obtain any provisional remedy, including without limitation, injunctive relief, orders for recovering possessions or similar relief, from any court of competent jurisdiction deemed necessary by either part to protect its property rights. The arbitrator shall award costs and reasonable attorney's fees to the prevailing party; in the discretion of the arbitrator, in making such award, consideration may be given to [state] law and case law discussing the interpreting [state] statutes.

<u>ACKNOWLEDGMENT OF ADDITIONAL CONTINGENCIES</u>: The parties acknowledge this agreement may not provide for all possible contingencies, and the partners agree with

one another to act reasonably to arrive at compromises necessary to the efficient operation of the practice, and enforcement of agreement provisions, and reasonable intentions of the partners. Further, any appropriate successors are directed to also act reasonably in arriving at necessary compromises.

GENERAL PROVISIONS: No significance shall be assigned to agreement headings or gender usage. Further, no significant is to be attached to the use of singular or plural designations. Each designation or gender shall be construed to include the others where appropriate.

This agreement may not be modified without the unanimous written approval of all existing partners. As a condition of transferring a partnership interest, any new partner shall sign an agreement the same as this agreement, or as modified by the agreement of the then existing partners. It is acknowledged depending upon the then existing number of partners, that, for example, percentages, such as relating to tax allocations and distributions, may need to be modified. The parties acknowledge an example of an event which would cause the need to modify the agreement, would be in the event a third partner is admitted to the partnership, in which case the parties acknowledge portions of the buyout provisions would need to be modified, to take into account the admission of the third partner. The partners further agree the partnership agreement shall be modified if required by law, such as to meet a requirement applicable to any audiology/hearing aid dispenser partnership.

This agreement constitutes the entire agreement between the parties, and no statements, promises or inducements made by either party or agent of either party that are not contained in this written agreement shall be valid or binding.

The partners agree in the event one partner reasonably requests that the other partner submit to a medical examination to determine disability or misconduct, the other partner shall consent to an examination followed by such determination by a medical doctor reasonably agreed upon by the partners (or an agent of one partner, such as a guardian or spouse of a partner). The partners (or an agent of a partner, such as a spouse) agree to reasonably cooperate to select the licensed [State] medical practitioner to make such disability determination. The partner to be examined shall have the right to select and pay for other independent examinations and reports. The parties agree if they are unable to agree as to a disability determination or length thereof, that such shall be submitted under the arbitration provision below.

It is agreed this agreement and related agreements shall be binding upon the heirs, personal representatives, lawful assigns and lawful successors of the shareholders.

If any provision of this agreement is declared void and unenforceable, such provision shall be deemed severed from this agreement which shall otherwise remain in full force and effect. Further, if any such provision may be reduced and/or narrowed in scope or the like, such provision shall be reduced, narrowed, and/or the like, and so enforced. Additionally, in the event any term or provision of this agreement is declared to be illegal or invalid, because of the duration or geographical scope, such term or provision shall be reduced to the extent necessary to become enforceable, and shall be enforced as so reduced. The parties to this agreement acknowledge and agree the geographical scope and time periods as to the respective restrictive covenants, are reasonable and necessary for the protection of the respective parties.

The parties agree in the event a breach of this contract, the breaching party will pay the other party's costs and reasonable attorney fees incurred because of a breach whether a lawsuit is instituted or not.

Each party to this agreement agrees to do all things and take such actions, and to make, execute and deliver such other documents and instruments as shall be reasonably required to carry out the provision, intent, and purpose of this agreement.

The parties acknowledge this agreement and related matters have been drafted and handled by Attorney [_____]. The parties acknowledge a conflict of interest exists, and that such conflict is waived. The parties acknowledge they have had the opportunity to have the agreement and related documents reviewed, at each partner's option, by any other accounting, legal or professional advisor.

EFFECTIVE DATE: _____

_____
Dr. A, Ph.D. CCC-A, Partner
(On Behalf of Her Marital Community Partner)

_____
Mr. B, M.A. CCC-A, Partner
(Currently Unmarried)

CONSENT OF PARTNERS' SPOUSES:
Each undersigned person acknowledges that he (or she, as the case may be in the future), is the spouse of an above partner. Each such undersigned person acknowledges he or she has read and approved the provisions of the partnership agreement, and agrees to be bound by and accept the provisions of such in lieu of all other interests he or she may have in the partnership interest, whether the interest may be community or otherwise. Each undersigned person agrees to be bound by the terms and conditions of the agreement, as surviving spouse or in any other capacity, and acknowledges such partnership interest may only be transferred under [State] audiology/hearing aid dispensing ethical standards, to another [State] licensed practitioner, as well as under the terms of the agreement and related agreements. Each undersigned person agrees to forego any and all management rights whatsoever.

Naming and Registering the Practice

This chapter outlines common regulatory steps associated with initiating or purchasing a practice. These steps are not unique to audiology. For the most part, they are required in most business start-ups except when one has purchased the stock of an incorporated practice. The steps are basic and assume the practice has no employees. Refer to Chapter 11 for a discussion of special governmental regulations that apply to employees.

NAMING THE PRACTICE

The name can create the image of the practice

Selecting the practice's name is a topic that might seem more appropriate under Marketing. Indeed, the name of the practice, like its location, can create a powerful image to the public about the services the company provides and how it provides them. Its alphabetical listing in the Yellow Pages may have a bearing, too, depending on the target markets and the number of competitors.

Surprisingly, experts advise that a *safe* company name should include words that are obscure, unrelated, nondescriptive, arbitrary, made-up or whimsical (Jenkins, 1993; Resnick, 1992)! The reason for this is to protect the practice's name as a trademark under state or federal law. A name that is too generic may not be legally protected from use by others (e.g., "The Hearing Center"), but a name that is too whimsical may confuse or turn off target markets (e.g., "Ears to You!"). Choosing the best name for a practice requires thought, research and informal survey, and an awareness of trademark laws. An initial error in the selection of a name can be costly, if not devastating to a new practice. For example, an audiologist selects "Micro-Ear" for a practice name. Shortly after opening the practice, the audiologist is sued by a large company with a similar name, and loses. It takes months to recover from this costly error.

The name can describe what the practice does

A good name should clearly describe the products or services provided by the practice. McCollom and Mynders (1984) recommend that the name should be "simple, spellable and memorable; have dignity; and not be catchy or faddish" (p. 76). On the negative, the authors recommend *avoiding*:

■ Acronyms (essentially "in-house" jokes that do not communicate much to the public)
■ Street or area names (what if the practice moves from Central Street to Park Avenue?)
■ Difficult personal names (McCollom and Mynder's example is the "Amos P.D.Q. Schwenksfelder Hearing Aid Service")

- The word "audiology" when "hearing" will do (after nearly 50 years many people still do not know the meaning of "audiology").

In addition to adopting a name that is descriptive of the services and products provided, the name must also be unique enough to qualify for protection under the law. This means that it cannot be *merely* descriptive of goods and services—it must also be arbitrary to the point that the name is not considered generic (e.g., Apple Computers). Finally, the name should be distinctive enough to avoid the costly legal entanglements associated with trademark infringement. As Resnick (1992) points out, "If you think your company is too small to get caught in the web of trademark litigation, think again. Lawyers say that ignorance of these laws can cost you dearly in terms of time, money, and customers, especially if you're forced to change a company name or logo you've spent years promoting" (p. 29).

Naming the Practice After the Owner

A strong lobby exists for using one's own name for the practice. This approach circumvents the legal concerns because the name is usually unique. A personal name does not describe services and products, but it does connote professionalism when degrees and certification are attached (hence, one of the marketing attributes of the professional doctorate). With proper marketing, the professional's name itself can take on a secondary meaning of "audiology and hearing aid dispensing." Paradoxically, therein lie the three main objections to naming the practice after the owner:

- Additional and repeated marketing efforts are needed to inform the public of the practice's products/services and make the owner's name synonymous with those products/services.
- Once the owner's name is indelibly stamped on the target markets, those markets tend to resist receiving services from nonowner audiologists employed by the practice.
- It poses a difficulty when selling the business to a new owner with a different name.

Jenkins (1993) raises a realistic, albeit extremely negative argument against naming the practice after the owner.

If you put your name on the business and the venture goes belly up, as so many new businesses do, many people in the community will automatically associate your name with the defunct or bankrupt business, which may make it very difficult if you try to start another business or to obtain credit in the same community in the future. (section 4.2, p. 2)

Registering the Name

Resnick (1992) recommends steps for selecting a good name and then registering it as a trademark.[1] According to the U.S. Patent and Trademark Office, a trademark is a work, name, symbol or device used to identify service and distinguish it from others. Steps 2 through 5 should be done together with an attorney.

1. *Scout out the competition* by searching the local yellow pages and checking library sources. For example, *The Trademark Register* is an annual publication that lists all federally registered trademarks.
2. *Run a name check.* For state trademarks, information is available from state offices (often by phone) on whether a name is available or is either the same or too similar to a trademark already in use in the state. Federal trademarks can be checked in the aforementioned *Trademark Register*. There also are search firms that will conduct a company-name and trademark search for a fee.[2] *Trademarkscan* is an on-line search service accessible via modem on Dialog or ·CompuServe. *Trademarkscan* is updated weekly or biweekly and contains comprehensive information on the names of trademarks registered federally in all 50 states and Puerto Rico.
3. *Test the name's legal viability* by asking three questions: Does it only describe the product or service? Is it "confusingly similar" to another trademarked name? Is it the same name as another company's but spelled differently or in a different language? Try a new name if one or more of the answers are yes.

---

[1]Having a federal trademark gives a company the right to sue in federal court for trademark infringement and for unflattering comparative advertising using the trademarked name. Trademarks may be preregistered and protected for up to 3 years by indicating an intent to use them at a future date on the application.

[2]Two sources are: (1) Thomson and Thomson, 500 Victory Rd., North Quincy, MA 02171, (800) 692-8833; and (2) Trademark Research Center. 300 Park Ave. S., New York, NY 10010, (800) 872-6275.

4. *Pick a "safe" name* that communicates to the public but is legally conservative; hence the recommendation for obscure, altered, or made-up words.
5. *Put it in writing.* A company name does not have to be registered, but registering it as a federal or state trade name protects the name nationally or in the state where the practice does business. However, a state registered trademark does not protect a company from out-of-state firms who choose to use the same name or logo, even within the state. Federal trademark application[3] costs as little as $175. State registration is often less than $20. Blank Affidavits of Trade Name Use are available in book stores with business sections.

Fictitious Names

Fictitious names are business names that do not contain the surname of the owner or all of the general partners. Even if the business name is that of the owner(s), it is still considered fictitious if it is used together with words like "company," "associates," "group," "brothers," or "sons" that suggest additional owners (Jenkins, 1993). Whether a fictitious name is registered as a trade name or not, the company must file and publish a fictitious business name statement for use of the name. Use of the name occurs if the name appears in advertising, on business cards or letterhead, or on products. Newspapers will often have filing forms and publish the notices. Filing of the affidavit or certificate is frequently done at the county recorder's office.

An individual or a company doing business under a fictitious name is referred to as "doing business as" (dba). For example, the mythical private practice described in the appendices of this book is owned and operated by Dr. A, who is dba Cardinal Hearing Services, Inc. If Cardinal Hearing Services decides to open a hearing aid repair shop called Cardinal Hearing Aid Repairs in another location, its official title is "Cardinal Hearing Services, Inc. (dba Cardinal Hearing Aid Repairs)."

---

[3]Contact the U.S. Department of Commerce, Patent and Trademark Office, Washington, DC 20231. (703) 557-4636 and request the free publication: "Basic Facts About Trademarks" which includes application forms and explanations of changes made to the trademark law in November, 1989.

Logos

Logos are treated in the same manner as names: They should not be generic, they should not be close copies of existing logos of other companies, and they can be trademarked federally or within the state in which the practice operates. Just as arbitrary or made-up words are recommended in the name, arbitrary symbols (e.g., twin arches, an apple, an alligator) are advocated for logos.

McCollom and Mynders (1984) wittily bemoan our profession's limited imagination and "slavish adherence of logo styles," opining that audiology logos should *avoid:*

- ears (too generic and too often repeated),
- ears with concentric circles (something of an inside joke, perhaps communicating something different to the public than to those in the profession),
- ossicular chains or cochleas (again based on inside information, communicating little or connoting something different to the general public).

BUSINESS LICENSES AND IDs

Local Licenses

One of the first steps after naming the business is to procure city and/or county business licenses and sales permits at city hall or county offices. There are usually fees for the initial applications as well as for annual renewal of the licenses.

Local licenses should be obtained before the business opens its doors to avoid penalty fines. Depending on the locale, businesses are taxed by the city or county based on gross receipts or some other measure of productivity. City sales tax may be collected on products sold.

State Licenses

It is illegal in almost every state to operate a hearing aid dispensing practice without securing a state license. The license is obtained by meeting the particular state's requirements for the profession, such as education, experience, examinations; submitting a detailed application; and paying a fee. It is kept by meeting that state's continuing education requirement (if any) and renewing the license periodically with an accompanying renewal fee.

A majority of states require state licensing of audiologists. If the state in which the practice is located has an audiology license requirement, the steps for obtaining the license are the same as those described for hearing aid dispensing.

It is important to get complete information on the specific requirements of the state in which the practice will be located. This should be done by consulting an attorney and an accountant. A basic overview of state and federal regulations is available through Jenkins' Starting and Operating a Business series, which is published for each of the 50 states (e.g., *Starting and Operating a Business in Arizona*).

Tax Identification Numbers

Each person or corporation doing business in a state must submit a tax application form to the state's department of revenue, along with a registration fee. After registration, the state issues the business an identification number and sends out necessary tax forms (e.g., state sales tax, payroll tax).

As early as possible, the business needs to apply for a federal employer identification number (EIN). An EIN is used to identify the business for most federal tax purposes (e.g., payroll and income tax returns). An EIN is obtained by filing a completed *Form SS-4*. To request an EIN application by mail, dial 1-800-829-1040. To receive an EIN over the telephone, or to mail an application, use the phone number or address of the Center shown for your state in Table 6–1. Allow 4 to 5 weeks if the application is done by mail. EINs can also be obtained over the telephone, but there is a long distance charge for the call.

SUMMARY

Before commencing business, an audiology practice must decide on a name and register the name. Naming the practice requires research and consultation with an attorney. Once a name is registered, the practice should next obtain various city, county, and state licenses and state and federal tax identification numbers in the practice's name.

Table 6–1. Regional IRS Centers for EIN Applications.

Region	Center
Florida, Georgia, South Carolina	Atlanta, GA 39901 (404) 455-2360
New Jersey, New York City & counties of Nassau, Rockland, Suffolk & Westchester	Holtsville, NY 00501 (516) 447-4955
New York (all other counties), Connecticut, Maine, Massachusetts, New Hampshire, Rhode Island, Vermont	Andover, MA 05501 (508) 474-9717
Illinois, Iowa, Minnesota, Missouri, Wisconsin	Kansas City, MO 64999 (816) 926-5999
Delaware, District of Columbia, Maryland, Pennsylvania, Virginia	Philadelphia, PA 19255 (215) 961-3980
Indiana, Kentucky, Michigan, Ohio, West Virginia	Cincinnati, OH 45999
Kansas, New Mexico, Oklahoma, Texas	Austin, TX 73301 (512) 462-7845
Alaska, Arizona, California (counties of Alpine, Amador, Butte, Calaveras, Colusa, Contra Costa, Del Norte, Eldorado, Glenn, Humboldt, Lake, Lassen, Marin Mendocino, Modoc, Napa, Nevada, Placer, Plumas, Sacramento, San Joaquin, Shasta, Sierra, Siskiyou, Solano, Sonoma, Sutter, Tehama, Trinity, Yolo, and Yuba), Colorado, Idaho, Montana, Nebraska, Nevada, North Dakota, Oregon, South Dakota, Utah, Washington, Wyoming	Ogden, UT 84201 (801) 625-7645
California (all other counties), Hawaii	Fresno, CA 93888 (209) 456-5900
Alabama, Arkansas, Louisiana, Mississippi, North Carolina Tennessee	Memphis, TN 37501 (901) 365-5970

REFERENCES

Jenkins, M. D. (1993). *Starting and operating a business in Arizona. A step-by-step guide.* Grants Pass, OR: Oasis Press.

McCollum, H. F., Jr., & Mynders, J. M. (1984). *Hearing aid dispensing practice.* Danville, IL: Interstate Printers & Publishers.

Resnick, R. (1992, August). What's in a name? Your livelihood! *Home Office Computing,* pp. 29–30.

Location

Everyone is familiar with the exhortation "Location, Location, Location!" Its ubiquity suggests that location is always the primary consideration of anyone contemplating a business start-up. Reality is otherwise:

> In finding a location . . . many owners take a passive rather than an active approach, stumbling more or less accidentally across a location, much as they drift into the decision to go into business in the first place. (American Speech-Language-Hearing Association [ASHA], 1985, p. 10)

> The practitioner should evaluate a potential location relative to the opportunities and demands for services rather than simply deciding whether it is a desirable place to live. (Cole, 1986, p. 127)

> Few entrepreneurs go through a logical process of site selection. Instead, they often permit personal preference to dictate their decision on where to locate. (Siropolis, 1990, p. 228)

Location is critical for audiology practice

Location may not be vital for businesses that can be done practically anywhere (e.g., consulting) or are unique (e.g., antique jewelry appraisal). But location *is* critical to the success of audiology practices. Equipment demands alone make it impractical for audiologists to go to patients. Patients must come to the practice, which means the practice must be easily accessible. Most practices do not have the luxury of being unique, nor do they lack worthy competitors. This means the practice must be placed in a location that is viable in terms of financial feasibility as well as accessibility.

PERSONAL PREFERENCES

Personal preference often plays an important part in selecting a location. Home towns are a popular choice, as are communities in which an audiologist has worked and established a good professional reputation. As Church (1984) points out, people who initiate their businesses in familiar surroundings usually do so at an advantage because "Their established credit gives them a better chance to get capital financing and credit and the developed reputation for integrity and dependability helps them create goodwill by attracting customers from among their acquaintances and others who have heard of them" (p. 153).

Weather, friends, academic associations, recreational opportunities, proximity, "trailing spouses," and other factors can and do color one's preference as to where to locate the practice. After all, this is where you are choosing to live your life as well as practice audiology!

Personal preferences have an immediacy that tends to obscure other more objective considerations. Little if any research is needed to know where you would *like* to practice, but a great deal of marketing research is needed to learn where you would *do best* to practice.

MARKETING RESEARCH FOR SELECTING A LOCATION

Siropolis (1990) identifies four steps of marketing research that are necessary to select the best location for a practice. In order, selection is made according to:

1. geographical region
2. a city within that region
3. an area within that city
4. a specific site within that area

The information gathered by doing this research is valuable not only for location and site selection, but also for formulating a business plan and developing marketing strategies for use once the practice is begun, as discussed in later chapters. The bulk of this chapter addresses what questions to ask at each of the four marketing research steps, and how to get the information to answer those questions. The chapter concludes with a brief discussion of facility types and psychological mapping characteristics of consumers.

Geographical Region

Regions refer to large areas, usually collections of states, that can be characterized along broad dimensions such as climate, cost of living, labor costs and availability, cultural amenities, transportation, academic institutes, industry, and general economic conditions. Typical regional divisions include New England, the Midwest, Southeast, Southwest, West, and Northwest. Studies on the relative "health" of one region versus another are often reported in business magazines and newspapers.

When looking at regional differences, the questions are broad:

■ Is the overall economy growing, faltering, or maintaining?

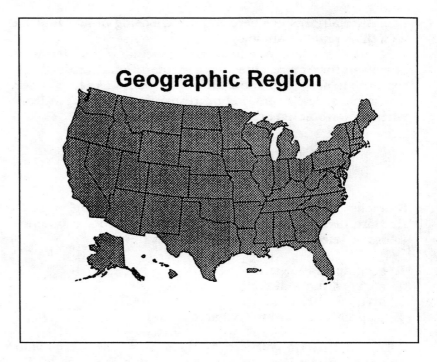

Geographic Region

- What are the main industries (e.g., service, manu-facturing, trade, farming)?
- Is there diversification?
- Is the population stable or transient?
- What is the unemployment rate?
- Are people moving in or moving out?
- What are the state licensing laws for audiology and hearing aid dispensing?
- What are the trends in managed care—are audiolo-gists recognized as providers?

Information sources for Step 1

If one is free to locate in any region of the country, the best approach is to use the public library to look up recent comparative reports of regional activity. Population statistics based on 10-year intervals are found in U.S. Bureau of the Census reports, which are also available at public libraries. A "Checklist for Locating a Practice" and Community Evaluation Chart are available from the American Speech-Language-Hearing Association (ASHA, 1994).

City Within the Region

Having identified a region of the country, the next step is to find the right city. In many cases, this may turn out to be

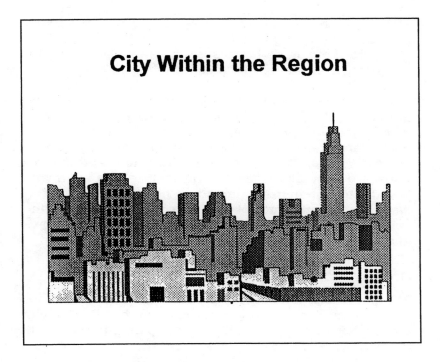

City Within the Region

the first step if personal factors (e.g., family, health, finances) dictate the region in which one must work. At this stage, the questions to ask are more specific:

- Is the city growing? If so, is the growth steady?
- What are the population demographics (age, marital status, income, occupation)?
- How is the real estate market (average cost of homes, length of time to sell)?
- Urban or suburban residents?
- Is the population stable or transient?
- How many audiologists, audiology clinics, and hearing aid dispensers are there? How are they doing?
- What is the availability and nature of the labor supply?
- What are the wage levels?
- What are the transportation modes?
- How is traffic?
- What are the city zoning ordinances?
- Is business seasonal?
- What are community attitudes toward health and education?
- Is there evidence of civic pride?
- What is the educational level of residents?
- What is the quality of the schools?

The answers to some of these questions can be found by perusing local newspapers. It is a good idea to subscribe to at least one of a city's newspapers before making a decision to move there. The local Chamber of Commerce is also a good resource.

Information sources for Step 2

Several annual publications provide information on cities in the United States. The "Survey of Buying Power" in *Sales and Marketing Management* magazine looks at major metropolitan areas. It reports information on population, income, and retail sales. The *Editor and Publisher Market Guide*, also published annually, reports on most cities. The information is quite comprehensive, including population, number of banks, registered automobiles, household statistics, principal industries, climate, retailing (outlets, department stores), and personal disposable income.

Area Within the City

The questions at this step are much the same as those asked in the previous section, except that they are limited to one or more areas of the city. In comparing the areas, the following questions should be addressed:

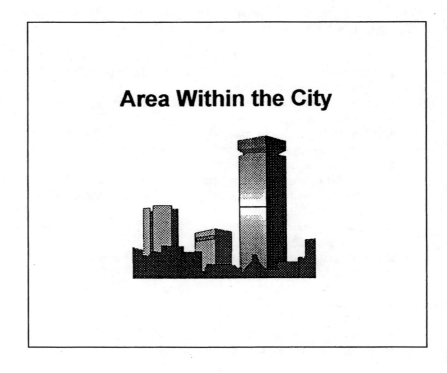

■ Is one area growing more rapidly than the others?
■ If so, is continued growth predicted?
■ Is public transportation comparable in each area?
■ What are the age demographics of the area?
■ Are there zoning or city tax differences between areas? (e.g., are some areas outside the city limits?)

Census tracts from the U.S. Bureau of the Census are available at county government offices. These data are updated every 10 years. Census tracts are available for all cities with populations of 50,000 or more. Each tract within a city comprises an average of 4 to 5,000 inhabitants and reports population density and distribution, along with many helpful descriptors. City planning reports can also prove useful in assessing potential changes in neighborhood conditions.

Information sources for Step 3

Specific Site Within the Area

The appropriateness of a potential site is rarely self-evident, even to an experienced analyst and the questions become numerous and highly specific at this last step. As Baxter (1994) points out:

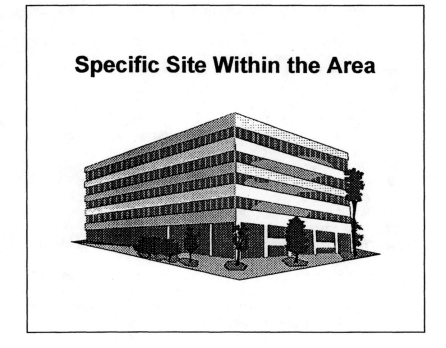

Specific Site Within the Area

> It is important to weed out undesirable sites and focus on sites that offer real potential. Collecting statistical data related to the particular market area can be an exacting task: however, selecting a practice location without knowledge of the potential consumers in the proposed area, the number and sizes of competing services, and the cost of occupancy can cause problems that might later necessitate moving to a new location. (p. 15)

Foremost are questions regarding accessibility, safety, convenience, competition, history, image, and cost (adapted in part from Baxter, 1994; Rizzo & Wilkins, 1993; Siropolis, 1990):

- Is the site on a main road?
- Is the site visible from the road?
- Can signs be seen from the road? At night?
- Is there visible parking?
- Is parking adequate and dedicated for each business?
- Is there a parking fee?
- Is parking convenient for patients with ambulatory difficulty?
- Is there covered parking?
- Are staff and public parking mixed or separated?
- Is public transportation available? If so, where is the nearest stop?
- Is the site on the right side of the street in terms of traffic flow? If not, does a divider in the road force U-turns?
- Is the site on the ground floor? Directly accessible or down a shared hallway?
- Is it close to a large population base?
- What kinds of business occupied the site previously? Were they successful? Why did they leave?
- How are neighboring businesses doing?
- Is the site near other professionals and potential referral sources?
- How close is the nearest competitor?
- Are nearby competitors effective? Well-known? Public or private?
- What are the zoning requirements?
- Is the neighborhood changing? If so, why?
- Will the site potentially be affected by city planning changes?
- Is the floor plan adequate with room for expansion?
- Is the site located in a controlled sound environment away from street traffic, main pedestrian areas, air conditioning systems, and other noise sources?

- Will the building support the weight of one or more sound booths in an interior space?
- Does the site meet the requirements of the Americans with Disabilities Act (1991)?[1]
- Are there environmental hazards on the site?
- Does the site meet safety and building codes?
- Are plumbing, electrical, and ventilation systems adequate?
- Is the site affordable? Rent or depreciation? Build-out or remodeling costs?
- What are the operating costs?
- What are the taxes (property, income, sales)?
- If leased space, what is length of lease? Ability to sublease? Renegotiation options?
- Is the building attractive, comfortable, and professional in appearance?
- Is the building located near easily recognized landmarks?
- Is it easy to give directions to the location?
- Does the site have good security? At night?

If the office is going to be located in a medical building, much of the site selection process is determined in advance by real-estate developers. Just as shopping centers and industrial parks dictate the locations of many businesses, hospital and medical center "campuses" are determining to a large extent where audiology services will be provided. In this case, the developers of the medical complex have already done much of the market research.

However, if one is constructing a stand-alone structure, or even remodeling or designing a clinic within a medical complex, the questions above and many more must be addressed (cf. Baxter, 1994; Katz, 1993; Rizzo & Wilkins, 1993). In all cases, it is a good idea to identify the most salient questions for the proposed practice and do a quantitative analysis along the lines of the sample Comparative-Cost Analysis Chart shown in Table 7–1.

---

[1]Title III of the Americans with Disabilities Act has been in effect since January of 1992. Title III prohibits discrimination on the basis of disability in "public accommodations," which include doctors' and lawyers' offices, etc. New public accommodations must be designed and built to be accessible to persons with disabilities. A new facility is defined as one with a state or local building permit issued after January 26, 1992 or a first certificate of occupancy issued after January 26, 1993.

Table 7–1. Comparative cost analysis chart for evaluating office locations.

Factors	Location 1	Location 2	Location 3
SITE FEATURES (in points[a])			
Location			
Parking			
Accessibility			
Physical suitability			
Room for expansion			
Safety			
Image			
Estimated value in 10 years			
Competition			
Zoning			
Community			
TOTAL POINTS:			
OPERATING COSTS ($)			
Heating			
Electricity			
Other utilities			
Rent or depreciation			
Wages			
Insurance			
TAXES[b]			
Property			
Personal property			
Income			
Sales			
Payroll			
City			
TOTALS ($):	$	$	$

[a]Rate as "good" (10 points), "average" (5 points), or "poor" (1 point).
[b]Use estimated or exact cost per year

TYPE OF FACILITY

The practice can be on a medical campus, in a business building, in a mini-professional mall (e.g., dental, nursing, physical therapy, etc), or stand-alone. It can be leased, sub-leased, or owned. Final selection of type of facility depends on the factors of image, availability, short-term cash flow, long-term goals and costs, financing arrangements, future zoning plans, and future of the surrounding community.

Medical campuses provide "a positive image as well as access to related services and referral sources. The layout (treatment rooms, waiting room, and reception area), plumbing, and electrical outlets are usually adequate without remodeling" (Baxter, p. 16, 1994). Offices in medical buildings can be purchased in some cases, but are more often available on a lease basis. In either case, the cost per square foot is usually high, but this may be more than off-set by access to referrals.

Medical office buildings offer a positive image but higher cost

Availability may be limited in areas that are growing and prosperous, especially if future zoning is promising. Availability may also be limited by protectionism clauses in the leases of previously established competitors (e.g., otolaryngologists, audiologists, or hearing aid dispensers) in the building or on the campus. Limited availability drives up the cost of space, sometimes to the point where cash flow demands in the start-up years cannot support an otherwise highly desirable location. In that case, the options are: (a) find less space in the same building or campus, (b) sublease, or (c) locate to a less desirable but more affordable facility.

Working with less space or subleasing within a facility can satisfy short-term cash flow needs, but may force relocation as long-term practice goals are achieved or if the sublease is not renewed. The flip side is to lease enough space for future growth and sublease to other professionals until cash-flow allows the practice to assume the full financial burden. The obvious threats in this arrangement are tenant vacancy or delinquency.

Stand-alone facilities can be leased, but more often are owned. Thus, start-up costs are usually much higher (Katz, 1993), although long-term savings may accrue if the property investment is made wisely. Stand-alone facilities are not always suitable to the image of a professional audiology practice. Pre-existing structures often require extensive remodeling and may be subject to zoning changes that have occurred since the building was constructed (Katz, 1993). These sites are usually not ideally located for access to other health professionals and referral sources.

Stand-alone offices require special considerations

In deciding whether to lease or buy, the initial cost of purchase tends to be overemphasized. However, this is a one-time charge which is amortized over the years of the loan. Over the long run, the business claims depreciation and gains a fixed asset. With an existing structure, one should weigh the cost of remodeling against the cost of constructing a new building. With an appropriately located facility, remodeling costs may be well worthwhile (Church, 1984). Whether one is building or remodeling, leasing or purchasing, another "cost" that is well spent is to put a good amount of time and attention into the construction (Baxter, 1994; Katz, 1993). Pay daily visits to the site to oversee the work, catch mistakes, and ensure that the final facility will meet the needs of the practice.

Assuming the structure is sound, there are three big obstacles to purchase:

1. *Obtaining financing.* In today's fiscal climate, it is unlikely that novice owners could obtain a building or office loan. Even established practitioners with excellent businesses and good credit histories have struck out on conventional financing (Katz, 1993).[2]
2. *Finding an appropriate office to purchase.* In high-rent areas, owners are not strongly motivated to sell their lucrative investment properties.
3. *Getting stuck with an undesirable location.* The facility may be available because it is in an undesirable area. Community demographics also may shift over the years, leaving the building in an undesirable area.

COGNITIVE MAPPING

Researchers in Behavioral Geography have demonstrated in numerous studies that consumers demonstrate "spatial choice behaviors" when selecting their destinations, and these choices are often based on subjective rather than physical realities (Cadwallader, 1981). Thus, "cognitive mapping" is an important variable at this point in the selection process (Parfit, 1984) because it addresses the "crystal ball" issues of image and desirability in the mind of the consumer.

As an example of cognitive mapping, the selection of one shopping point over another equidistant one is not based simply on a time versus distance trade-off analysis (Halperin, Gale, Golledge, & Hubert, 1983), but more likely on the relation of the destination to a customer's perceptual "anchor point." Site selection must include an analysis of anchor points in the cognitive mapping of consumers in the market area.

Anchor points are shared by large groups of people in cities, so that effective directions are given in relation to the anchor point (e.g., "Go past the hospital one block and our

---

[2]If the practice is a corporation or Limited Liability Company (LLC) with multiple professional shareholders/members, the facility should not be brought into the business as an asset, because it is then exposed in the event of negligence lawsuits brought against the business. See Chapter 5 for further discussion of this issue.

office is on the left"). Often, anchor points are "indistinguishable physically from other such places . . . made special by some extra shared knowledge that exists only in the minds of the people, in the same way that everyone used to know the one tree among thousands that was used for hangings" (Parfit, 1984, p. 128).

Anchor points are learned by living in a community over a period of time—at least 6 months according to Parfit's report. Obviously, site selection can benefit enormously from knowledge of local residents' perceptual mapping, suggesting that one is wise to live in a community for some time before selecting a business site.

Locate the office relative to community "anchor points"

SUMMARY

Location is crucial to the success of most audiology practices. Choosing a location begins with marketing analysis of regional and city statistics, followed by comparisons of different areas within the city of choice. Finally, a specific site is chosen for the practice. In addition to marketing analysis, personal biases, financing, and cognitive mapping have an effect on the selection process and the success of the selected site. Answers to specific questions need to be found at each step as the location search narrows to a single site. Numerous sources of marketing information are available to aid the audiologist in answering these questions. The resulting marketing analysis is valuable not only for helping in site selection, but also in developing business plans and marketing strategies once the practice commences.

REFERENCES

American Speech-Language-Hearing Association. (1985). *Planning and initiating a private practice in audiology and speech-language pathology*. Rockville, MD: Author.

American Speech-Language-Hearing Association. (1994). *Development and management of audiology practices*. Rockville, MD: Author.

Americans with Disabilities Act in brief, focus on employment, public accommodations, transportation, telecommunications. (1991, July 26). *Federal Register*, Parts I, II, III, IV, and V.

Baxter, J. (1994). Locating and equipping an audiology practice. In H. Hosford-Dunn, J. Baxter, A. Desmond, G. Jacobson, J. Johnson, P. Martin, & E. Cherow (Eds.), *Development and management of audiology practices* (chap. 4, pp. 15–24). Rockville, MD: ASHA.

Cadwallader, M. (1981). Towards a cognitive gravity model: The case of consumer spatial behavior. *Regional Studies, 15*(4), 275–284.

Church, O. D. (1984). *Small business. Management and entrepreneurship.* Chicago: Science Research Associates.

Cole, P. R. (1986). Selecting the location and site for a private practice. In K. G. Butler (Ed.), *Prospering in private practice* (chap. 7, pp. 127–134). Rockville, MD: Aspen.

Halperin, W. C., Gale, N., Golledge, R. G., & Hubert, L. J. (1983). Exploring entrepreneurial cognitions of retail environments. *Economic Geography, 59*(1), 3–15.

Katz, K. R. (1993). So you're thinking about buying your own office building. *The Hearing Journal, 46*(9), 27–29.

Parfit, M. (1984, May). Mapmaker who charts our hidden mental demands. *Smithsonian,* pp. 123–131.

Rizzo, S. R., Jr., & Wilkins, J. E. (1993). Planning and designing audiology and speech-language pathology (ASLP) facilities. In S. R. Rizzo, Jr. & M. D. Trudeau (Eds.), *Clinical administration in audiology and speech-language pathology* (chap. 3, pp. 65–92). San Diego, CA: Singular Publishing Group.

Siropolis, N. C. (1990). *Small business management. A guide to entrepreneurship* (4th ed.). Boston: Houghton Mifflin.

Leasing or Subleasing Office Space

*Leases should never
be signed without first
consulting with a realtor,
an accountant, and
an attorney.*

Having gone through the steps in the previous chapter to locate the desired site for a practice, the next step is to obtain it. In most cases, this means securing a lease or sublease on the office space. This chapter discusses how this is done.

TIES THAT BIND

A lease or sublease is the legal document that binds the tenant to certain restrictions and limitations (Church, 1984). Leases should be negotiated with the needs of the tenant and the owner and should *never* be signed without first consulting with a realtor, an accountant, and an attorney.

Signing a binding legal contract commits the lessee to pay rent for the length of the lease. Neophytes should not sign long leases, because there is risk in predicting how successful the practice will be or whether conditions will prompt a need to move within the first few years. Most businesses tend to start off with rapid growth or they fold quickly (Jenkins, 1993).

Whenever possible, it is important to sign a lease that allows one to sublease or assign the lease to someone else. If the space looks as though it may be too small as the practice grows, the landlord may be receptive to a 1-year lease with the option of moving to another facility the landlord owns.

Short-term leases have risks, too. Failure to renew a lease can devastate a practice. The more often the lease is renewed, the higher are the chances for the rent to increase (Breske, 1993). Long-term leases often lock the tenant into a good price for a longer time, but then one is gambling that the location will remain desirable and spacious enough to accommodate a growing practice. A good lease or sublease requires much thought and many questions should be asked in the negotiating stage.

BASIC QUESTIONS TO ASK

What is the term of the lease?

For start-up practices, it may be wise to start by leasing on a month-to month basis, even if the rent is higher, with options to renew. This way, the financial obligation of a long-term lease is avoided if the practice should falter, expand too quickly, or even perhaps turn out not to be the audiologist's cup of tea.

For established practices, long-term leases or multiple renewal options are usually desirable to secure the location and keep a cap on rent increases. Five-year leases are common.

In a subleasing arrangement with physicians, especially otolaryngologists, a long-term lease with options and a cap on rent increases is usually essential. The lease protects the audiology practice in the event that the physicians desire to take over the practice for reasons of control and profit.

What is the rental cost?

Rent is usually calculated in dollars per square foot annually[1]. For example, a 1000 square foot office with a rental cost of $20 per square foot means an annual rent of $20 × 1000 = $20,000, yielding monthly payments of $1666.66.

Total monthly rent may be more than this simple calculation due to "triple net" items that are added to the base rent (insurance, taxes, common area expenses). Be sure to get the initial total monthly rent charge *in writing* prior to signing a lease. Control increases in triple net items by getting the landlord to agree to a "cap" on total monthly rent—not to exceed a specified dollar or percentage amount.

What about build-outs?

Find out if the structure can be altered to meet the needs of the practice. If so, find out what building allowance comes with the lease, who does the build-out, and how it is paid (i.e., paid directly to subcontractors of the landlord, subtracted from the rent, or reimbursed to tenant). Depending on the

---

[1]Avoid percentage rent based on some measure of productivity (e.g., number of hearing aid sales), which is generally added to a base rent. The exception is when the landlord will accept a lower base rent in return for a higher "ceiling" at which percentage rent begins.

extent of remodeling, build-out charges are paid by the land-lord, by the tenant, or shared jointly.

Ask for the right to terminate the lease in the event that build-out is not done by a specific date. Long delays that prevent the practice from opening its doors or operating normally can be devastating to cash flow.

What are the options in the lease?

There are *many* options that can make the lease more favorable to the tenant. They can be added as addenda to a standard lease, if the landlord agrees. Although the landlord may not agree to all of the following (suggested by Chaney, 1994), the best way to get favorable terms is to ask for them!

"Ghost town" option to terminate. The tenant has the right to terminate the lease in the event of loss of an "anchor" tenant (e.g., a primary referral source to the practice), or if total occupancy of the site goes below a specified percentage.

Small firm escape hatch. The lease can be terminated if the owner is disabled or dies. This is especially important for professional tenants such as audiologists where revenues are solely dependent on their ability to practice.

"Preservation" escape hatch. The tenant can terminate the lease if revenues/collections fall below a specific average dollar amount per month for a specified number of consecutive months.

Rent offset for landlord default. The tenant can withhold or offset rent if the landlord is slow to reimburse the tenant for maintenance that the landlord failed to perform.

Multiple renewal option. At the end of the lease, the tenant has the right to renew again. For example, the tenant may ask for one or two 5-year renewal options when the lease is first negotiated.

First option for adjacent space. The tenant has the first option to lease unoccupied space for expansion purposes.

Option to sublease. The tenant has the right to sublease a portion of the space with consent from the landlord not to be unreasonably withheld or delayed.

Option to assign the lease. Standard lease forms often allow assignment only at the sole discretion of the landlord. This option allows the tenant to assign the lease to another party, again with reasonable and prompt consent by the landlord.

What about parking and signage?

Parking needs to be designated, preferably on a drawing of the site, and guaranteed. Be sure parking charges are specified or included with total monthly rent quotes.

Ask for exact and specific agreements on the availability and location of indoor and outdoor signs. Find out if there are restrictions on size, wording, and types of signs.

How have things gone in the past?

Ask other tenants about their lease experiences with the landlord. Are outside grounds well maintained? Are repairs done correctly and promptly? Is the property manager responsive and reasonable? Does the property manager keep tenants informed of changes (e.g., new tenants, new property ownership, etc). Do other tenants get along well?

TIPS FOR NEGOTIATING THE LEASE

As in any other negotiation, the best agreement is one with which both sides can be satisfied. A few very basic rules are important in achieving that goal.

RULE 1. Always Use an Attorney

Regardless of which side drafts the lease, each party should use its own attorney to go over the draft and make suggestions and changes to shape the final document.

RULE 2. Don't Leave "Money on the Table"

This is an old saying that means one of the parties negotiated poorly. It is difficult to explain exactly what it means, mainly because it manifests in so many different ways. "Money on the table" does not literally mean that someone puts money forth, but it figuratively means that one of the parties ends up acquiring a negotiable at a higher cost than was necessary.

Money on the table usually turns up when one of the parties has not done all of its homework beforehand and then tries to be accommodating and agreeable in the early stages of the negotiations. For example, the potential landlord might throw out a rental figure that appears reasonable to an audiologist who is new to the area. The audiologist quickly agrees to the price and moves on to other questions, only to find out a few months down the road that the agreed-upon price is twice the going rate for the locale.

RULE 3. Don't Leave Loose Ends

Again, this comes from being agreeable rather than careful. For example, in a subleasing arrangement with a physicians' group, the physicians may casually mention that the minor operating room is "available" for the audiologist to do evoked potential and ENG tests. Availability is not spelled out in the sublease. In reality, "availability" means that the equipment must be stored elsewhere and the room is free on such an unpredictable basis that appropriate scheduling is not possible.

RULE 4. Don't Negotiate With Anyone but the Top Person(s)

This is especially true in situations where audiologists share space with physician landlords. Not infrequently, the physicians have their office manager negotiate the lease. This is fine for basic issues like rental rate, but it is very important to discuss the "living" arrangement in detail with the physician(s) before signing an agreement. The operating room example in Rule 3 is illustrative.

As another example, the space arrangements negotiated between an audiologist and a medical office manager might be acceptable to all parties, but the physicians might balk at the audiologists practice procedures (e.g., hours of operation, on-call availability, marketing approach), with the result that the lease is not renewed. There is absolutely no substitute for talking to the real people in charge when making decisions that affect the livelihood of the practice.

THE LEASE

The following items are some of the items that should or may be addressed in a lease or sublease (cf., Baxter, 1994):

- *The parties to the lease:* landlord and tenant, or tenant and audiologist in a sublease
- *Date of lease*
- *Description of the premises:* Address, square footage, and a sketch of the space (blueprints whenever possible)
- *Use of leased premises:* This describes what business the lessee will be conducting on the premises.

- *Term and renewal options*
- *Additions and alterations by landlord and by tenant*
- *Assignment or subletting*
- *Rent:* annual rent, due date, late charges, interest, first and last
- *Other charges:* taxes, common areas and operating costs, utility charges, janitorial, building improvements
- *Security deposit*
- *Signs, awnings, and canopies*
- *Inspections, repairs, maintenance*
- *Indemnification and insurance of landlord and tenant*
- *Designated parking*
- *Amending the lease*
- *Default by tenant*
- *Damage, destruction, or condemnation of the leased premises*
- *Restriction of access to area by competing professionals*

Appendix 8-A contains a sample sublease for an office sharing arrangement between an audiology and otolaryngology practice. It illustrates the wording attached to many of the items listed above, as well as other items negotiated for the particular situation. In addition, it illustrates some of the standard legal terminology attached to leases and subleases of this type.

The final version of the lease should be reviewed carefully, with both parties initialing each page and then signing and dating the last page. This should be done on two copies, one for the landlord and the other for the tenant.

SUMMARY

A lease is a legally binding document that commits the audiology practice to a potentially long-term financial obligation. There are many questions and considerations that audiologists must address when negotiating a lease. To achieve a satisfactory arrangement, negotiations must be conducted with deliberation and legal consultation.

REFERENCES

Baxter, J. (1994). Locating and equipping an audiology practice. In H. Hosford-Dunn, J. Baxter, A. Desmond, G. Jacobson, J. Johnson, P. Martin, & E. Cherow (Eds.), *Development and management of audiology practices* (chap. 4, pp. 15–24). Rockville, MD: ASHA.

Breske, S. (1993, November 22). Leaving home: Checklist for moving private practice to office setting. *Advance for Speech-Language Pathologists & Audiologists*, p. 5.

Chaney, A. D. (1994). Closely held business law in Arizona: *Business owner guide and attorney/CPA desk reference*. Tucson, AZ: Author.

Church, O. D. (1984). *Small business management and entrepreneurship*. Chicago: Science Research Associates.

Jenkins, M. D. (1993). *Starting and operating a business in Arizona*. Grants Pass, OR: Oasis Press.

APPENDIX 8-A

Sample Sublease for Office Sharing Arrangement

This sublease, made and entered into as of the [day/month/year], by and between _____, hereinafter referred to as "Tenant," and _____, hereinafter referred to as "Audiologist."

Whereas, Tenant is the lessee under a certain lease for space located at _____, which Audiologist desires to sublease for the practice of audiology and the sale of hearing aids.

WITNESSETH:

In consideration of the mutual covenants, conditions, agreements and stipulations contained herein and each and every provision hereof, the parties hereto agree as follows:

Section 1. Term and Grant.

1.1 Sublease. Tenant does hereby warrant and represent that she has the right under her lease to lease space to Audiologist. It shall be the responsibility of Tenant to obtain any consent necessary to sublease to Audiologist from Tenant's landlord or lessor.

1.2. Premises. Tenant hereby subleases unto the Audiologist and Audiologist hereby subleases from Tenant [addresses of sublet space], consisting of a reception room, waiting room, office, laboratory and audiology suite. Exclusive use by Audiologist of the reception room, waiting room, office, laboratory, and audiology suite is granted.

1.3 Term. The initial term of this Lease shall be for a period of one (1) year commencing as of the 1st of [month/year], such date being hereinafter referred to as the "commencement date" and terminating on the 31st day of [month/year].

1.4 Renewal Options. If Audiologist shall not be in default in performing any of Audiologist's obligations under this Lease, and with the approval of Tenant, Audiologist shall have the option to extend this Lease on the same terms and conditions, except as to rental, for one (1) year periods ("renewal periods"), to begin on the 1st of [month/year]. In order to exercise this option to renew, Lessee shall give Lessor written notice of exercise of the option not later than [day/month/year], with respect to the first renewal period. Tenant may terminate this Lease with a thirty (30) day written notice prior to the renewal period.

Section 2. Fixtures. All construction and alterations, additions, improvements and fixtures, other than trade fixtures and professional fixtures of the Audiologist, shall remain the property of the Tenant. It is expressly agreed by and between the parties hereto that all trade fixtures, office supplies, cabinets installed in the office and laboratory and inventory which are used particularly by the Audiologist in relation to audiology services which may be brought upon or installed by Audiologist upon the premises, shall remain the sole property of the Audiologist, and Tenant agrees to surrender the same to the Audiologist upon termination of this Lease. There will be no structural alterations or improvements made without the Tenant's approval. Upon termination of this Lease, Audiologist shall remove all fixtures, cabinets installed, office equipment and furniture from the leased premises and return the leased premises to its original state, ordinary wear and tear excepted.

Section 3. Rental. The Audiologist agrees to pay as rent during the term of this Lease the sum of $_____ in advance, on the first (1st) day of each and every calendar month during said term and any renewal period, subject to increase in the rental charge as provided in Section 1.4, said monthly rental to include all rental taxes, which taxes shall be the responsibility of Lessor, utilities and electricity, excluding telephone services.

Section 4. Use of Premises.

4.1 Activities. That portion of the demised premises subleased to the Audiologist shall be used for the sale of hearing aids and other related audiology items and performance of audiology services. Audiologist shall not use the demised premises or any part hereof for any purpose contrary to law or the rules of regulations of any public authority or in an any manner so as to increase the cost of hazard insurance maintained.

4.2 <u>Signs</u>. Audiologist shall have the right to advertise the location and nature of its business facilities and/or offices with a sign on the door to the office and on each Directory with the [name of office complex] subject to Tenant approval.

4.3 <u>Indemnification and Insurance</u>. Each party hereto agrees to carry adequate liability insurance to provide coverage in the event of any third part liability claim. Each party, therefore, agrees to indemnify and hold harmless the other part from any claims, demands, damages, expenses, fees, costs, liabilities, actions or causes of action arising as a result of the indemnifying party, its employees or agents. Audiologist agrees to carry a minimum of One Million Dollars ($1,000,000.00) single limit professional liability insurance.

Both the Tenant and Audiologist agree to carry at their own expense throughout the term of this Lease public liability insurance covering their portion of the demised premises, and their respective professional equipment, inventory and fixtures.

4.4 <u>Maintenance</u>. Subject to obligations of the Audiologist Tenant shall keep and maintain the subleased premises in good tenantable condition during the entire term of this Lease and all subsequent terms. Should any portion of said premises be damaged through the fault and/or neglect of the Audiologist, or the Audiologist's officers, agents, employees, invitee or customers, then the Audiologist shall promptly and properly repair the same at no cost to Tenant.

If there is a material noncompliance by the Tenant with the provisions hereof, then the Audiologist may deliver a written notice to the Tenant specifying the acts and omissions constituting the breach of Tenant's agreement to keep, repair and maintain the entire premises. Tenant shall have not more than thirty (30) days after receipt of said notice to remedy the breach, and failing the remedy of the breach by the Tenant, then the Audiologist may terminate this Lease.

4.5 <u>Taxes, Assessments and License Fees</u>. Tenant agrees to pay when due all taxes levied against the premises, as required by Tenant's lease.

Tenant agrees to pay all personal property taxes, assessments, license fees or public charges levied, or assessed or imposed, or which become payable during the term hereof, upon the demised premises and upon Tenant's fixtures, furniture, appliances or personal property installed or located in the premises. Audiologist is responsible for payment of his personal property taxes on furniture, equipment, appliances or personal property installed or located in the premises.

Each party further agrees to pay its own sales or transaction privilege taxes levied or assessed before they become delinquent.

4.6 <u>Additional Obligations</u>.

4.6.1 Tenant will assume the cost of janitorial services for [subleased office space] to the same extent as provided for [Tenant's space]. Additional services will be paid for by the Audiologist.

4.6.2 Tenant shall pay the rental and comply with all obligations assumed by Tenant in Tenant's lease with [office building complex] except for default occasioned by Audiologist. In the event Tenant shall receive written or verbal notice of the breach of any provision of Tenant's lease, Tenant shall, within three (3) days, provide a copy of such written notice, if any, to Audiologist or inform Audiologist of such declared breach within three (3) days of receipt. Audiologist shall have the right to cure any breach of Tenant, but shall have no obligation to do so, and shall have the right to deduct reasonable expenses incurred in curing such default of Tenant from future rental payments.

4.6.3 In the event that Tenant assigned her lease or terminates Tenant's lease with [medical office building], or Tenant's lease is terminated, Tenant shall provide

Audiologist sixty (60) days prior written notice of such assignment or termination. Audiologist shall have the right to negotiate a new lease with the new tenant or [medical office building] or other owner of the [medical office building].

4.6.4 Audiologist shall be responsible for all costs associated with maintaining the audiology equipment and sound chamber, and ensuring that the audiology equipment is properly calibrated at least once yearly.

Section 5. <u>Default</u>.

5.1 <u>Tenant's Remedies</u>. Upon default of Audiologist in the performance of any provision hereof, Tenant shall provide Audiologist with written notice of said breach and if Audiologist fails to remedy said breach within fifteen (15) business days after notice if the breach is a failure to pay rent or within thirty (30) days after said notice for any other breach, then Tenant shall have the right to immediately re-enter and take possession of the leased premises, and declare this Sublease to be terminated, in which event this Sublease, all rights of the Audiologist and all duties of the parties shall immediately cease and terminate, and the Tenant may possess and enjoy the leased premises as though this Lease has never been made, as Tenant's sole liquidated damages.

5.2 <u>Audiologist's Remedies</u>. Upon default of Tenant in the performance of any provision hereof, Audiologist shall provide Tenant with written notice thereof. If any default of the Tenant continues uncorrected for a period of thirty (30) days after receipt of written notice thereof from the Audiologist, stating with particularity the nature and extent of the default, the Audiologist may cancel this Lease by written notice of cancellation served upon Tenant; provided, however, that the Audiologist shall have no right to cancel this Lease if within thirty (30) days after receipt by Tenant of any notice of Tenant's alleged default, Tenant corrects such default, or in good faith commences the remedying thereof and diligently proceeds therewith.

Section 6. <u>Partial or Total Destruction of the Premises</u>. If the building in which the premises are situated is partially or totally destroyed by fire or other casualty, whether insured or not, so as to become partially untenantable for the business conducted by Audiologist, the Audiologist's performance under this Lease shall be suspended and as soon as possible after such repair or restoration Tenant will give possession to Audiologist, and a proportionate reduction shall be made from the rental, corresponding to the time during which and to the proportion of the demised premises which Audiologist be deprived of the use on account of the damage, restoration or repair. Audiologist agrees that Tenant shall have no absolute obligation under this section to see that the Premises are repaired or restored. If the premises remain partially untenantable and the Tenant or other person does not complete repairs to the premises to make it tenantable within thirty (30) days, the Audiologist may elect to cancel and terminate this Lease. If this occurs the Tenant shall refund to the Audiologist prepaid rent on a pro rata basis for the period after the date of the happening.

If the premises are at any time destroyed or substantially damaged by a casualty which makes the premises untenantable and such casualty substantially interferes with the business conducted by Audiologist, the Audiologist or the Tenant shall have the right to cancel and terminate this Lease as of the date of the happening of such event, by the giving of notice to the other party of the election to do so within fifteen (15) days after the happening of such event.

Section 7. <u>General Provisions</u>.

7.1 <u>Notices</u>. Any notices or demand required or permitted by law or any provision of this Sublease shall be in writing and may be completed by mailing such notice to the Tenant or Audiologist, or any agent designated by either to receive such notices by certified or registered mail, return receipt requested, postage prepaid, at the addresses listed below. Notice delivered personally shall be effective as of delivery and notice which is mailed shall be effective seventy-two (72) hours after deposit in the mail.

Notice to Tenant shall be made to:
[Tenant's name and mailing address]

Notice to Audiologist shall be mailed to:
[Audiologist's name and mailing address]

7.2 <u>Additional Parties Bound by Provisions of this Lease</u>. Any person, corporation, partnership, joint venture or entity of whatever type or nature, purchasing or procuring by any means whatsoever any interest in this Sublease, unless otherwise provided for, shall become a party to this Lease and be bound by the provisions herein.

7.3 <u>Word Genders and Numbers</u>. Whenever words are used herein in any gender, they shall be construed as though they were used in the gender appropriate to the circumstances. Whenever words are used herein in the singular or plural form, they shall be construed as though they were used in the form appropriate to the circumstances.

7.4 <u>Topic Headings</u>. Headings and captions in this Lease are inserted for convenience and reference; and in no way define, limit or describe the scope or intent of this Lease, nor constitute any part of this Lease and are not to be considered in the construction of this Lease.

7.5 <u>Governing Law</u>. This Lease shall be subject to and governed by the laws of the State of _____.

7.6 <u>Counterparts</u>. Several copies of this Lease may be executed. All executed copies constitute one Lease, binding on all parties even though all parties have not executed the original or the same copy.

7.7 <u>Entire Agreement</u>. This Lease contains the entire understanding between and among the parties and supersedes any prior understanding or agreements between and among them respecting the subject matter. No representations, arrangements, understandings or agreements oral or written, relating to the subject matter of this Lease, except those fully expressed herein, are or shall be binding upon the parties. No changes, alterations, modifications, additions or qualifications to the terms of this Lease shall be made or be binding unless made in writing and signed by each of the parties.

7.8 <u>Holding Over After Terms</u>. If Audiologist holds over and remains in possession of said premises after the term of this Lease or any renewal thereof, Audiologist will from that date forward, unless the parties by written agreement stipulate to the contrary, be a tenant from month to month at the same monthly installment rental rate and on the same terms and conditions as in existence at the time of the termination of the then existing Sublease or any renewal thereof until premises are vacated by Audiologist.

7.9 <u>Laches</u>. Any failure of either party to enforce rights or to seek remedies upon any default of the other part hereunder or the delay of said enforcement or the seeking of remedies shall not prejudice or affect the right or remedies of the non-defaulting party in the event of any subsequent default or attempted enforcement at a later date.

7.10 <u>Waiver</u>. No waiver of any condition or legal right or remedy shall be implied by the failure of either party to declare a default or for any other reason, and no waiver of any condition or covenant shall be valid unless it be in writing and signed by the party to be charged.

7.11 <u>Eminent Domain</u>. In the event the demised premises, or any part thereof, or any of the land of which the demised premises is a part, shall be taken or condemned for public purposes by any competent authority, each party shall have the right to pursue its own legal remedies, and either party shall have the right to terminate this Sublease.

7.12 <u>Surrender of Premises</u>. Upon termination of this Sublease, whether by lapse of time or otherwise, or upon the exercise by the Tenant of the power to re-enter and repossess the lease premises, as hereinbefore provided, Audiologist shall at once surrender the possession of the same to Tenant in good order and repair (ordinary wear and tear expected) and at once remove all of Audiologist's property therefrom.

7.13. Quiet Enjoyment. Tenant hereby covenants and agrees that if Audiologist shall perform all the covenants and agreements hereinbefore stipulated to be performed on Audiologist's party, Audiologist shall at all times during the continuance hereof have the peaceable and quiet enjoyment and possession of its part of the premises without any manner of let or hindrance from Tenant or any person or persons lawfully claiming the premises.

7.14 Invalidity of Any Provision. The invalidity or unenforceability of any particular provision of this Agreement shall not affect the other provisions hereof and the Agreement shall be construed in all respects as if such invalid or unenforceable provisions were omitted.

7.15 Amendment of Agreement. This Agreement may be altered or amended only in writing, signed by both parties.

IN WITNESS WHEREOF, the Tenant and Audiologist have signed this Agreement as of the day and year indicated below to be in force the day and year first above written.

TENANT:
[name of Tenant]   [name of Audiologist]
By: [Signature of Tenant]   By: [Signature of Audiologist]
Date:_____   Date:_____

9

Creating the Office

The previous two chapters were concerned with finding and securing a site for the practice. This chapter extends the discussion by examining factors that affect functionality, safety, livability, and "looks" of the practice, once the site is obtained. Equipment needs are then addressed in the same context.

CRITERIA FOR DESIGNING THE OFFICE SPACE

Efficient Function

Efficient office arrangements are paramount to the long-term success of a practice. An *inefficient* office arrangement is costly and frustrating to staff and patients. Employee morale, productivity, and customer service are affected negatively. The end result is that the practice's bottom line suffers from higher expenses and lower revenues. *Size, physical layout, and technical requirements are important factors that contribute to office efficiency.*

Office Space

Office space must be efficient but inexpensive in the embryonic stage of the practice, but must also remain sufficient *and* efficient as the business grows. When looking at office space, it is a good idea to always assume the practice ultimately will require more space than is needed initially. For optimum efficiency, strike a balance between present and future space needs (Kishel & Kishel, 1993). As always, a comprehensive business plan will help predict space needs and costs.

If the practice is an integral part of an existing clinic, hospital, or ENT practice, space will likely be allocated based on some combination of availability, productivity, and turf lines. Growth and efficiency are often at odds in such situations, as additional space must be "won" from competing services rather than allocated according to a business plan for growth. Because "winning" is usually based on demonstrations of growing revenues which must be produced in cramped quarters, this is often a "Catch 22" situation. To succeed, the owner/manager must strive for innovative ways to maximize efficiency while maintaining employee morale. In some extreme cases, there comes a point where this is no longer possible, with the result that the practice either begins to fail or relocates to a more autonomous environment.

Office Layout

Plan Layout According to:

- *Office Flow*
- *Space Value*
- *Accessibility*
- *Confidentiality*
- *Lighting, Plumbing, and Ventilation*
- *Electrical and Communication Lines*
- *Kitchen and Bathroom Facilities*
- *ADA Requirements*

A good layout facilitates the processing and flow of work and patients (Church, 1984). Layout encompasses the physical design of activity, support, and administration spaces (Rizzo & Wilkins, 1994) as well as the physical arrangement of furniture, fixtures, equipment, merchandise, and supplies (Kishel & Kishel, 1993). Rizzo and Wilkins' (1994) discussion and diagrams of design considerations for physical layout are especially helpful for large clinics and offer many useful pointers for small practices as well.

Church (1984) discusses layout requirements in terms of "work flow" (products and information), "traffic flow" (patients, staff, deliveries, visitors, and people asking for directions), and "space value." According to Church, traffic flow is greatest in the front and to the right, so front space is most valuable, back space is least valuable. The overall "office flow" is facilitated by a layout that arranges functionally related spaces together (Rizzo & Wilkins, 1994), minimizes walking back and forth, minimizes lines, prevents the need to dodge fixtures or people, prevents environmental sound interference, ensures confidentiality, guarantees some personal space to each staff member, and uses space according to its value (e.g., product displays, educational materials, and greeting area in front; storage in back).

Other layout considerations are: adequate, energy-efficient lighting to enhance staff productivity while containing energy costs; comfortable heating, cooling, and ventilation systems that are consistent in each room; full use of each piece of equipment; and easy access to the information environment (books, mailing lists, filing systems, software support, etc).

Test rooms should be directly accessible from the waiting room. They should be large enough to: (a) maneuver wheelchairs and gurneys into the test booth, (b) allow room for history taking, and (c) accommodate at least one family member or aide during testing. At all times during testing, the patient should be visible to the tester, and the patient should have some view of the tester and the room encompassing the test booth.

Whenever possible, keep different types of equipment in separate areas. A one-person practice may function best with all test equipment in one test suite. However, as the practice and staff expand, this arrangement makes equipment unavailable to other staff and does not allow for several procedures to be performed at the same time (e.g., real ear equipment in the same room as a sound booth).

Consultation rooms should be close to test rooms, but acoustically insulated. They should have direct access to the waiting room and hearing aid laboratory. They should be large enough to house consultation tables and accommodate the patient, one or two clinicians, and several family members or helpers.

The layout should meet the requirements of the Americans with Disabilities Act (1991).[1] For example, entrances, exits, and interior doors should have wheelchair access; ramps should replace stairs, or be in place where the floor level

---

[1]Some of the costs associated with addressing public access requirements of Title III of the ADA are deductible or can be claimed as a tax credit. For more information on the ADA, contact: Equal Employment Opportunity Commission, 2401 E. St., Washington, DC 20506 (202) 663-4264; or U.S. Department of Justice (202) 514-0301.

changes more than one-half inch; elevator buttons, sinks, public phones, and so forth, should be placed at heights within reach of people in wheelchairs.

Layouts, like everything else about the practice, are best if they are methodically planned rather than allowed to "happen" as the practice acquires equipment, furniture, and staff. Scale drawings should be made of different areas, with equipment, furniture and fixtures either drawn in or represented by cutouts that can be arranged in different ways on the drawing. Computer programs can also assist with designing the layout. A good rule of thumb for designing operator spaces (e.g., audiology control rooms, consultation/fitting areas, repair benches) is that they should be as compact as the cockpits of airplanes: all necessary controls are within easy reach of the clinician or support staff member (Whitmyer, Rasberry, & Phillips, 1989).

Technical Requirements

Sound booths should be constructed and situated to meet ANSI standards for permissible ambient noise levels (American National Standards Institute, 1986) and large enough for accurate sound field testing (American Speech-Language-Hearing Association [ASHA], 1991). Equip sound booth doors with in-swinging or out-swinging hinges, depending on their positions in the layout and clearly mark door thresholds if they are raised. Eliminate resonating surfaces inside sound booths (e.g., children's formica topped table for Play Audiometry). Ventilation system ducts must be appropriately sized to minimize vent noise. Electrical outlets should be plentiful. Electrical lines must be free of 60 cycle interference for electrophysiologic testing. The number of telephone lines needs to accommodate all incoming calls and faxes. Install telephone jacks, computer cables, and modem lines that are needed or may be needed in the future. Use surge protectors with computers to preserve data and minimize down time. Place printers (especially noisy ones) in accessible locations away from patient areas and use noise-isolation covers.

Safety

ASHA guidelines state that the facility must meet ". . . applicable building and safety codes, including those for adequate fire protection, indoor and outdoor lighting, elevator safety, walking surfaces, electrical safety . . ." (American Speech-Language-Hearing Association [ASHA], 1989).

Steps and raised thresholds should be clearly marked (e.g., painted red, marked with electrical tape) and "Watch Your Step" signs posted. Carpets must be appropriately installed and maintained. Commercial dense pile carpets should be used to allow easy perambulation by patients with walkers and clinicians pushing equipment (Rizzo & Wilkins, 1994). If padding is used, it should not vary in thickness from one room to another. Equipment cables and electrical cords should be tacked down against wall boards or floor edges.

Heavy things should be lifted up, not down: never store heavy boxes or other objects high up where they could fall and injure people. Make sure chemicals and cleaning supplies are correctly and clearly marked. House them in closed storage areas that are inaccessible to children. The latter may seem unnecessary, but in small practices the following scenario is unfortunately not unusual: a mother arrives with three children, one of whom is scheduled for a pediatric audiologic evaluation. The audiologist, test assistant (often the front office person), and mother work with the child in the test room while the oldest child is "in charge" in the waiting room.

The nightmare scenario of unsupervised children in the practice prompts another rule of thumb: treat the practice like a home when the grandchildren visit. Put away breakables (e.g., coffee pots, cups) and other potentially dangerous objects (batteries, ear plugs, hard candies). Move chairs away from tables or other high surfaces that invite climbing and do not encourage climbing by placing food invitingly out of reach. Close off hearing aid repair areas containing razor blades, motors, pointed tools, glues and other dangerous chemicals. Finally, be sure that a bell or buzzer on the exit(s) will ring if any child decides to leave.

Restrooms should be neat and clean with handicap access and safety railing. Sinks in treatment rooms should be kept clean and uncluttered. Trash should be emptied and disposed of daily. Food and beverages should be consumed in a kitchen or dining area, never in patient areas. The staff must clean up after themselves and observe sanitary procedures at all times. Janitorial services should clean floor and wall coverings, furniture and equipment on a regular basis.

Observe infection control procedures

Infection control procedures as described by OSHA and Centers for Disease Control (CDC) should be implemented and observed (Jacobson, 1994; Kemp, 1994). The following require sterilization: ear impression tools (e.g., ear lites, otoscope speculae), stock ear molds, cerumen management instruments, probe microphone tubes, immittance and otoacoustic emission probe tips, foam ear tips (if reused), and needle electrodes. In addition, surgical gloves and other barrier controls should be worn by the audiologist as needed. Finally, audiologists and other staff should thoroughly wash their hands between patients, using sinks installed in each treatment room.

Livability

Kishel and Kishel (1993) describe a "livable" facility according to the purpose of the business: "The same building that's a dream come true for an automobile repair shop would probably be a nightmare for a jewelry shop" (p. 36). An "Audiology Practice Livability Index" is composed of many of the factors that have already been discussed in other sections, but it is worthwhile to group them together under this rubric to get a "feel" for the day-to-day livability of the office space:

1. Construction

   - strong enough to support test booth(s)
   - sound enough to guarantee acoustically insulated test and counseling environments (see Rizzo & Wilkins, 1994, p. 86, for a description of building materials)
   - sound enough to provide good climate insulation
   - able to resist heavy wear and fire

2. Design—does it allow a layout that is compatible with the practice's needs?

3. Accessibility

   - easy to find (so office staff are not constantly giving complicated directions or trying to find lost patients)
   - close, safe parking for patients, staff, and delivery persons
   - easy to walk in (e.g., not through an entry way, up an elevator, and down a long hallway!)
   - easy ingress: few or no steps, well-marked entrance(s) for patients (front) and deliveries (side or back)
   - easy egress in emergency situations

4. Happiness

   - enough light, space, and quiet for everyone to co-exist
   - water fountains and restrooms conveniently located for staff and patients
   - kitchen facilities for busy days (at least a microwave and small refrigerator)

■ close enough to post office, office supply stores, bank, accountant, and so on, for outside business needs to be met without impacting office efficiency
■ close enough to restaurants, schools, shopping, health facilities, and so on, for employees to satisfy personal needs without impacting office efficiency

Lighting is both a livability and efficiency factor that deserves special attention. Placement and quality of lighting are the important issues. Indoor lighting should be adjustable and movable. Close-up work surfaces (e.g., hearing aid modification bench) should receive direct light, but work stations (e.g., computer entry) should focus the light from behind the worker's head. According to Whitmyer, Rasberry, and Phillips (1980), outdoor light is essential for normal health—at least 45 minutes per day. Yet even workplaces with an abundance of natural light are ineffective because the glass and plastic coverings screen out most of the ultraviolet (UV) light that provides essential Vitamin D. These authors suggest using full spectrum lighting (fluorescent or incandescent) which provides missing UV and presents "true" colors because "Studies conducted for over a decade have indicated that people who work under full spectrum lights experience improvement in visual acuity, more energy, and fewer colds or illnesses than people who don't" (p. 103). Full spectrum lighting is more expensive but is more efficient to operate.

Looks

Image exerts a great influence on the success of a practice (cf. Jelonek & Staab, 1994). There is general agreement that a practice must "look" professional, starting with the neighborhood image. As McCollom and Mynders (1984) playfully point out "there are no hearing aid dealers on Bourbon Street, New Orleans" (p. 37).

Think of the *building's exterior* as the book cover by which the practice is judged. Thus, the penchant for locating in a medical office complex, which yields instant credibility to bypassers. "Even those who never come inside and know next to nothing about your business will form opinions about it on the basis of its outside appearance—its looks alone. As such, the exterior of your building should be thought of as a communications medium, capable of transmitting messages about your business" (Kishel & Kishel, p. 34, 1993). These and other authors (Church, 1984; McCollom, & Mynders, 1984) warn

Avoid sending the wrong message

against unintentionally sending the wrong message: marble and brass create an image expressing exclusivity, class, and high prices which may not be consistent with the socioeconomic strata where the practice is located. Stucco or brick communicate reassuring ordinariness, economy, and practicality. The overall impression should bespeak pleasantness. Landscaping should be attractive, tidy, and create an image of spaciousness without clutter.

Exterior signs are a practical means of helping people find the practice, but they also imprint an idea of what the business is and what kind of person owns it. Like the building's exterior, signs are a powerful first impression and care must be taken to insure that they communicate the intended message.

A good looking sign attracts the interest of people passing by without demanding their full attention. People are subconsciously affected by the mood and atmosphere of a sign, forming opinions about the practice based on what the sign conveys (Church, 1984). Rizzo & Wilkins (1994) enumerate basic rules for designing effective signs to ensure that they are noticeable and readable.

A few principles of esthetics and comfort apply to all customer service situations. All *interior designs* need to maximize staff morale and productivity. Decor should put patients at ease and instill them with confidence about the staff. Upholstered arm chairs allow older patients to get up and out easier. Age-appropriate chairs, tables, toys, and books are important for children. The value of appropriate lighting has already been discussed in the "Livability" section.

Color is an important consideration for wall and floor coverings, furniture, and fixtures. Dark colors depress, bright colors stimulate, greens and blues sooth. Rizzo and Wilkins (1994) recommend soothing colors and earth tones for waiting areas and brighter colors for clinical and administrative areas. Church (1984) recommends light, unobtrusive colors (e.g., beige, pale lemon, cream) accented with bright color touches.

The "looks" of the practice should be professional, but they must also project a personal image—how are this practice and this audiologist unique? An office can project almost any image the owner desires, so long as the exterior and interior decor are harmonious. The exterior establishes the "look" of professionalism, but it is in the interior that the professional image is carried out and indelibly stamped with the personal image of the practice. If the decor and layout are compatible, patients perceive a harmonious theme that blends the physical environment to the actions of the staff, in much the same

Use interior decor that blends with exterior look and projects a personal image

way that props and actors capture the imaginations of theater-goers.

Like a good layout, interior decor deserves careful planning for each area, starting with "Act I," the waiting room.

Act I: The Waiting Room

In a narrow sense, waiting rooms are nonproductive space—an overhead item that is not income producing (McCollom & Mynders, 1984). In a broader sense, waiting rooms are probably the most important area in the entire office. They almost always occupy the front, most valuable, space. They receive the most traffic flow and can also support a great deal of information flow. The personal image of the practice is strongest in the waiting room, which sets the stage for all that follows. In their excellent 1984 book, Herbert McCollom and Joel Mynders have different ideas of what their respective waiting rooms should convey. McCollom recommends using the waiting room to create moods and images that are

Contemporary . . . yet stable

Successful . . . yet conservative

Comfortable . . . yet not Sybaritic. (p. 65)

Mynders' office, in a more urban area, recommends a waiting room "designed in such a style that your 'carriage trade' clients are at home, and your other clients think 'it's nice' but don't know how much it costs" (p. 67).

The current authors, having designed, visited, or been patients in a variety of waiting rooms, have identified several image "types" with their corresponding props and scripts:

1. Gracious Living

Props. The mood is quiet and subdued. Furnishings are conservative, comfortable, perhaps antique. Lighting is natural or indirect. Amenities (e.g., coffee service and small cakes) are obvious, attractive, and adequate. Today's newspaper and the most recent copies of a few informative magazines (e.g., New Yorker, Sunset) are set out neatly. Professional cards, brochures, newsletters and other practice information are displayed prominently. Seating is limited (chairs, not couches) with scheduling arranged to minimize overlap and overcrowding.

Script. The patient is greeted by an informed employee immediately upon entering the office, helped if possible, or informed of the time until he or she will be seen. Preregistered information is confirmed and additional questionnaire information is obtained. Staff are busy but polite. The nature of the office layout makes staff activities apparent but discreet while the patient waits.

2. Modern and Efficient

Props. The mood is bustling and active. Furnishings are contemporary, designer fabrics, colors, and lighting are used. There are no food amenities. News and human interest magazines are fresh (e.g., *Newsweek, People, Life*). Brochures and educational information are in a display rack. There is plenty of seating (couches and chairs) to accommodate tight scheduling and early arrivals.

Script. The patient goes to the front desk and signs in upon arrival. A receptionist behind a sliding glass partition confirms preregistration information. The patient is seated until called. Staff activity occurs out of sight of the waiting area.

3. Spare and Basic

Props. The mood is relaxed or even lethargic. Furnishings are nondescript but adequate. Fluorescent overhead lighting is used. A Mr. Coffee, styrofoam cups, and a water fountain compose the amenities. Magazines are a hodgepodge of types and ages, as are educational and professional brochures. Seating may or may not be adequate, depending on who shows up.

Script. The patient will be greeted and registered as soon as someone is available, but otherwise feels content to sit and wait, as directed by a sign on the front desk. Staff activities are audible (but not discriminable) from back rooms.

4. Cold and Untouchable

Props. The mood is distant, disinterested, but clinical. Furnishings and lighting fixtures are angular and metal. Color is lacking. There are no food amenities. Glossy magazines (e.g., *Architectural Digest*) are carefully arranged in a rack display. Educational and professional brochures are absent. Seating is more than adequate and patients are seen promptly (and quickly).

Script. The patient is acknowledged at front desk registration by being asked for method of payment and insurance information. The patient is seated until called. Staff activity occurs out of sight of the waiting area.

With the exception of Waiting Room 4, each of these waiting room types projects an image that will be acceptable to a reasonable number of patients and practitioners, depending on the degree of formality demanded by their personal styles. The type will also be dictated to some degree by clinic size—Waiting Room 3 is much more likely to occur in a small practice, Waiting Room 1 could work in a larger practice, while a very large practice may necessitate Waiting Room 2. *If Waiting Room 4 is ever required, it is probably time to rework the business plan.*

The point is that successful offices can and probably do vary as much as the individual practitioners. They project images that are quite different from one another, but all share common bonds of professional and considerate treatment of their patients.

Acts II and III: The Examination and Counseling Rooms

Just as the transition from exterior to interior must follow suit, it is important that transitions from waiting room to test and counseling rooms appear natural and in keeping with the overall image of the individual practice. Thus, one would not expect to step from a "gracious living" waiting room into a "spare and basic" examination room, or from a "modern and efficient" waiting room into a "gracious living" counseling room.

The audiologist plays the biggest role during testing and counseling, and the role must be compatible with the surroundings. If the image of the office is "modern and efficient," the audiologists must be that too. Perhaps more obviously, practitioners who lean toward the quantitative rather than the counseling aspects of the profession will do best if they are not working in what "looks" like a gracious living environment. It is too much to ask patients who were treated gently in the waiting room to turn around and respond positively to a dry and brusque clinical treatment in the examination room.

CRITERIA FOR EQUIPPING THE PRACTICE

Substance Over Image

Test and office equipment are very expensive and can place an enormous overhead burden on new practices. As always, a good business plan is essential in deciding what services will be offered and what equipment is needed.

Part of the business plan is to define the practice's marketing "niche." In light of the previous discussion, it probably comes as no surprise that decisions about equipment are weighed not only in terms of function, efficiency, safety, and ergonomics, but also in terms of practice image. Although image is certainly not a compelling reason to purchase or not to purchase a piece of equipment, it is also true that practices with high tech images have high tech equipment, whereas more low profile practices often function just as effectively with fewer bells and whistles.

Neophytes, especially those enamored of electrophysiologic procedures, sometimes purchase expensive new equipment without adequately analyzing their professional goals or their bottom line. The results are often disastrous to both. The image *must* fit the pocketbook, and fiscal responsibility is one of the best images a practice can develop in a community. When considering equipment purchases, a few questions along the following lines are helpful:

- Is it necessary?
- Is there room for it?
- Will it generate revenues? Five years from now?
- Is it priced competitively?
- Is it available secondhand?
- How long until it pays for itself?
- What is its resale value?

Capital Equipment

When all equivocal purchases are eliminated, there remain a number of pieces of office equipment and test equipment that really are essential to the operation of the most basic audiology practice. Other equipment items are optional in the sense that the practice could perform basic functions without them, but the marketing plan may target them as "essential" purchases as the practice develops. For another listing of equipment, supplies, furniture, and fixtures for audiology practices, see Baxter (1994).

Office Equipment

These items are purchased or leased locally at costs that vary substantially from one community to another and within the community. The costs to the individual practice are best determined when constructing the business plan.

Purchase a telephone system that can handle electronic communications and office expansion

Telephone systems are sold by many different communications companies. They are priced according to the number of available lines and outlets, as well as extra features (intercom, automatic dial, programmed dialing, conference calling, fax, modem, etc). The cost may or may not include installation and service contracts. Additional costs are usually associated with connecting the installation to the telephone carrier's lines. Always purchase a system with enough lines to accommodate electronic communications and allow for expansion as the practice grows. Be sure the system has an excellent internal communication system.

Copiers and fax machines can be purchased from discount office supply warehouses or from dealers. Dealers offer purchase or lease programs. They also provide service support contracts that can be very worthwhile in the long run. Personal copiers are not fast enough or sturdy enough for routine office demands and their replaceable cartridges are very expensive. Office copiers are more cost effective in the long run and they have useful features such as enlarging, reducing, front/back copying, and collating.

Fax machines no longer require a dedicated telephone line. Instead, some are equipped with sensors that determine in the first few seconds of a call whether the caller is a person or another fax machine. Letter quality fax machines are available, or the fax can be connected directly to a computer. In the latter case, only information in the computer can be faxed out, not pictures and other hard copy. This is easily remedied, however, by attaching an inexpensive optical scanner to the computer.

Computers and peripherals can be purchased by mail order, through office or computer discount supply warehouses, from the manufacturer, or through a computer consultant. A *laser printer* is necessary for letter quality items, and a *dot matrix printer* is required when printing multiple-part forms or serial mailing labels. For more information on computers and peripherals, see Chapter 10.

Minor but necessary office equipment includes: microwave oven, coffee maker, refrigerator, tool set, pencil sharpener, calculator with print-out, heavy duty two- and three-hole punches, postage scale, and cash box.

Arguably necessary office equipment includes: typewriters, dictation equipment, Rolodexes, account posting systems, adding machines, and receipt dispenser. None of these is necessary in a computerized office. Besides the cost of purchase, these items are undesirable because: (1) they occupy horizontal work space, and (2) only one person can use them at a time.

Optional office equipment includes postage meters, credit card machines, paper shredders, and other items that individual practices may deem important for efficiency.

Test Equipment

Most basic audiometric equipment can be obtained, new or used, from medical equipment supply companies or some large hearing aid manufacturers.[2] Equipment manufacturers and suppliers usually exhibit at professional conventions such as AAA, ASHA, and larger state meetings. This is a good time to shop and get detailed information on the various features of instruments.

Used equipment can be purchased directly from clinics, audiologists, or hearing aid dispensers who are upgrading or liquidating their practices.

When purchasing or leasing test equipment, it is very important to obtain quotes from different companies and solicit advice from colleagues who have experience with similar equipment. If possible, obtain the equipment on a trial basis to ensure that it performs as expected and is operator friendly. (Be sure to keep the original packing materials in case it needs to be returned!)

Interview local companies that sell and service audiometric equipment to learn about their product lines, years of experience, and their warranties and repair policies (e.g., How long for a service call? Do they repair other brands? Do they provide loaner equipment? Is their staff oriented and trained toward sales or repairs?). If a company is selected, identify an honest, responsible *individual* in the company to familiarize with the practice's operation and equipment needs. Treat the individual as an outside consultant who will: (a) periodically demonstrate new equipment advances to keep the practice current, (b) advise the practice on new purchases, (c) find reliable used equipment to meet the practice's needs, (d) check out used equipment from other sources before the practice purchases it directly, (e) main-

Good equipment consultants are a valuable resource

---

[2]Some hearing aid manufacturers offer "co-op" arrangements in which the purchase price of equipment is partially offset by discounts applied to future hearing aid purchases from the company. This can be an effective cost-saving method of equipment purchase. However, there are several factors to consider: (1) the sale price typically is higher than from a equipment sales company, 2) the total sale price is often due at the time of purchase, or the practice must sign a lease commitment for the full amount, (3) cost recovery can be very slow unless the manufacturer's hearing aids meet the amplification needs of the practice, and (4) obtaining local equipment service can be a problem.

tain practice equipment, and (f) perhaps do calibrations. A consultant of this type can save the practice thousands of dollars in start-up and long-term operating costs. It is not always possible to find such an individual in the local community, but they *do* exist . . . they are worth the search effort, and they deserve cultivation, even if they leave the equipment company and relocate.

Necessary Test Equipment

Table 9–1 estimates the costs of the following necessary audiology equipment, purchased new and used. As these data demonstrate, it is expensive to set up even the most basic audiology practice. Paring down to the bare essentials and going with used equipment whenever possible, the cost is still around $15,000. Compared to purchasing all new equipment, however, this number represents a savings of over $10,000.

Table 9–1. Cost of new and used necessary audiometric equipment.

Equipment	Cost if Purchased New	Cost if Purchased Used
Single-walled sound booth (including freight and installation)	$7,000	$5,000
1.5 or 2-channel audiometer, including sound field	$3,500–5,000	$2,000
Speakers	$400	buy new
Tape/CD Player	$250	buy new
Acoustic Immittance plus XYT Plotter	$6,000	$4,000
Hearing Aid Analyzer with printer and Real Ear	$6,500	$4,000
Visual Reinforcement Audiometry equipment	$250–900	buy new
Total Cost Range:	$23,900–26,050	$15,000

A *sound booth* is necessary, despite occasional claims that someone is getting by with insert earphones and real-ear equipment. Used sound booths may be as good as new sound booths, if they have been carefully disassembled and stored. Even used sound booths are expensive, however, mainly due to the cost of freight and installation.

Affordable sound booths that fit in available spaces are usually single-walled. A sound booth must be constructed and situated so that its interior meets the ANSI standard "Criteria for Permissible Ambient Noise During Audiometric Testing" (ANSI, 1977). Internal dimensions must be large enough to allow sound field testing without interference from standing waves and room furnishings must be selected and arranged to minimize their effects on the sound source (ASHA, 1991).

A *1.5 or 2-channel diagnostic audiometer* is necessary for diagnostic testing and sound field assessments of hearing aid performance. New audiometers usually are equipped with sound field amplifiers and computer compatible plugs for exporting data. Used audiometers may require additional purchases for sound field testing, and are rarely computer compatible.

Any audiometer purchased for general clinical use must have the following minimum features: air and bone conduction, pure tone and warble tone capability, speech channel, tape or compact disc channel, narrow-band and speech masking, talk-over and talk-back, response button, and external output channel. Whenever possible, the audiometer should be capable of mixing two channels (e.g., speech and taped noise) into one output (e.g., earphone or speaker).

Tape or compact disc players can be purchased in any stereo equipment store.

Acoustic immittance with XYT plotter, new or used, is available from the same sources as are audiometers. For *diagnostic* purposes, it is wise to purchase equipment with capabilities for: ipsilateral and contralateral acoustic reflex testing, plotting on a time base for reflex latency and decay testing, and putting out hard copies of the data.

Hearing aid analyzers with printers and real-ear capability, are also available new or used. New equipment is computer compatible so that real-ear data can be displayed on-line to patients on a VGA monitor. Old equipment is usually limited to tape printout or monochrome displays on small screens.

Excluding Veterans Hospital Audiology Clinics, it is difficult to imagine a diagnostic audiology practice that never has occasion to test a young child. For that reason *Visual*

Reinforcement Audiometry (VRA) equipment is included as a necessary purchase. This is a specialty item that may be purchased from a few companies that build the equipment themselves. The most effective (and expensive) VRA comes with Plexiglas cubes equipped with chaser lights and movable toys that can be replaced.

Optional Test Equipment

Table 9–2 estimates the costs of the following optional audiology equipment, new and used. It is immediately apparent that optional equipment purchases dramatically affect operating capital and cash flow. Once again, a careful business plan is the best guide when considering such purchases. Table 9-2 also shows that some of the items are much less expensive if they can be purchased used.

Before buying optional equipment, be aware of several market observations:

■ Optional equipment, by its nature, is used less frequently than the practice's "work horses." This almost always means that the time required to recoup purchase costs through equipment-generated revenues is longer for optional equipment than it is for necessary equipment.

Table 9–2. Cost of new and used optional audiometric equipment.

Equipment	Cost if Purchased New	Cost if Purchased Used
Portable audiometer (air/bone)	$1,500	$300
Portable audiometer (air/bone/speech)	$2,000	$750
Insert earphones	$500	buy new
ABR	$10,000–20,000	$5,000–10,000
ENG Hardware	$5,000	$1,500
ENG software	$20,000	buy new
Otoacoustic Emissions	$9,000–15,000	buy new
Total Cost:	$46,000–$62,500.00	$16,300–$46,250.00

- Some pieces of optional equipment are very large, difficult to move, and require a good deal of dedicated space for their operation. Indirect costs for storage, operation, and shipping (at purchase, for repair, and when sold) need to be calculated and added to the purchase cost.

- The more exotic and rare the piece of equipment, the fewer qualified repair people, the higher the cost of repair or service contracts, and the riskier it is to purchase the equipment used.

- The more specific the equipment application, the lower the resale value and the greater the chance for obsolescence.

These caveats are not intended to dissuade practitioners from purchasing and using equipment to expand their practices. On the contrary, the appropriate and frequent use of specialized test equipment by well-trained practitioners is very important in establishing and maintaining the scope of practice in our profession. Autonomous practitioners need to determine whether their practice settings are or can become appropriate sites for such equipment.

Portable audiometers are useful in practices where patients must be evaluated off-site (e.g., bedside in hospitals or nursing facilities; satellite "clinics" of the practice; industrial screenings). Some clinicians who work alone prefer to test young children with a portable audiometer. Portable audiometers may also be used as marketing tools by offering free screenings at health fairs, and other public events, so long as extreme care is taken to ensure that screenings are performed only in appropriate test environments. Portables that are equipped with speech channels can be used as backup audiometers if a regular diagnostic audiometer fails or requires off-site servicing.

Insert earphones can be used for general testing, but are especially useful when testing patients with collapsible ear canals, to avoid masking dilemmas, or for infection control. They can be used to attenuate background noise, if occasional testing must be performed in undesirable ambient noise situations. They are more expensive than regular earphones, not only because of the initial purchase price, but because disposal ear tips must be replaced periodically.

Auditory Brainstem Response (ABR) equipment is very useful in hospital-based practices or practices that have a high percentage of physician referrals, especially if the physicians are otolaryngologists, neurologists, neurosurgeons, neonatologists, or pediatricians. ABR requires a room large enough to house a bed or reclining chair for adults and a crib for infants.

Electronystagmography (ENG) equipment consists of a variety of hardware (e.g., caloric baths, OPK drums, gaze lights, graphic recorders) and software. The hardware has been available for years and can be run and analyzed "by hand." Used hardware is available at low cost because much of it is obsolete by modern standards. Modern ENG testing relies on software-driven peripherals and computer analysis. The systems are expensive and not readily available as used equipment. Used equipment might be a questionnable purchase anyway, because the systems depend on software support and are subject to software upgrades from the original manufacturers.

Otoacoustic emissions (OAE) equipment will likely become a necessary item in the audiology practice of the very near future. Although OAEs are relatively new, this technology is one of the fastest growing areas of clinical audiology, so it is included in Table 9–2. OAE testing is relatively expensive for stand-alone practices, and third party reimbursement schedules are still being developed. Like the high technology "silver bullet" marketing approach described in Chapter 13, OAEs offer a novel way for an audiology practice to provide new, useful diagnostic services to its referral sources and distinguish itself from its competitors.

OAE equipment requirements include a suitable computer and printer, an OAE preamplifier and probes, and OAE software. In some cases, the computer used for OAEs can be shared for other diagnostic procedures (e.g., ABR or ENG) or office management functions.

Undoubtedly, more OAE systems will become available and prices may come down in the future as other manufacturers gear up for this new market. Because this is a new area of audiology, used equipment is not likely to be available for some time.

Tools and Supplies

With the exception of otoscopes and cerumen management tools, most of the small equipment has to do with fitting, modifying, and repairing hearing aids. Every dispensing practice will have its own list, depending on what types of aids are dispensed and which manufacturers are used, but the following list is basic to most practices.

- Fiberoptic otoscope(s) and tips
- Cerumen management instruments
- Magnifying light
- Battery tester and ohm meter
- Hearing aid listening device (stethoscope or ear mold)
- Hot and cold air blower
- Fan (for working around tubing cement and other chemicals)
- Loaner aids
- Screw Drivers
- Cleaning tools and supplies
  Surgical gloves
  Ultrasonic cleaner and ear mold cleaning solution
  Wax loops
  Pipe cleaners
  Forced air blower
  Disinfectant spray
  Sterilant, sterilization tub, and heavy gloves
- Impression tools and supplies
  Earlites
  Oil-based impression material
  Silicon impression material
  Syringes (for both types of impression material)
  Mixing cups
  Spatula
  Otoblocks (several sizes in foam and cotton)
- Modification and repair equipment
  Dental drill
  Grinder/buffer
  Chuck, burrs, and bits
  Buffing compound
  Safety glasses
  Tubing (several thicknesses, diameters)
  Ear hooks
  Tube puller
  Tube expander
  Blunt nose scissors
  Methylethylketone
  Jeweler's forceps
  Needle-nose pliers
  Reamer
  Linoleum knife
  Crochet hook
  Tweezers (blunt and pointed)
  Loctite

Tubing cement
Receiver tubing
Contact cleaner
Patching material
Battery door and volume control replacements
Razor blades (single edge)
Clothespin (for holding reattached faceplate)

■ Shipping Supplies
Mailing boxes
Glue (Elmers or rubber cement)
Preprinted mailing/Airborne/Fed Ex labels

■ Sales Supplies
Batteries
Phone pads
Desiccator kits
Air blowers
EAR plugs
Binaural equalizers

Furniture and Fixtures

The style of furniture and fixtures is dictated by the practice's desired image (see Substance Over Image) and does not require further discussion in this section. It is a good idea to visit other offices to see how arrangements and selections have been made. Visiting hearing aid manufacturing facilities can be very helpful in getting ideas for the hearing aid dispensing lab. Necessary acquisitions include:

■ Lateral file cabinets, with locks, for patient charts
■ Standard file cabinets
■ Audiometer desk(s) and chair(s)
■ Front office station
■ Computer station(s) and chair(s)
■ Waiting room chairs/tables/lamps/display and magazine racks
■ Test booth chair(s)
■ Consultation room table and chair(s)
■ Hearing aid analysis station(s)
■ Hearing aid repair station(s)
■ Storage units

Pay attention to ergonomics

Ergonomically designed furniture and functionally efficient arrangements will help maintain the health and productivity of staff members. The analogy of the work station to an airplane cockpit was already mentioned: frequently used supplies and tools should be stored within easy reach and at a convenient height to prevent frequent standing and sitting (Church, 1984). Use adjustable shelving and avoid built-in desks or other fixtures.

It is easier to look down than up: set computer monitors about 17 inches in front and below eye level when sitting in a normal chair (Whitmyer, Rasberry, & Phillips, 1989). Use supports in front of keyboard pads and set them low enough to minimize wrist strain that could lead to carpal tunnel syndrome. Some computer desks are available that set the monitor and keypad below desk level. The monitor is viewed through a glass top built into the desk top and the keypad is on a sliding shelf below the desk top.

Chair backs should fit firmly into the lumbar part of the back and be adjustable to a height that places the sitter's feet flat on the floor. Chair height should also coordinate to desk height:

> Sit upright in your chair and let your arms drop relaxed at your side. Then bend your arms at the elbow. Your hands should be resting on the surface of your desk as you hold your lower arms, from the elbow to your hands, straight out from your body. At worst, there should be only a slight upward bend. (Whitmyer, Rasberry, & Phillips, 1989, p. 105)

For very short people, this may require placing a stool under their feet when the chair height is properly adjusted.

SUMMARY

Office design begins with an exterior theme that must be carried out by the interior decor and demeanor of office staff. The theme must be professional, but also must convey the unique, personal image of the practice. Signs, office space, layout, walls, doors and ceiling colors, floor and window coverings, equipment, furniture and fixtures, and lighting must all be designed or purchased according to guidelines of functionality, efficiency, safety, "livability," and affordability.

REFERENCES

American National Standards Institute. (1977). *American National Standard Criteria for permissible ambient noise during audiometric testing*, ANSI S3.1-1977 (rev. 1991). New York: Acoustical Society of America.

Americans with Disabilities Act in brief, focus on employment, public accommodations, transportation, telecommunications. (1991, July 26). *Federal Register*, Parts I, II, III, IV, and V.

American Speech-Language-Hearing Association. (1989). *Professional services board accreditation standards and manual. Standard 23—Physical plant.* Rockville, MD: Author.

American Speech-Language-Hearing Association. (1991). Sound field measurement tutorial. *Asha, 33*(Suppl. 3), 25–37.

Baxter, J. (1994). Locating and equipping an audiology practice. In H. Hosford-Dunn, J. Baxter, A. Desmond, G. Jacobson, J., Johnson, P. Martin, & E. Cherow (Eds.), *Development and management of audiology practices* (chap 4., pp. 15–24). Rockville, MD: ASHA.

Church, O. D. (1984). *Small business. Management and entrepreneurship.* Chicago: Science Research Associates.

Jacobson, G. (1994). Infection control. In H. Hosford-Dunn, J. Baxter, A. Desmond, G. Jacobson, J., Johnson, P. Martin, & E. Cherow (Eds.), *Development and management of audiology practices* (chap 13, pp. 89–90). Rockville, MD: ASHA.

Jelonek, S., & Staab, W. J. (1994). Utilizing your dispensing office as a marketing tool. *Hearing Instruments, 45*(4), 27–28.

Kemp, B. (1994). Practicing office safety in the 90's: Infection control for audiologists. *Audiology Today, 6*(5), 23–25.

Kishel, G. F., & Kishel, P. G. (1993). *How to start, run, and stay in business.* New York: John Wiley.

McCollom, H. F., Jr., & Mynders, J. M. (1984). *Hearing aid dispensing practice. Planning—starting—operating.* Danville, IL: Interstate Printers & Publishers.

Rizzo, S. R., Jr., & Wilkins, J. E. (1994). Planning and designing audiology and speech-language pathology (ASLP) facilities. In S. R. Rizzo, Jr. & M. D. Trudeau (Eds.), *Clinical administration in audiology and speech-language pathology* (chap. 3, pp. 65–92). San Diego, CA: Singular Publishing Group.

Whitmyer, C., Rasberry, S., & Phillips, M. (1989). *Running a one-person business.* Berkeley, CA: Ten-Speed Press.

Computers in the Office

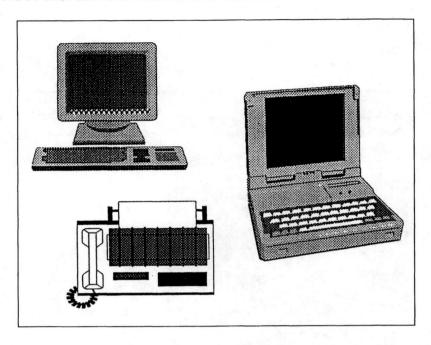

Computers are ubiquitous— embrace them!

Dispensing audiologists use computer technology every day, even if they do not use computers. The micro-processor technology that runs personal computers also forms the core of new generation audiometric test equipment and programmable hearing aids. The challenge for audiology/dispensing practices of the 1990s is to formulate strategies that maximize the power of these technology applications by tailoring their use to the individual needs of different practice settings. This involves laying the groundwork to integrate the technologies that reside in the practice today and planning for future growth and expansion.

The decision to integrate computers into the practice should not be made capriciously. Effective use of these new tools requires allocation of much time and many dollars to planning, purchasing software and hardware, converting existing procedures, and staff training. The decision also involves risk. Successful practice automation produces a better practice, but a poorly conceived integration attempt translates to diminished quality of care and subsequent loss of business. Selecting the wrong computer hardware and software mix means money lost on unusable or unwieldy products, time lost trying to run the practice while recovering from the debacle, confidence and enthusiasm lost among staff members, and patients lost due to errors, miscommunications and sheer frustration.

Computers can provide practices with valuable information and operating skills. The key is not to lose sight of the primary purpose of the practice, which is patient service. For instance, computers should smooth out and speed up service delivery, not function primarily as data base generators, or force a certain type of scheduling because of limitations in the scheduling program. Making a patient wait 15 minutes to purchase a package of batteries because of complex data entry procedures to meet a bookkeeping requirement is another example of taking the wrong approach to integrating computers into the practice.

Computer integration undergirds quality care and economic health

This chapter starts with a glossary for audiologists who are not familiar with some computer terms. It goes on to survey computers uses for practice management. The discussion is divided into two sections. The first considers general business uses of computers. The second addresses computer applications that are unique to the hearing health care industry.

GLOSSARY OF COMMON COMPUTER TERMS

Applications. Programs that do things such as word processing, graphics, accounting, data base management, and spreadsheets.

BIOS. **B**asic **I**nput/**O**utput **S**ystem. This is a chip in your computer that determines the compatibility of your system to various software packages and add-on hardware. A brand name BIOS generally ensures compatibility.

Bit. Smallest unit of measure. 8 bits make up a byte.

Byte. Made up of eight bits. A byte is equivalent to a single character such as a letter or a number.

Cache. High speed memory located on the mother board that runs about five times faster than normal memory. It speeds up the operation of programs by maintaining the most recently used information in this faster memory.

CD-ROM. **C**ompact **D**isk, **R**ead **O**nly **M**emory. Very similar in appearance to audio CDs. Used to distribute large data bases. Data cannot be changed.

CPU. **C**entral **P**rocessing **U**nit. Usually, a single chip about 1 inch square that does the main computing work. All the rest of the hardware is just a way of getting data to and from that chip. When reference is made to "386" or "486" it is referring to the generation of this chip.

Databases. Store and retrieve information. Allow users to sort on specific fields in the data base to create files of unique information.

DOS. **D**isk **O**perating **S**ystem (see Operating Systems). A common operating system found on almost all IBM-compatible computers. Microsoft created the standard version which is referred to as MS-DOS. This software handles the basic functions of the computer and is required by almost all software that runs on an IBM-compatible computer. There are many versions of DOS, the most recent are versions 5.0 and 6.0. Version 5.0 introduced a program called DOS Shell which is a series of pull down menus that eliminated the need to remember all the DOS commands. Version 6.0 incorporated many useful utility programs for the system environment (e.g., backup, anti-virus, disk compression utilities).

DX / SX. See *Math co-processor.*

Fields. An area where information is stored. It can be a dialog box in an application or a location in a data base. Fields can be fixed (e.g., a 6 digit patient ID number) or they can be almost unlimited (e.g., journal entries in a patient file). Some fields are user-defined, but usually most fields are set by the application. Programs can be written to search and sort on fields.

Floppy Disk Drive. Like the hard drive, a magnetic storage medium. Unlike the hard drive, the storage medium is removable from the computer, allowing transport of magnetically stored data from one location to another. Data can be programs or files. Programs or applications are often loaded onto the hard drive via floppy disks. The media for floppy disk drives are 5.25 inch and 3.5-inch diskettes with capacities commonly ranging from 360KB to 1.4MB. The 3.5 medium is replacing the 5.25.

Gigabyte (GB). It equals roughly a billion bytes. New hard drives are coming available in this size.

Hard Disk. Can be referred to as hard disks or hard drives. A magnetic storage medium in the computer for programs and files. Unlike RAM, which is erased when power is removed, information is physically recorded on the computer's hard drive. 200 MB hard drives are considered adequate in today's environment, and sizes have reached a gigabyte in capacity.

Integrated Software. See *Suites.*

Keyboard. Like a typewriter, the keyboard provides a direct means of communicating with the computer.

Kilobyte. Basically a thousand bytes. A common measure of storage or memory.

LAN. Local Area Network. A system that connects multiple computers, printers, or other peripheral devices, for the purpose of sharing of hard drives, files, devices, and software. Local generally refers to the same room, rooms in the same building, or buildings that are in close proximity. The network is made up of the server, work stations, and the connecting interface. LANs require both hardware and software and can service anywhere from two to thousands of work stations.

Macro. A single command that activates a series of actions. A very efficient way to use many applications. The user does not have to remember complex strings of commands. Powerful macros that automate whole tasks are sometimes referred to as **Agents.** Consultants can help with writing macros and agents.

Math coprocessor. Special circuits that allow a computer to perform math functions faster. A designation of 386DX or 486DX indicates that a math coprocessor is installed. A designation of 386SX or 486SX indicates that there is no coprocessor installed.

Megabyte (MB). A more common measure of memory or storage size. It equals slightly more than 1 million bytes.

Megahertz (MHz). The speed of the CPU is measured in MHz. Generally the higher the number the faster the CPU speed. This is useful only to compare like CPUs. For example, a 486 running at 25 MHz is faster than a 386 running at 33 MHz.

Menu. A good example would be DOS Shell or Windows where selection of an option from a menu bar across the top of the screen "pulls down" a secondary menu related to the first selection.

Modem. A device that can be either externally or internally installed that allows one computer to communicate with other computers over a telephone line. Some modems also can send or receive faxes.

Monitor. Or display. Provides the visual medium for communicating with the computer. Today, super VGA (vector graphics array) is considered the standard for part of the system. From a human factors' point of view there are several monitor features to consider such as size, dot pitch, refresh rate and interlacing.

Mother board (or system board). The large circuit board in the system unit that the CPU and feature boards plug into.

Mouse. A device used with Windows and numerous other applications that allows quick communication by moving a pointer to make selections and activate commands.

Operating system (OS). System software that translates the commands from the applications into commands that the computer can understand. DOS is the dominant operating system. Windows is not really an operating system but an interface that allows the quick switching between applications by changing Windows. IBM's OS/2 is the newest operating system and allows running of DOS and Windows applications simultaneously.

RAM. **R**andom **A**ccess **M**emory. Where the computer stores the data and programs that are in use. The more memory, the better and faster programs run. With limited memory, overhead is incurred to constantly update RAM. A DOS environment can run in 1 MB of RAM but Windows applications require a minimum of 4 MB, with 8 to 12 MB closer to ideal.

RISC. **R**educed **I**nstruction **S**et **C**omputer. An emerging technology that achieves faster throughput by using graphical-based instruction sets (as opposed to character-based sets in existing technologies). Improves speed only for software revised for use with RISC-based computers. Does not run existing non-RISC software applications any faster. Cannot run standard Windows without a special software emulator, but can run Windows NT (see below).

RS-232 Interface. The serial standard interface connecting peripheral equipment through the serial port of a computer.

Spreadsheets. Useful in keeping track of quantitative information such as financial or inventory data. Allows forecasting by changing specific values to see the effects on the bottom line of changing a variable

Suites. Integrated packages of software that offer a fully bundled package of software for little more than any one of the software programs would cost individually. Offered by major software companies, they usually include word processing, spreadsheets, graphics, and perhaps scheduling and accounting software. All the software is integrated and capable of moving files from one application to another.

Tape cartridge. A common medium for archiving or backing up the computer. Requires a tape drive which is usually an external unit that can fit into a floppy disk port. Tapes resemble cassette tapes and cost about $20 apiece. Their storage capacity is about 220 MB.

Windows. A Microsoft product that provides the user with a more flexible method of using PCs by graphically interfacing with DOS. Version 3.1 is the current standard. Windows NT is a new version that supports the new generation of RISC-based computers. Common features are the ability to start programs by pointing and clicking on them with a mouse, running two or more programs simultaneously, viewing documents as they will look when printed, and selecting commands from pull down menus.

Word processors. Create and store documents, allowing users to insert and delete words, move whole sentences and paragraphs. Most word processors come with spell checkers, some also provide grammar checking and thesauruses.

COMPUTERS IN GENERAL BUSINESS

The Decision

Computers are for everyone. It is no longer a question of "Should the practice get a computer?" The decision now is "What role will the computer(s) play in the practice?" At the most basic level, every practice can benefit from replacing the typewriter with a computer's word-processing capabilities. Attaching a letter quality printer to a computer gives correspondence a professional appearance. Word-processing programs range from simple "what you see is what you get" (WYSIWIG) programs to very complex text editing programs used for desktop publishing. Likewise, every practice can benefit from replacing the 3×5-inch card index with a computer data base system. Database systems range from simple, dedicated programs with a few fixed data entry fields to large-scale relative data bases. Deciding where to start and what will work now and with future expansions usually requires advice from an outside expert.

Get rid of paper, use a computer

Most audiologists readily see the advantages of hiring an attorney and an accountant as consultants to the audiology practice. They also see the benefits of consulting with bankers and insurance agents. Relying on professionals to provide legal, financial, or insurance services and advice makes the practice more efficient, even when the owner/manager possesses the necessary skills to do the tasks for which these outside profes-

Use a computer consultant as you would an accountant

sionals are hired. The same is true for computer consultants. Once the decision is made to incorporate computers, hiring a computer consultant wisely is a good investment for the practice. The adverb "wisely" is stressed because computer consultants are an unregulated profession. Select a computer expert with the same care used to recruit and hire an employee. The wrong choice can lead to almost unbelievable expense, lost time, and frustration.

The Consultant

There are three types of consultants in the computer industry. Each provides services in a unique area of expertise. Over the long term, an audiology practice may eventually employ each type.

General consultants specialize in finding out the requirements of the practice and recommending hardware and software solutions to meet those requirements. The right general consultant may be the only computer consultant a practice ever needs.

Training consultants provide training on particular products. This type of consultation may take the form of a software course offered to the general public, or a consultant may come on-site and tailor the training to the needs of the practice. General consultants sometimes provide this service.

Programming consultants design custom software. Practices should do extensive research before embarking on this avenue to meet or resolve their system requirements. There are three reasons for this. First, paying for development and support of custom programs is very expensive. Second, finished software is not always delivered on, or anywhere near, the promised date. Third, the "final" product is not always what the audiologist envisioned, prompting the need for further programming development or cancellation of the project.

The obvious costs of custom software are paying by the hour or project to get the project designed and built. The cost of keeping the software upgraded and compatible with other products is less obvious and may be difficult to project. Costs depend on how responsive the programming consultant is to resolving problems and providing documentation. There are also the questions of who supports the product or even who owns the object code if the programming consultant goes out of business or moves.

Finding a Consultant

Selecting a consultant is much like hiring an employee. Determine what type of consultant is required and begin the search process, using the following guidelines:

- *Referrals are very important.* Solicit recommendations from colleagues, people in the business community, and/or computer stores.

- *Check to see how long the consultant has been in business.* Like audiology, computer consulting is a service business that cannot survive if the practitioner fails to deliver or if the quality of the work is poor.

- *Check out the business location and environment.* Many people enter consulting because it has low start-up costs. Most new consultants work from home at first. A consultant with an office and professional telephone answering service usually has enough sustained business to support a business away from home.

- *Ask for referral clients.* A good consultant is eager to provide referral customers. Ask the referrals about the types of services they required, the responsiveness of the consultant, and their satisfaction with the consultant's service. It is important to determine that services are delivered on time, as promised, and supported when and if problems arise.

- *Discuss fees and get written quotes* from potential consultants. Determining the costs is an important part of the final selection process. Does the consultant plan to bill on a per hour or per project arrangement?

Working with a Consultant

Once a consultant is selected, spell out every detail of the discussions in a project agreement to avoid misunderstandings; also to ensure that the costs cover the project the practice envisions and match the budget. The more detailed the agreement, the less frustration and add-on expense near the end of the project. A successful and experienced consultant can avoid most misunderstandings regarding the scope and cost of a project. Both parties should have their respective attorneys review a project contract.

Defining Practice Needs

In most cases, start out with a general consultant. Time spent with the consultant on up-front planning and definition pays large dividends in user satisfaction once the systems are installed and running.

Before meeting with the consultant, develop a "wish list" by brainstorming *everything* that automation could improve in the practice, if computer systems could do everything. Go over the wish list with the consultant in detail to arrive at realistic expectations and cost estimates that are in line with the practice's budget.

Establish a support plan for whatever systems will be purchased. When planning the systems, important questions are: Who is going to assemble the hardware? Who is going to install and customize the software programs and applications? Who is going to fix problems when systems fail or applications do not work? Are these services part of the purchase contract or are they additional charges? The practice needs to answer these questions and document the action plans in advance. Doing so ensures that no time is lost in getting a call into the right resource when things go wrong, and every effort is made to reduce the impact on the practice.

Finally, determine the training requirements. Don't put off training or relegate it to a low priority. The success of the practice in adapting to the new environment is greatly enhanced by a well planned and supported training program.

Many audiologists shy away from these tasks, deferring to the consultant and excusing themselves on the grounds that (a) they are too busy to indulge in wish list fantasizing, (b) they have no idea what computers can do, and/or (c) that is why they hired a computer consultant. Invoking these excuses is a huge mistake that almost certainly dooms the project before it is off the ground. Computer consultants know computer systems, they do not know audiology/dispensing needs. Only the audiologist knows the automation needs of the practice. Audiologists who "leave it to the experts" have only themselves to blame when expensive and powerful systems are installed and eventually left to gather dust because they did not meet practice needs, cannot be expanded to accommodate new applications, or lack support.

Understand the needs of the practice before asking for help

The Wish List

Clearly describe the modus operandi of the practice

The best way to start a wish list is by observing office operations, noting each type of task that is performed on a regular basis. Many of these tasks are itemized in staff job descriptions. Next, step back from the list and look for task "connections" that may serve as logical transitions in the automation process. Note these connections on the wish list. For example, if the consequence of every failed hearing screening is a letter and referral card sent to a primary care physician, it makes sense to try to automate the sequence.

Finally, look at the list from the owner/manager's perspective, grouping wish list items according to management activities that could be automated. For example, if the practice sends out a quarterly newsletter to all physicians or birthday cards to patients on a monthly basis, the wish list could request updated mailing lists at specific intervals.

Good wish lists take time, imagination, and patience. Like any brainstorming exercise, the end result should reflect desires and possibilities, regardless of feasibility. The consultant's job is to ground the wish list in reality by creatively using the best technology available within the budget to address as many items as possible on the list. Usually, a sizable portion of the list remains in the wishing realm, waiting for future money, new technologies, and projected developments in the practice. Appendix 10-A is a wish list for a small audiology/dispensing practice. As this chapter was written in 1994, there were no systems available that come close to meeting this wish list. Although the capabilities exist, they are not available in a single, integrated package. The cost of customizing all of the required applications is prohibitive. However, more and more of the items on the wish list are becoming feasible as new hardware and software solutions come to market each year.

Choosing Applications and Technologies

Having defined immediate and future practice needs, attention is now directed to figuring out what systems approach best meets the needs. It falls to the general consultant to ensure that all hardware and software system components are compatible with each other and meet the expectations of the practice, today and for several years to come.

Software Applications

The first step in building a system is to select software applications and then choose hardware that best matches those products. This approach is less expensive and time consuming than buying hardware first and then trying to figure out what will run on it. Srebnik (1993) posits several humorous corollaries for the consequences of doing it the other way around:

> Corollary 1. The hard drive space required to install your new software is one megabyte more than you have on your system . . . .

> Corollary 2: The microprocessor required to run your new software at reasonable speed is one level faster than the one you have in your system . . . .

Corollary 3: The amount of free RAM or operating program memory required to run your new software is only slightly more than you have in your system. (p. 29)

Major software applications that dispensing audiologists need to consider are:

■ Word processing
■ Bookkeeping
■ Billing
■ Scheduling and planning
■ Record keeping
■ Importing test data
■ Desktop publishing (marketing)
■ Networking (local & remote)

With the right software-hardware mix, computers can perform these individual applications with ease. A large selection of general business programs is available from major software houses. Different programs support different combinations of word processing, bookkeeping, scheduling, data base, networking, and desktop publishing applications. The more integrated the program, the more applications it supports.

Several companies now offer bundled "suites" of integrated applications that feature their flagship word processor coupled to some combination of spreadsheet, graphics, office mail, scheduling, and accounting applications. The products are neatly tied together, and the suites are reasonably priced. A bundled suite of software applications is often a good value, especially for computer novices who want to start with several of these applications in their practices.

Whenever possible, use off-the-shelf software. To some extent, packages can be adapted to practice needs by using macros that are written by the audiologist or by a consultant. Custom software or heavily modified software exposes the practice to the dangers of getting locked into a technology or having serious service problems emerge as the expertise that created the work fades away or disappears.

Use custom software as a last resort—explore off-the-shelf packages first

Hardware Technologies

There are two basic hardware technologies, one provided by Apple Computer, the other that is "IBM-compatible." The two technologies are incompatible, although Apple is making strides to accommodate IBM-compatible software on Apple systems. In 1994, Apple announced a new family of products with two computers in one chassis. One computer runs

Apple-based software, the other runs limited IBM-compatible software. These new systems have a significant price tag.

IBM-compatible systems are made by manufacturers all over the world. At present, they dominate the personal computer (PC) market. IBM-compatibility means the computers use an operating system called DOS. DOS is designed to operate with the INTEL 8086 processor hardware architecture developed for the first IBM PC. INTEL and IBM left the technology open to encourage growth, choosing not to restrict its use as Apple did. That strategy was very effective: almost 90% of all personal computers are IBM compatible, about 10 percent are Apple- or Macintosh-based systems. Succeeding generations of IBM compatibles use 80286, 80386, and 80486 processor technologies. They are commonly referred to as 386 or 486 systems as an abbreviation of processor chip technologies (Magid, 1993).

The newest generation of PCs is powered by the INTEL "Pentium" 80586 processor. But, for the first time INTEL is facing competition. Motorola, in cooperation with Apple and IBM, is now producing the "Power PC Chip." Based on RISC technology, the Power PC Chip is in the new generation of Apple systems and the new family of PCs produced by IBM. Motorola touts this technology as superior to the 80586 generation in speed and performance.

Purchasing Hardware and Hardware Support

Computer components can be purchased from computer stores, discount stores, electronic stores, and mail order catalogs. Computer stores have higher prices but usually provide support options that are not available through the other purchasing avenues. These options may include preinstalling software and customizing software installations. Systems purchased from computer stores often are accompanied by basic operating classes that are included in the purchase price (Magid, 1993). When the practice saves money by buying at a discount house or from a catalog, part of the savings is the loss of this local support. If the practice is using a consultant, or these services are not required, then shop at a discount store or electronic store, or have the consultant order system components from mail order suppliers.

It is rarely cost effective to settle for basic requirements. The extra expense of additional capacity is less than the cost of interrupting the practice to upgrade systems and debug new applications. The capacity decision is based not only on estimates of practice growth, but also on expansion capability. It is imprudent to purchase a system that can handle additional workload but lacks the capacity for expansion to handle new applications (e.g., networking, peripheral test or hearing aid equipment).

System Components

1. System. Buy the largest and fastest system the budget can afford. Beginning in 1995, Microsoft's operating system, coded named "Chicago," will be the operating system on new IBM-compatible systems. Chicago places higher demands on computers (e.g., higher processing speed, more RAM, and more hard drive capacity).

Choose a 486 processor.[1] Processor speed is measured in MHz: chose a processor with a clock speed of 66 MHz. If math requirements are minor, select an SX model without a math coprocessor. A 486SX-66 computer has a 486 processor without math co-processor and operates at 66 MHz.

Purchase as much RAM as possible. Windows runs poorly on less than 8 MB of RAM, and 12 MB is recommended to handle future system requirements. Get a large capacity hard drive. New audiology and hearing aid applications software demand a large hard drive capacity. The computer adage is apt: "Hard drives are like closets, once you've had them it's hard to give them up." A 500 MB hard drive is a better buy than a 200 MB hard drive for a dispensing audiology practice.

2. Monitor. Purchase a super VGA adapter and a display that is capable of taking advantage of it. The extra expense is minimal in light of better graphics and the human factor of reduced eye strain. Standard displays are 14 inches measured diagonally, the same as television sets. Larger displays are more pleasing to work with, but much more expensive. Other aspects of display quality are "dot pitch," which is a measurement of screen pixils, and refresh rate. The lower the dot pitch number, the higher the quality. A dot pitch of .28 or lower is acceptable. Refresh rate measures how frequently the screen is refreshed. The higher the number the better. Another aspect of screen refresh is whether the screen is updated in interlaced or noninterlaced mode. Interlaced screens refresh every other pass. A noninterlaced screen with the same refresh rate will refresh twice as often as an interlaced screen.

---

[1]The reason a 586 processor (Pentium) is not recommended is because few applications were available to take advantage of the increased power and speed of the 586 in 1994. New 486 processors can be upgraded to 586 later, and they are much less expensive.

3. Keyboards. Find one that is comfortable. The interface is standard so different brands of keyboards are interchangeable. Only laptop computers limit keyboard selection.

4. Mouse. A necessary accessory for working in Windows or OS/2 environments. A mouse is attached to the computer in one of three ways: (1) through an expansion slot on the mother board, (2) commonly, by using the serial port (RS-232 interface), and (3) via an integrated mouse port available on some systems.

The connection is important for dispensing audiologists because some hearing aid applications require a mouse as well as a serial port. In these cases, the computer must have a nonserial port method for attaching the mouse.

5. Modems. A wide variety of modem speeds are available today. But equally important as the modem speed is the port to which the modem connects. Modems that connect to the serial port and standard serial ports are unbuffered. This means that each time the computer sends or receives data it must change information from a parallel format to serial or from serial to parallel. This stops the system for each byte of transfer. In effect, a faster modem stops the system more often. Buffered serial ports can be purchased to reduce these system interruptions and are a wise addition to a modem purchase.

6. Tape Cartridges. A sound and economical investment for archiving or backing up system data on a regular basis. The drive itself and the tape cartridges are solid technology and reasonably priced. Units can be purchased to stand alone or to mount into a floppy disk drive bay.

7. Printers. A wide variety is available today. Laser and ink jet print technologies provide superb quality at a price most businesses can afford.

8. CD-ROM. An increasing number of applications are being delivery on this medium. If purchasing this component, make sure it is rated as "double speed" and has an access time of less than 350 msec. Whenever possible, purchase the entire system with CD-ROM integrated, if this feature is desired.

Networks

Networks allow co-workers to share hard drives, printers, modems, and other hardware, as well as system and application software and data files. In audiology/dispensing practices, networks provide an efficient means of sharing scheduling calendars, patient files, PC-based hearing aid fitting applications, as well as expensive peripherals. Planned carefully and established with foresight and discipline, networks improve service delivery and patient satisfaction.

Local Area Network (LAN)

The most common networking approach for audiology applications is the LAN. A LAN is a hardware and software configuration that connects computers and peripheral equipment in a localized area for purposes of sharing resources and information. A basic LAN configuration involves a main computer (the server) and one or more "slave" computers or peripherals (the work stations), all connected by network hardware and software.

There are two types of LAN networks: peer-to-peer and client-server. In peer-to-peer arrangements, all work stations have equal communication status and can exchange data with any other station. Client-server arrangements reduce data transfer over the network by not sending whole data bases back and forth when executing tasks. In a client-server arrangement, the updating or task is done on the server and only the results move across the network.

Network configurations generally follow three formats: the star, ring, and the bus. The most popular is the bus configuration in the form of what is called "ethernet." A large percentage of LANs use this format because it is economical and high speed. A computer consultant versed in networks can provide the best advice for determining the form of a practice's network.

LANs add expenses to the computer budget. Network interface cards must be purchased and installed in every server and work station. These cards physically attach the components to the network. Network software must be purchased and installed to allow communications between the servers and work stations. Another expense is purchasing network (as opposed to single-user) versions of applications software.

LANs can provide considerable savings that more than offset the expenses of installing a network. Although network versions of applications are more expensive, only one copy needs to be purchased. In non-network environments, copies of software need to be purchased for each work station. It is generally illegal to use a single copy of an application on multiple computers. Networks allow sharing of expensive peripherals such as laser printers, CD-ROMs, and Fax modems, as well as a large data bases on the server hard drive.

Hooking Up Networks

Networks are connected using a variety of technologies and configurations. Common cabling options are coaxial, shielded twisted pair, unshielded twisted pair, and fiber optic. Coaxial and shielded twisted pair provide shielding against electromagnetic interference and can move data over long distances. Often, unshielded twisted pair is used for very close environments (e.g., small offices or single departments). It is easy to use but offers no protection against interference. Fiberoptic cable provides the highest degree of reliability and is the most expensive (Hsu, 1993).

Training

Tailor the amount and type of training to the computer literacy and job requirements of each employee. For continuity as employees come and go, owner/managers need more in-depth training on all aspects of the systems than most of the staff. *The owner/manager also needs to know how to use accounting and financial management applications that good business practices dictate are privileged above normal staff access.*

Training options are: (1) consultants, (2) classes, and (3) self-study. General consultants may offer training as part of the overall project cost or on an hourly basis. Training consultants are available to teach specific products. Universities, community colleges, local computer groups, and computer stores offer classes in most common software products. There are also self-study courses available for common products such as word processors, data bases, and spread sheets.

HEARING HEALTH CARE SOLUTIONS

A number of software programs on the market offer dispensing audiologists some degree of practice management control. The range of offerings is broad in applications and varied in origin. Some are basic office business systems that individual audiologists developed and tested in their offices. Other systems developed by individual audiologists offer business, clinical record management, and equipment control applications (e.g., PC/MACHear). Equipment manufacturers and hearing aid manufacturers such as Madsen (HearWare) and Starkey (Pro-Hear) support systems that do office management, hearing aid tracking/marketing, and interfacing with computer compatible audiometric equipment or hearing aid systems.

These companies and systems are not named as endorsements, only as examples of what is available. There are other products on the market at the time of writing, and there are sure to be a number of new and spin-off companies and products in the next few years to meet the computer needs of audiologists/dispensers. Refer to the "products for sale" sections of *The Hearing Journal, Hearing Instruments,* or *Hearing Review* for products, names, and telephone numbers of different companies.

Dispensers and audiologists owe a debt to the hard-working and talented practitioners who have toiled in their offices and back rooms to pioneer custom software solutions for our practice management needs. The same is true for equipment and hearing aid manufacturers who have shouldered the research and development costs of developing practice management software applications. Without these efforts, office automation would still have little application to audiology/dispensing practices.

Naturally, the sources that created the present applications have left their stamp on the products in the form of personal biases and industry goals. The results are that, as of this writing (1994), none of the management software products available offers a full solution to the office automation wish list. Most of the products are heavily weighted toward hearing aid management, with less attention paid to patient management and quality assurance measures. In most cases, data fields are limited, and there are few if any user-defined fields available. Some products lack schedulers; others lack sophisticated accounting packages; some are difficult to install, awkward to use, or expensive. All are proprietary at present, so buying into one system "marries" the practice to that vendor and that approach to practice management.

Until recently, a general business configuration of hardware and software did not adequately support further integration of programmable hearing aid systems, real ear, or diagnostic test equipment. Software for these systems was limited and proprietary. Audiologists who wanted to integrate all of their service operations had to purchase "computer compatible" test equipment, and individual systems from different hearing aid manufacturers, design and build their own hardware and software interfaces, and develop custom software to handle the data after it was transported from the equipment to the computer! Few, if any, audiologists were able to accomplish these tasks, much less afford them. Although unique system tailoring can be very satisfying when successful, it is never cost effective and can turn into a support nightmare.

Industry Solutions

Since 1994, the American hearing aid industry has taken steps to provide reasonable solutions for practices trying to integrate practice management, test, and hearing aid applications. Through the Hearing Instrument Manufacturers Software Association (HIMSA), a not-for-profit coalition of American and European hearing aid manufacturers,[2] efforts are under way to establish standards that allow unique hearing aid systems and test equipment to communicate with normal PC-based integrated systems over common interfaces.

HIMSA's approach requires large capacity computers, a common interface, and software interfaces. The advantages to the hearing health care infrastructure of having standardized hardware and software integration are:

- establishes a global communication standard in the hearing industry,
- offers start-up and traditional audiology/dispensing practices a reasonable way to initiate computer use,
- allows computer literate practices to upgrade their office automation by integrating hearing aid fitting procedures from different manufacturers into one computer system,
- data from "computer compatible" test equipment are treated in a clinically useful manner (e.g., audiograms, reports),
- provides practices with opportunities to render higher quality hearing health care services more quickly and at reduced costs.

The Software Platform

HIMSA-America introduced Noah in the second half of 1994. Noah is written in C++ with a Paradox data base. It functions as an extended operating system that operates in a DOS/Windows environment. Noah links hearing aid fitting systems, some office management software,[3] and computer interfaced test equipment with the computer and the normal operating system.

Noah provides six basic functions that are selected from a pull down menu. Functions currently available are:

---

[2]Currently, HIMSA efforts are supported in America by 10 hearing instrument manufacturers: Ascom Audiosys, GN Danavox, Oticon, Phonak, ReSound, Siemens, Starkey, Unitron, Widex, and 3M.

[3]When this chapter was written in 1994, several companies that offer hearing care office management software packages (e.g., PC/MacHear, HearWare, and Pro-Hear) were planning to support Noah with their products.

Client. This menu is for entering client and hearing aid information into a very basic data base (a couple of dozen fields). The information is compatible for all supported hearing aid manufacturers. Unlike individual systems the data only have to be entered once.

Audiogram. This menu is for entering audiometric test data into a spreadsheet format. Data can be entered manually or transferred from newer model audiometers that interface directly with the computer via an RS-232 interface.

Select Manufacturer. This menu provides access to the proprietary software offered by hearing aid manufacturers who are Noah licensees.

Fitting. Selecting this module allows the programming and fitting of programmable hearing aids using a hardware interface programming device.

Insertion Gain. This function can be used to transfer real ear test data to the computer if real ear test equipment has an RS-232 interface to the computer.

Journal. This function provides extensive note capability that is tied to the patient file.

Noah System Requirements

Noah requires an operating environment of MS-DOS version 5.0 or higher with Microsoft Windows version 3.1. Its hardware requirements are an IBM-compatible 486 processor with 8 MB of RAM, and a very large hard drive. A 300 MB hard drive will not be too much once software applications from different hearing aid manufacturers are loaded. It is also important to note that the system mouse must be integrated or controlled via a mouse driver in an expansion slot. The serial port is consumed by a hardware interface such as HI-PRO (discussed in the next section) and one additional serial port is required for each piece of test equipment that is interfaced to the computer,[4] in addition to any modems on the system.

---

[4] In a network approach, test equipment can be spread among work stations, reducing the number of expansion slots required for serial ports on a single machine. When this chapter was written in 1994, a network version of Noah was not available yet.

The Hardware Interface

HI-PRO (**H**earing **I**nstrument **PRO**grammer) is an interface box that connects hearing aid manufacturers' proprietary fitting modules to the serial port on PCs.[5] It was developed by HIMSA, is manufactured by Madsen, and is supported by Noah (Bisgaard, Christensen, & Morrison, 1993). HI-PRO is sold through hearing instrument manufacturers.

This physical interface allows the practitioner to program hearing instruments from different manufacturers without having to switch between systems. Participating hearing aid manufacturers provide their own fitting software and cables. The advantages for dispensing practices are:

■ elimination of numerous proprietary systems from different hearing aid manufacturers,
■ programmable and nonprogrammable hearing aid fittings are automated by using general purpose computer systems that may already be in place,
■ reduced costs and space requirements for fitting programmable hearing aids, and
■ better ergonomics (e.g., enhanced graphics, easier handling) by substituting PC system for hand-held processors.

Cost savings are a major advantage for all concerned (Jelonek, 1994). Participating manufacturers no longer must face the expenses of developing their own processors and hardware interfaces. They need only concentrate on creating application software that is compatible with HI-PRO. Hearing aid returns and circuit change requests should plummet, reducing manufacturers' costs even more. These significant savings to the industry will be passed on to practitioners. As capital expenses and dispensing costs decline, practitioners can offer patients a wider range of products and services.

SUMMARY

Full computer integration should be an objective for every practice that is intent on improving service quality and economic survival.

Combining planning, training, and the judicious use of consultants, even inexperienced purchasers can design and

---

[5]Other proprietary interface boxes will also connect to Noah (e.g., Pro-Connect and Resound).

build systems that streamline day-to-day operations, simplify complex operations, and introduce new standards of consistent service delivery. Computerization involves a commitment of intent, time, and money. These resources are well spent if automation reduces costs and magnifies the contribution of each employee.

The future looks bright for full automation of audiology/dispensing practices. Wish lists are becoming feasible with the recent introduction of integrated software suites for general business applications and the emergence of standardized hardware/software interfaces for specific audiology/dispensing applications.

REFERENCES

Bisgaard, N., Christensen, C., & Morrison, P. (1993). Order from chaos: A PC-based universal programming interface. *Hearing Instruments, 44*(1), 20.

Hsu, J. (1993). All about networking. *PC Today, Premium Issue PCT3,* 42–46.

Jelonek, S. (1994). Noah/Hi-Pro system offer industrywide standard for fitting programmables. *Hearing Journal, 47*(5), 21–22.

Magid, L. J. (1993). *The little PC book.* Berkeley, CA: Peachpit Press.

Srebnik, J. A. (1993). Murphy's laws of computing. *Hearing Instruments, 44*(9), 29.

SUGGESTED READINGS

For novices, there are courses and books available that can eliminate the mystery and magic that seems to surround computers.

Burnard, P. (1993). *Personal computing for health professionals.* London: Chapman & Hall.

Magid, L.J. (1993). *The little PC book.* Berkeley, CA: Peachpit Press.

Williams, R. (1993). *The little Mac book.* Berkeley, CA: Peachpit Press.

"Dummies" books published by IDG Books Worldwide, San Mateo, California. They include various titles such as "PCs for Dummies," "DOS for Dummies," "Windows for Dummies."

APPENDIX 10-A

Automation Wish List for Cardinal Hearing Services, Inc.

(A working document prepared by Dr. A and Mr. B for XYZ Computer Consultants, in preparation for meeting set for January 2, 19--)

VII. C.

I. Patient/Customer Care Activities—Audiology Functions
   A. Chronologically organized chart-type documentation of all encounters (scheduled appointments, drop-ins, phone calls)
   B. Computerized forms for patient history, communication handicap self-report questionnaires, medical clearance, product contracts.
   C. "Hands-free" audiograms recorded, configured, and printed by the computer. Audiogram options include masked and unmasked air and bone thresholds, MCLs, UCLs, acoustic reflex thresholds, aided and unaided sound field thresholds. Audiogram print options to include: left and right ears separately, or combined; referenced to dB HL or dB SPL; "right side up" or "upside down."
   D. Computerized word list selections with automatic correct/incorrect counter. "Hands-free" recording and printing of speech audiometry results.
   E. "Hands-free" acoustic immittance recording and printing.
   F. "Hands-free" special testing (ENG, ABR, OAEs).

II. Scheduling/Record Keeping/Planning
   A. Computerized patient scheduling for two or more professionals, denoting time of appointment, length of appointment, patient's name, type of service, referral source, telephone number.
   B. Daily, weekly, monthly, and trimonthly schedule views.
   C. Automatic updating and cross-referencing between schedule and patient charts and rolodex to eliminate duplicate data entry by scheduler. New patient information "shared" between schedule and patient records, referral information "shared" between rolodex, schedule, and patient records.
   D. Daily schedule printouts.
   E. Automatic dialing for appointment reminders.
   F. Search/listing/merge capabilities by patient name, referral source, audiologist, test type, or number of appointments.
   G. Archival storage of past schedule information.
   H. Daily, weekly, monthly, and annual planning schedules for each practitioner (e.g., To-Dos, appointments, projects).

III. Correspondence
   A. Standard formats for professional reports (e.g., screening and diagnostic reports to referrals sources), modified for individual patients. Report formats to include graphic and tabular descriptions of audiometric, speech, and acoustic immittance data.
   B. Standard formats for product contracts, modified with individual information on type of product, sale price, amount paid, balance due, payment plan, nonrefundable amount, and any other terms and conditions of the contract.

    C. Standard formats for hearing aid orders, hearing aid repairs, hearing aid warranties, with custom notes section for individual comments. Computer merging of formats with each manufacturer's information.

    D. Standard formats for patient notification letters, modified with individual patient information (e.g., warranty renewal letters).

    E. Correspondence type and date "shared" between patient chart notes, product contracts, and hearing aid order/hearing aid history logs.

IV. Hearing Aid Fitting/Product Logs/Product Reports

    A. "Hands-free" hearing aid fitting protocols for different products and product settings, including real-ear measurements.

    B. Automatic calculation of Articulation Index.

    C. Product logs, according to manufacturer, model, date of order, invoice date, invoice amount, payment records (patient payments, manufacturer payments), date of dispensation, patient name, warranty expiration, repair history, patient satisfaction measure(s), and staff member that performed the service.

    D. "Sharing" between correspondence, product logs, and patient records to eliminate duplicate data entry or missed data entry. For instance, each hearing aid order, hearing aid repair, or warranty renewal correspondence should automatically generate an appropriate log entry and a chart note (e.g., "1/1/95 warranty renewal ltr to X Mfr by Dr. A").

    E. Maintain inventory of hearing aids, batteries, supplies.

    F. Link battery purchases to battery inventory and battery club information in patient charts.

    G. Generate hearing aid performance reports for individual instruments, or by model type, date of manufacture, manufacturer, degree/type of loss, etc.

V. Accounting and Billing

    A. Complete accounts management system with check register, chart of accounts, general ledger, accounts receivable, accounts payable, statement, check writing, and report capabilities.

    B. Automatic billing for insurance reimbursement, including modem communications and computer-printed insurance forms.

    C. Automatic direct-patient billing (e.g., single or multiple part forms, envelopes) at scheduled intervals.

    D. "Sharing" between patient chart information, product contracts, hearing aid repair/warranty logs, and accounting to eliminate duplicate data entry and avoid missed billings.

    E. Generate daily, monthly, quarterly, annual, and budgetary (proforma) income statements, based on user-defined intervals and account categories. Generate Balance Sheets. Graphic and/or comparative-interval representations of report data.

VI. Marketing

    A. Desk top publishing of newsletters, special promotions, letters, etc.

    B. Automatic generation of mailing or contact lists according to specific criteria (e.g., birthday, warranty expiration, age of patient, date of last test or hearing aid purchase, type of hearing loss, etc.).

    C. Marketing "log" available for each patient or client, showing dates and types of promotional contacts.

    D. "Sharing" of patient record information, accounting, and product log information to generate marketing reports that indicate whether practice goals were met, should be adjusted, etc.

VII. Communications
   A. Data base rolodex with automatic dialing capability.
   B. Computer fax.
   C. Off-site network connection (e.g., Dr. A's home office or laptop when traveling).
   D. Scanner.
   E. Voice-to-text dictation.

11

Staff Planning

Effective staff planning, staff recruitment, and staff retention are essential to the long-term success of any audiology practice.

Effective staff planning, staff recruitment, and staff retention are essential to the long-term success of any audiology practice. Finding and keeping the most capable, creative, and energetic people is one of the highest priorities of good businesses; and it requires attention, ingenuity, and initiative on the part of management (Kishel & Kishel, 1993).

Even in the smallest viable practice there will come a point where the audiologist cannot do it all and must add support personnel or other audiologists. In hospital- and clinic-based practices, help is often available from the human resource department. In stand-alone practices, the owners/managers are usually responsible for the majority of recruiting and training, often when they have the least time to give.

This is a "reality paradox" of staff planning for most autonomous practices: when business demands on existing personnel are reasonable, it is difficult to justify creating new positions, nor are there likely to be staff vacancies due to job stress. When business demands go up and everyone is working too hard, a need suddenly emerges to create new positions and fill vacant ones, just when resources are scarce and it is most important to match the best person with the job.

Few audiologists have sufficient training in human resource management to effectively address staff planning issues while running their practices. Excellent staff planning information is available for directors of hospital and clinic-based audiology programs (Welch & Fowler, 1994), but how can human resource management be done effectively in smaller practices? This chapter is a "nuts and bolts" description of basic procedures, regulations, and pitfalls associated with staff planning, recruiting, and training in situations where the owner/manager is the main resource.

ORGANIZATIONAL STRUCTURE

For the owner/manager, the best solution to the "reality paradox" is advance planning. Just as cash flow projections and market analysis are part of the business plan, organizational planning should take place when the business plan is being written. Before the first patient walks through the door, the practice should have a planned and documented approach to the growth of the organization. Key sections of the business plan such as organizational structure should be treated as working documents which are reviewed, revised, and integrated into the operational plans for the organization on an ongoing basis.

Defining Skills

An organization is a team of people working together to meet common objectives. An audiology practice is an organization. As such, the practice needs to define itself in terms of skills rather than individuals. A practice that defines itself on the basis of skill requirements rather than individuals will do a much better job of meeting the requirements of the practice and delivering quality care to patients. Kishel and Kishel (1993) itemize the following important questions that need to be answered at this juncture:

What work has to be accomplished?

Do I need additional help to do it?

How many people do I need?

Would part-time help be sufficient?

What skills am I looking for?

How much experience is required?

Is the labor market favorable?

How much am I able to pay? (p. 126)

A simple matrix built from the business plan can assist in this process. Make a list of the skills that the practice requires. Opposite the skills indicate where the skills are acquired. Some skills, notably those within the scope of audiology, usually are addressed by hiring employees, but other skills require talent from outside the practice. See Table 11–1 for an example.

Creating Skill Based Job Descriptions

Once the skills in the practice are defined, it is time to identify positions and build job descriptions to satisfy these skill requirements. A job description documents major elements of the position, thereby avoiding confusion and conflict as the practice grows and matures (Siropolis, 1990). Appendix 11-A contains examples of job descriptions for a small audiology practice. Other examples for larger practices are available in Welch and Fowler (1994).

Table 11–1. Skills required to manage a practice.

Skill	Owner	Other
Define practice	X	
Set up accounting system	X	Accountant
Establish legal entity of practice	X	Attorney
Legal services	X	Attorney
Financial advice		Accountant Banker Financial planner
Direct patient care	X	Professional staff
Patient contact	X	Staff
Insurance	X	Insurance agent Financial planner
Billing and collections	X	Staff collection Agency[a]
Marketing	X	Staff consultant[a]
Monthly books	X	Bookkeeper[a]
Computer Installation, Upgrades, Maintenance	X	Consultant

[a]If necessary

Typical items for a job descriptions include:

- **Title:** One or two identifying words such as Audiologist or Receptionist.
- **Job Statement:** A sentence or two that defines what skills this position provides to the practice.
- **Major Duties:** A list of the major aspects of the position as well as an indication of acceptable standards. Examples would be "Greets patients cheerfully" or "Files charts accurately and in a timely fashion."
- **Minor Duties:** An example might be that an audiologist "Answers the telephones when the office staff is away or tied up."
- **Relationships:** Establishes the organizational structure. For example; "Reports to office manager."
- **Education and experience:** States minimum requirements for educational degrees, licensing, certification, and years of experience.
- **Skills:** Specific skills needed.
- **Experience.**

Including relationships in the job description is an important part of defining the organizational structure. Even if the "practice" is only the founder, it is wise to lay out the structure of the organization in advance. As the practice grows and positions open, the reporting structure remains clear. Often, when the organizational structure is not defined, existing staff are resentful when a supervisorial position is filled. This is because the staff has become used to reporting directly to the owner and not to a *position*. When it is clear from the beginning that they report to the office manager (a position originally filled by the owner) there is less resentment when the position is filled from the outside.

Layout lines of communication for each position, even if the position is not filled

Hiring or Contracting

Constructing skill-based job descriptions keeps a practice flexible and competitive. Just as major corporations are "downsizing" to stay competitive, small businesses need to ensure that everyone employed in the practice is involved in delivering the patient care product. Support staffs may not meet this requirement, regardless of size. Many businesses are discovering that contracting for these services is more efficient and profitable. The process, dubbed "outsourcing," works because contractors that specialize in support services are motivated financially to provide cost effective service (Calabresi, Van Tassel, Riley, & Szczesny, 1993; Drucker, 1992).

"Outsourcing" helps businesses stay lean and competitive

For example, when a practice grows and expands its support staff, the founder needs to be concerned with maximizing the use of this nonpatient care resource. Plainly put, it is a question of "how do I keep these people busy and contributing?" On the other hand, if the practice contracts for the work, the concerns about contribution and efficiency shift to the provider of the service. Clerical employees of a business are often treated and act like second class citizens. Paradoxically, the same individuals will dramatically alter their approach in a contractual situation where the business (in this case an audiology practice) becomes their customer rather than their employer (Drucker, 1992).

Temporary Employees

A practice can resolve some of its supporting staff requirements by using temporary employment services. These services provide employees on an hourly basis or for periods that range from weeks to months and even years.

Examples of situations suited to temporary employees are: moving furniture or offices; labeling newsletters or stuffing envelopes; covering telephones during a promotion; converting an office from paper to computer. Terms and conditions vary with job requirements and the agreement with the temporary service provider. Hiring temporary employees provides an audition process for potential staff additions. If someone special appears, arrangements can be made with the service to hire the individual. Usually, the service requires the equivalent of 2 to 6 months of contract fees to release the employee for hire.

Temporary agencies charge more but can offer long-term savings and an opportunity to audition future employees

Temporary services are more expensive than one's own employees on a per-hour cost, but there are often significant savings and advantages gleaned from the arrangement. Temporary help report to the practice but are not employees of the practice. The service or agency pays their salaries, withholding taxes, and social security contributions. If the practice is unhappy with their work, it can send them back without going through termination procedures. The practice incurs the expense of additional staff only for as long as they are needed, with no long-term commitment. Temporaries address a "bubble" of demand in the work and are then returned to the service.

Outside Skill Support

The exercise of constructing a matrix like Table 11–1 to identify outside skill categories is helpful to the practice.

These categories include attorneys, accountants, insurance agents, computer or equipment repair, computer consultants, and financial advisors. Once the need is identified, the practice must find and then hire or contract for these skills. The practice can interview skill providers and proactively establish relationships rather than searching for the service when a crisis arises. Table 11–2 describes various types of outside professional assistance the practice might need, how to find sources, and arrange liaisons with these services.

State and national associations are another source for locating some services. For example, information on accountants is available from the American Institute of Certified Public Accountants (1211 Avenue of the Americas, New York, NY 10036).

The practice can also look to agencies and organizations to meet some of its outside skill requirements. These resources allow new businesses significant cost savings and education in areas outside of audiology. Typical resources are the Small Business Administration (SBA), the Internal Revenue Service (IRS), U.S. Department of Commerce, Federal Trade Commission, Government Printing Office, local Chambers of Commerce, and workshops and seminars offered by colleges, business groups, and professional associations.

For example, the SBA offers four counseling programs to help small enterprises:

1. **SCORE (Service Corps of Retired Executives)**. Helps launch new ventures. Members are retired executives with successful business histories. The SBA attempts to match the expert to the needs of the practice.
2. **ACE (Active Corps of Executives)**. Acts much like SCORE, but its members are still actively engaged in business.
3. **SBI (Small Business Institute)**. Utilizes student talent from colleges and universities to help small organizations. Graduate students in business receive credit hours based on how successful they were in helping resolve issues for the requesting small businesses.
4. **SBDC (Small Business Development Center)**. Modeled after the extension services provided by agricultural colleges to the agricultural community. The college or university provides technical and professional extension services to the small business community (Siropolis, 1990), as well as seminars on market research and business plans. The SBDC Connection (800-633-6450) operates as a clearinghouse for all the centers (Greco, 1992).

Develop liaisons to bring important professional skills into the practice

Use agencies like the SBA to find outside professional assistance

Table 11–2. Types and sources of outside professional help.

Advisor	Types of Assistance	How to Locate
Accountant	Recommendations regarding tax advantages of business decisions Setting up record keeping and financial control systems	Other practitioners Bankers Attorneys Interview[a]
Attorney	Assist in choosing form of organization Help draw up agreements, file government forms, interpret contracts and leases Arbitrate disputes General counsel	Other practitioners Consultants and other business contacts Interview[a]
Banker	Set up business accounts Provide loans Financial guidance Credit services	personal bank Other practitioners close to practice Interview
Insurance Agent	Advise on insurance needs and set up best package	Comparison shop Other professionals Interview[a]
Computer consultant	Design and install software and hardware for practice needs Sell or recommend hardware purchases Maintenance	Other professionals Computer stores Computer groups Interview[a]
Marketing consultant[b]	Develop marketing strategies Set up advertising	Other professionals Interview[a]
Management Consultant[b]	Help with business plan Advise on management of the practice	Same as marketing consultant

[a]Get fee quotes as part of the interview. Negotiate final fee arrangements as part of hiring process.
[b]This type of advisor is not essential to the practice. Use on an as-needed basis.

RECRUITING EMPLOYEES

There are many different ways for a practice to find potential applicants. As a start, the SBA offers a pamphlet entitled "Employees: How to Find and Pay Them" (available for $1.00 by calling 202-205-6740).

Organized and aggressive recruiting approaches use active networking, advertising (direct and blind), or employment agencies. Passive approaches rely on serendipitous walk-ins, write-ins, and low-key networking that may produce referrals from friends, employees, and acquaintances.

Active recruiting is "a commitment by the program administrator to expend valuable resources to attract qualified candidates" (Welch & Fowler, 1994, p. 98). The owner/manager of the practice needs to tailor the search process to the demands of the practice, taking into consideration time, money, efficiency, and probability of success. The latter is optimized by careful and accurate presentation of the position, timing of the job search, and compliance with Equal Employment Opportunity (EEO) and Affirmative Action legislation. Welch and Fowler (1994) provide a good description of the issues related to these Acts.

Networking

The practice that uses active networking will have more success in recruiting than one that relies solely on advertising. Drake Beam Morin, Inc., a firm that specializes in career enhancement and candidate placement, has found that 70% of positions are filled by networking and only 5% through advertisements. A combination of networking and advertising is usually the most effective means of filling a position and minimizing search time (Siropolis, 1990).

Networking is efficient because it gets the new opening out before a much wider audience than the practice would normally reach. When networking a position one typically contacts colleagues, local educational institutions, the alma maters of current staff members, and industry contacts (e.g., hearing aid manufacturers or other suppliers).

Networking often turns up candidates that have not actively been searching for positions. It also puts many people to work for the practice at no cost. As an example, there are usually a number of part-time or even full-time potential employees available at area trade schools and local colleges and universities, if only they can be alerted to the existence of positions. Taking the time to meet college administrators and requesting that

Networking is most successful way to recruit employees

position announcements be posted or distributed can be a highly effective and inexpensive form of active networking.

Passive networking can also be effective. Family, friends, and employees are a good source for applicants, partly because they are familiar with the particular business, its operating style, and its needs. However, applicants are often close friends or relatives of employees, which can pose problems down the road if personal loyalty conflicts with company loyalty (Tway, 1992).

Advertising

Help wanted ads in selected local or regional newspapers are often a quick and effective means of filling support positions, particularly when used in conjunction with networking. They typically generate a large number of responses, especially if unemployment is high in the area (Tway, 1992). The ad needs to clearly state job specifications to discourage unqualified respondents. To be effective, the ad must be interesting and concise, give adequate details about the job, and state required skills, education, and experience (Kishel & Kishel, 1993).

State job specifications clearly in the ad

Blind advertising is used when the practice does not want to reveal its intentions to competitors, or when the practice wants to assess the interest or talent available in the community. Blind ads do not identify the practice and use either the publication running the ad or a post office box to receive correspondence.

Local advertising is usually effective when searching for nonprofessional employees, but a national search may be required to find the right audiologist. Openings for Clinical Fellowship positions can be posted at universities or colleges with audiology curricula. Experienced, certified audiologists are often hard to find, because they usually already have positions with employers who wish to keep them. A practice can use direct advertising at conventions (e.g., *ASHA Daily* published at the annual national convention). Professional and trade journals (e.g, *Advance Magazine, Hearing Instruments, The Hearing Journal*) are another avenue. This recruiting method is usually quite lengthy. Publication lead time runs up to 90 days in the journals. Respondents often live in other regions of the country and require a good deal of lead time themselves to arrange time off for travel and interviews. If they accept the position, further time is required for relocation.

Employment Agencies

State and federal employment agencies often maintain lists of unemployed workers in the area, according to job category. This can be a rich source of applicants, especially for nonprofessional positions (Tway, 1992).

Private agencies (also known as "head hunters") will search and do initial screening of candidates. They are most effective for jobs requiring special or professional skills. Private employment agencies are appealing, because if they do not have the right person to fill the position, they will go out and find such people. Agencies demand a premium price for their services, usually 10–30% of the first year's salary when they successfully fill a position. This fee varies with the job, and the agency and is paid either by the applicant or the employer. The ASHA Buyer's Guide lists organizations that specialize in providing temporary and permanent employees for audiology and speech pathology practices.

Only when time demands exceed the concerns for controlling expense should an audiology practice consider using a private employment agency. The size of the practice, however, should not be a deterrent. These agencies can be just as effective for small as for large businesses. If this option is chosen, the owner/manger should interview the agency to find out how reputable they are, ascertain the terms and expectations of the agency and of the practice, and meet with the "head hunter" assigned to the account. Provide this person with as much information as possible about the practice, the position, and the kind of person that is sought for the job (Tway, 1992).

Walk-ins and Write-ins

Sometimes a resume will arrive unexpectedly when an opening has occurred. This is most likely for clerical and front-office positions, where turnover is usually highest. Unsolicited audiology applications and resumes come along also, occasionally at just the right time, but more often in a group just as spring graduation nears. Even if there are no positions available, it is prudent to respond to each applicant, if for no other reasons than to acknowledge them as colleagues, wish them well, guide them to other job openings, and incorporate them into the practice's network. Let them know that their application will be kept active and encourage them to contact the office if they move or get another position.

EMPLOYEE SELECTION

Coincident with the search process, the practice needs to devote time and thought to the screening process. How will applicants be screened? Will they *all* be interviewed (an imposing task if the search process is a help wanted ad)? Will there be a prescreening process? What are the job requirements?

Screening Tools/Procedures

- *Resumes*
- *References*
- *Credit Checks*
- *Application Forms*
- *Skill Tests*

Industry and larger corporations incorporate many tools and procedures in the screening process. These include resumes; references (personal and professional); credit checks; application forms to document work history, possible felony arrests, or substance abuse problems; skill tests; and specific physical examinations to verify health and/or substance use and abuse. Audiology practices need to be aware of these tools and apply those that meet the specific needs of the practice and observe guidelines promulgated by the Equal Employment Opportunity Commission (EEOC).

Blind advertisements used as part of the search process can be useful in screening. Applicants are screened on the basis of resumes and references prior to learning the potential employer's identity. Once this screening reduces the applicant pool to a manageable number, the practice can proceed with a more detailed screening process.

Resumes

Initial screening can be handled very objectively based on resume information. Resumes provide a summary of the applicant's work history, educational background, personal and professional affiliations and accomplishments, as well as any specialized licensing or expertise. A resume also provides insight into an applicant's employment stability, job progression, career motivation, and competency (Desmond, 1994). As Solomon (1991) points out, the resume's style reflects on the candidate's skills and motivation: neat and concise resumes reflect positively, sloppy and disorganized resumes reflect negatively.

Resumes provide source information for probing questions during an interview. The screener needs to review the resume for gaps in the work or educational profile (Croghan, 1993) and obtain explanations for unaccounted for blocks of time when interviewing an otherwise viable candidate.

References

Professional and personal references need to be contacted and asked for letters of reference. Unfortunately, businesses often refuse to provide any more than the dates of employment, last position held, and the last salary the applicant was paid. This is a matter of policy to protect themselves from the threat of lawsuits (Weiner, 1993). Desmond (1994) suggests that "carefully thought-out telephone interviews with reference sources can yield information that they might be hesitant or unable to put in writing" (p. 67). If the telephone interview yields negative information, care must be taken subsequently to protect the source. One question that may elicit a written or oral answer from a reference source is: "Would you hire this person back?" Sometimes, a failure to respond to this question is as meaningful as a response.

"Would you hire this person back?"

Application Forms

These forms are used to develop profiles of applicants so that viable candidates are identified and others are disqualified early in the process. The forms are designed to obtain relevant information allowed by law, such as:

- a list of previous residences,
- social security number,
- arrests and convictions,
- illegal substance use,
- credit history,
- current and expected compensation.

For example, a standardized release signed by the applicant can allow the practice to run a credit check through the same agencies that banks, other lenders, or major corporations use.

It is prudent to identify potential problems that information from the application form may reveal. Employees, associates, or partners with financial, legal, and/or addictive problems can have a devastating effect on the reputation or finances of a small practice (Croghan, 1993). However, application forms must be structured to protect the legal rights of applicants. For example, Title I of the Americans with Disabilities Act bans questions on the application or in the interview about an applicant's physical or mental condition (e.g., "Do you have any mental or physical conditions that would prevent you from performing your job functions?").

ADA bans some questions

Samples of application forms and other standardized forms can be found in the business sections of libraries and some bookstores. One example is contained in Appendix 11-B. An attorney can review and modify these sample forms to meet the specific needs of an audiology practice.

Interviewing

The interview is the final screening performed on a reduced list of candidates. Ideally, viable candidates should be interviewed by several people in the practice. Welch and Fowler (1994) provide a good overview of interviewing techniques. The interview should be conducted in private, in a quiet location without interruptions. The screener should get the applicant to do most of the talking, rather than dominating the interview.

The screener needs to be aware of all the facts when screening candidates. Use a quick check to verify the credit report against the resume. Most people need jobs to maintain their credit obligations. If the applicant's credit weakened coincident with being out of work, the candidate may still be a strong contender for an open position (Walberg, 1993).

The interview should be designed to gather more information about the candidate, such as:

■ Is the candidate organized and concise?
■ What is his or her level of maturity and self-awareness?
■ What are the candidate's motivators, values, or attitudes?
■ Does the person match the job and criteria?
■ How does the person handle stress and what is this candidate's market value?

Questions designed to help the interviewer obtain this information are given in texts on interviewing (Yate, 1987).

The following are a few examples of interviewing questions designed to elicit different kinds of information:

1. Is the person organized, concise, and prepared?
   - *Tell me about yourself.*
   - *Define success and have you been successful?*

2. What is this person's sense of awareness and maturity?
   - *What are your weak points?*
   - *Has your work ever been criticized and how did you handle it?*

3. What are this person's motivators, values, and attitudes?
   - *How would your co-workers describe you?*
   - *What are you looking for in this job?*
   - *What kind of hours do you work?*
   - *What was the last book you read?*

4. Is this person a match?
   - *What can you do for us?*
   - *What are your goals?*
   - *Can you work under pressure and meet deadlines? Describe situations.*

5. What is this person's confidence level and ability to handle stress?
   - *How would you structure this job?*
   - *Why should we hire you?*

Caution must be exercised in the screening and interview process. The process (and questions) should be applied consistently to all candidates. The EEOC statutes and the Americans With Disabilities Act, specifically limit or eliminate questions that could be construed as discriminatory (Jenkins, 1993; Welch & Fowler, 1994). Questions that ask about age, race, religion, marital status, child care arrangements, transportation, or handicaps are prohibited by law. Appendix 11-C gives examples of acceptable and unacceptable questions. The interviewer can use open-ended questions to afford the candidate an opportunity to provide restricted information on a voluntary basis.

Tests

Finally, the practice may use tests to evaluate candidates. Clerical skills can be assessed by typing, math, filing tests, or observation of computer use. Professional skills can be observed by having the audiologists work with patients, or by posing clinical questions (Desmond, in 1994).

Under certain highly restricted conditions,[1] applicants may be asked to take simple health examinations to ensure that they have no communicable diseases that pose a threat to patients (although this cannot be used as grounds for not hiring). They may also take a urine test to determine substance use or abuse. The audiological practice often operates in close proximity with other health care providers. It is very detrimental to the practice's reputation if an employee or associate is suspected or caught abusing substances illegally in the medical environment.

HIRING

Negotiating

When the selection process is completed, the best candidate is contacted for a final interview. A variety of topics is addressed in the final interview to tie up any loose ends, check the focus of the candidate, answer questions the candidate may have, and be as sure as possible that this is the right person for the position.

Discussion topics at this appointment include the job description, terms of employment, probationary period (if applicable), future career development, noncompetition agreement, and expectations of the candidate. If the owner/manager has any lingering doubts at this point, it is better to schedule another interview than to proceed with an offer.

Tway (1992) suggests waiting at least 24 hours after the final interview before making an offer, even if the offer is sure to be made. She reasons that an immediate offer suggests desperation on the part of the business and shifts the onus for succeeding from the employee to the business. Tway suggests that employees who feel lucky to be hired are more personally motivated to succeed.

If all goes well in the final interview, an offer is made to the candidate. The offer includes a reiteration of the job

---

[1]Title I of the Americans with Disabilities Act places severe restrictions on the use of health examinations in the screening and hiring process. Pre-offer examinations are prohibited but the ADA does not prohibit voluntary tests. An offer may be contingent on satisfactory results of a medical examination, but results cannot be used to withdraw the offer unless they show that the potential employee is unable to perform tasks required of the job. The ADA includes people with AIDS, HIV virus, and rehabilitated drug abusers (including alcohol) in its definition of "disabled." The ADA does not require, however,that employers hire persons who are known drug users or who have contagious diseases. The ADA leaves regulations on drug testing of employees to the individual states (Jenkins, 1993).

description, followed by discussion of basic office policies, and the proposed salary/benefits package. Compensation levels vary from one community to another and also according to current market conditions in the community (e.g., need, economy, number of qualified applications). This places the burden on the practice to determine current market conditions and make an appropriate offer. There is often some trial and error in the procedure, and additional negotiations are not uncommon before the practice and the candidate agree to a final package.

Most private practice employer-employee arrangements in audiology are "at will" agreements, meaning that the employee can be discharged at any time without cause due to the "needs of the business" (i.e., a downturn in the practice). If a position is at will, it is very important to make this clear in the negotiations and avoid any verbal or written promises about longevity, promotion, or salary increases. Failure to do so could result in wrongful discharge claims.

"At will" employment

If the applicant accepts the offer of employment, the employer is required under federal law to check for alien status. The new employee must complete a Form I-9 (Employment Eligibility Verification) showing proof of United States citizenship, a certificate of naturalization, an alien registration card, or an unexpired INS Employment Authorization with proper passport identification.

Employment Agreements

Once an offer is accepted, the employee should be informed of a start date, told what time to come, how to dress, and who to see upon arrival (Tway, 1992). Most importantly, the employee should be provided with a written version of the final package, known as a service contract or employment agreement. The service contract should state whether the employee is "at will," and describe compensation, termination provisions, restrictive provisions, time to be devoted to the business, vacation and sick days, and any fringe benefits that will be provided. A simple example of an "at will" employee agreement is shown in Appendix 11-D for Cardinal Hearing Services, Inc. The agreement should be reviewed by the employee and signed by the employee and owner/manager.

Restrictive Provisions

Restrictive provisions in an employment agreement are meant to protect the employer by:

- ensuring that while the employee works for the practice, and for some time after termination, the employee will not interfere with the practice's patients (a nonsolicitation clause) and
- protecting and ensuring return of confidential business information, including patient data, pricing, and "trade secret" types of information and intellectual property (e.g., forms, correspondence, proprietary software, marketing formats) (an anti-piracy clause).

At the same time, employees must be protected from entering into restrictive agreements that prevent them from earning a living in the community. In the same vein, restrictive covenants cannot prevent terminated employees from using skills they have learned or exercising talents they have developed on the job.

Restrictions must be narrow and fair

For these reasons, restrictive provisions must be narrow in scope as to time and geographical location. In practical terms, the agreement must be fair to both parties to prevent lawsuits and ensure compliance. Reasonable geographical boundaries need to be specified and noncompete time should reflect the time it would take to fully train another employee, or no longer than 1 year.

Finally, a restrictive covenant needs a "comprehensive severability clause." Such a clause allows the scope of the agreement to be narrowed by legal decree but still enforced.

Orientation

The hiring and training process are essential to the early success of the employee and the long-term success of the practice. As the first few months are usually probationary, a comprehensive orientation gives the new employee the best chance to become a contributing member of the staff. It allows the owner/manager an opportunity to monitor the employee's progress. If an obvious mismatch has occurred, it is the responsibility of the owner/manager to correct the situation quickly. Sometimes in large organizations this means finding another position within the organization where the person can still contribute. In a small practice it usually means letting the person go. *It is much easier to let someone go during the probationary period than it is to keep a marginal employee too long and have to go through termination procedures later.*

Orientation provides an opportunity to demonstrate leadership and to coach the new employee. Careful orientation procedures help maintain an employee's confidence, communicate and reinforce practice policies and procedures, and address positive as well as negative behaviors. Employee confidence and satisfaction increases as the knowledge of the job expectations are communicated and reinforced (Welch & Fowler, 1994).

As part of the hiring process, clearly defining the training objectives and responsibilities must be done during orientation. Start with a broad outline of the operational, administrative, and interpersonal objectives that are desired and begin defining the specific goals and objectives under each heading. Assign responsibilities for each item, set target dates and document the plan. Discuss the Performance Evaluation form (an example form is shown in Appendix 11-C) and how training goals relate to performance evaluation. Again, avoid making verbal promises such as "You seem to be picking this up quickly. I'm sure you'll have a long future here" that could result in a disaster (e.g., the employee purchasing a new home) if the practice declines unexpectedly.

Well documented orientation procedures define objectives and set goals

TRAINING

Training is vitally important in bringing the new employee or associate into the practice. Training provides an early opportunity for the practice to demonstrate that what it states as important and what it does in reality are one and the same. If a practice states that training is important, but its actions relegate training to a low priority, then much of the practice belief structure will be questioned. This does not put the full burden of training on management. New employees or associates have an obligation to aggressively avail themselves of opportunities during business hours and on their own to become contributing members of the practice. The manager of the practice needs to convey that obligation clearly.

Training is a responsibility of management and the employee

For the practice, a well-trained individual becomes effective more quickly, thereby reducing frustration on the part of the new members as well as existing staff. Training can also ensure long-term employee effectiveness by anticipating and preventing problem employee situations. Preventive personnel policies are achieved by clearly communicating policies during orientation and posting office policies prominently in the workplace (Gardiner, 1990).

Training often brings to light existing procedures that have become inefficient, redundant, or are no longer needed. An enterprise that declares it is a quality organization needs to constantly search for ways to improve itself and the delivery of its service to the patient.

All practices need Procedures Manuals

Management input is key to employee training. Only management can adequately convey what is truly expected from the candidate (Walton, 1986). A Procedures Manual facilitates the training process. Large clinics almost always maintain Procedures Manuals, but small practices may not have one, on the premise that it is unnecessary to document the actions of a few employees who do "everything" in close proximity. Indeed, it is often quite difficult to persuade employees to document actions that they have come to take for granted. The error of this premise becomes obvious immediately upon hiring a new person for whom nothing can be taken for granted. If a practice does not have a Procedures Manual, it may be a wise investment to have the new employee create one during the training process and review and correct it with management. Creating the document reinforces the employee's new knowledge. It also gives the owner/manager insight into the employee's perception of the tasks associated with the job. Once more, however, care must be taken that the manual does not contain performance-related language that makes apparent "promises" relating skill acquisition with longevity, promotion, and salary increases. Such language may be interpreted as contractually binding.

Scenario 11–1 describes a situation in which a practice's normal operating procedure is criticized by a new employee and scrutinized by management, eventually requiring either reorientation of the employee or procedure changes that need to be documented in the procedures manual.

SCENARIO 11-1

Ms. C has come forward with a complaint. She has only been with CHS a short time, but feels she is not getting a fair shake on her patient contacts. Mr. B has been with CHS much longer, but to Ms. C it seems unfair that Dr. A and Mr. B get a much more varied and financially rewarding patient mix.

It is common at CHS to start out new staff members with a patient mix heavily weighted toward patients on public assistance. The advantage to this approach is that the services are fairly standardized, and the staff member gets experience dealing with agency protocols. From a compensation point of view this approach makes no difference in the first year. But, after the first year employees can augment their salaries with commissions by achieving certain performance criteria. At this point, patient mix is important because revenues from private patients are usually higher.

ANALYSIS:

CHS, for whatever its reasons, assigns public assistance patients to its less-experienced staff. On the surface this provides a captive population for training and familiarization with procedures, leaving the rest of the patient base for the more experienced staff members. This approach ensures that the higher revenue-base patient population is seen by staff members who, through experience, represent the corporate culture of the practice.

Questions and Management Suggestions for Dr. A

Question 1: Does Ms. C's complaint have merit? Is she being discriminated against in her patient contacts?

Suggested Answer: Ms. C's complaint is probably without merit. It is a form of discrimination only in the context that a choice is made, but it is made only on the basis of experience and training. If the patient mix continues past its normal time frame, Ms. C may have a more valid complaint or management may have a performance issue with the staff member in question.

Question 2: Should Dr. A look at how CHS assigns appointments and determine if this approach to patient management is in the best interest of the patients and CHS?

Suggested Answer: This question is valid in any situation. Any quality conscious organization needs to periodically review how it conducts its business to ensure that it is always striving for a "constancy of improvement," particularly where patient service is involved.

Question 3: Should Dr. A review this training approach and determine how rigid or flexible it really is?

Suggested Answer: Reviewing this training approach for its rigidity or flexibility may have some validity. Generally, the practice will find that its quality people are ready for more challenging assignments before any stated calendar time. The demands of a growing and healthy practice tend to bring people along just slightly faster than they feel ready to go. Ms. C may be exceptional, or she may need counseling on what she needs to accomplish at this point in her career and how she fits into the overall view of CHS.

Question 4: Based on the overall assessment, how should Dr. A proceed?

(continued)

SCENARIO 11–1 *(continued)*

Suggested Answer: Dr. A should look at a couple of factors in this situation. First, Dr. A (perhaps together with Mr. B) needs to review how she feels about this approach to patient service and staff training. If she is comfortable with this approach, she should so state. If she is not, she should solicit and introduce modifications.

Second, if Ms. C has a valid complaint, Dr. A needs to rectify the situation and determine how it happened. If the complaint is not valid, then Ms. C needs to be apprised of the findings and reoriented to the goals and policies of CHS.

The worst possible situation is having employees teaching employees, especially if they are teaching without management-developed training materials. This situation is much like the game of "gossip": an employee teaches his or her own edited version of the position to someone who will further edit because there is no basis being taught for performing tasks. It is important that the philosophy and reasoning behind the procedures are taught with the procedures.

Operationally, the modern practice may have many pieces of diagnostic equipment from a number of manufacturers. Unless the new employee is proficient on specific equipment, an orientation on each piece should occur. Of course, the orientation must be tailored to the overall experience level of the new employee. A check off list of current equipment should be used to document this aspect of the training process.

The practice needs to maintain a centralized file that contains manuals and documentation for all installed equipment to serve as a ready reference when questions do arise. The new employee should be indoctrinated into the use and maintenance of this file. That means new manuals are added when new equipment is installed and old manuals removed when equipment is replaced. Individuals or groups that receive old equipment are generally amazed and pleased to receive the original documentation with the equipment.

Computers are used in many aspects of the modern practice. They are used in direct patient care as well as the administrative portions of the practice. Training in the use of the hardware as well as familiarity with the various software products used to run a modern office will require time. The training period needs to reflect this obligation. Again, prior background can make this transition period vary from a matter of hours to many weeks. The search and screening process provides indications of the training requirements.

Each practice has numerous unique procedures. Many actions taken each day are habitual to the existing staff. The new person often feels overwhelmed even answering the telephone or getting the mail. For example, how does the practice handle the mail? Is it delivered? Where? When? Who should pick it up? How is it sorted? How does mail go out? How are hearing aids handled? Are the same procedures used for new aids as those returned from repair? How are they shipped? How are they received? Are they checked out once they are received? Are they logged in and where? When is the patient notified? These are simple questions when one knows the answers. A new employee or associate assimilates quickly when provided with a ready reference that answers these questions. Again, a Procedures Manual that documents some or all of these procedures is vitally important. It relieves stress on new employees and keeps them from constantly interrupting office flow to ask how to do simple tasks such as how to sell batteries to a drop-in patient.

WILLING WORKERS

The principal responsibility of management is leadership. Modern experts on management, such as W. Edwards Deming, stress that leadership means that management provides an environment in which employees take pride, and that management has discovered and eliminated barriers to the success of the employees and the organization. This is the basis of point seven of the well-known 14 points[2] outlined by Deming for effective management (Walton, 1986). With few exceptions, failure on the part of an employee is usually failure in the system. For further discussion on management styles and leadership, see Chapter 20.

Periodic performance evaluations (see an example in Appendix 11–E) are useful, but their purpose should be to provide feedback and coaching, not to keep employees "in line."

Problem Resolution

Problems can arise even with the best of employees and it is the manager's responsibility to identify, address, and resolve these problems in a dignified and fair manner. Gardiner (1990) sets forth a series of steps for management solution of employee problems and problem employees. Gardiner briefly summarizes the steps in the following quote, but it is well worth reading Gardiner's entire book before implementing them.

---

[2]See Chapter 13 for a list and discussion of Deming's 14 points.

Step I: Act and Set Up the Interview

1. Intervene early—take action when the problem becomes apparent.
2. Ask for (do not demand) a private meeting with the employee.
3. Ask the employee to be seated, either face to face with no desk intervening, or with the employee seated at the corner of a desk.
4. Treat the employee courteously, as an adult.
5. If it will help relax the employee, start with a short period of work-related small talk.

Step II. State the Problem

1. State the problem specifically, objectively, and factually in a calm and matter of fact manner.
2. Rehearse the statement of the problem.
3. Don't preach, accuse, intimidate, or tell the employee you're the boss.
4. Use an open-ended question to get the employee talking (e.g., "Could you tell me what happened?")

Step III. Be Fair and Clarify the Problem

1. Do not appear judgmental. Use repetition, paraphrasing, and summarization to clarify what the employee is saying.
2. Listen to the employee rather than talk.
3. Ask direct factual questions to get the employee to talk.
4. Do not agree or disagree with the employee. If disagreement occurs, stop and set a time to talk again.

Step IV. Get a Promise of Action from the Employee to Solve the Problem

1. Depending on the severity of the problem and the employee's attitude, the employee can either volunteer to take action that will clear up the problem or suggest an action plan. If the employee is reluctant to take action, ask or tell the employee to take action. If necessary, spell out the consequences of not taking action, including termination.
2. If formal disciplinary action becomes necessary, follow the sequence of steps required by [the] organization and make genuine offer to help before firing the employee.
3. When all other interventions fail, you terminate the employee. You always terminate because of the employee's *failure to perform satisfactorily*. You terminate because you were *left with no choice*, and you terminate with regret, but with finality. (Gardiner, 1990, p. 118)

Terminating an employee is emotionally one of the hardest tasks an owner/manager can undertake. Once the decision has been reached, the employer needs to act decisively. The employer needs to schedule an interview period that is not to be interrupted. The time should be during business hours, preferably early in the day and no later than mid-week. The employer needs to be prepared at the interview to discuss the reasons for firing, financial matters such as severance pay and accumulated vacation pay, and the effective date of termination. There are situations when the date is immediate and the person is terminated and escorted out the door at the conclusion of the interview. The employer is the judge of when these situations exist.

When terminating an employee, employers must heed basic rules to protect themselves against potential defamation suits:

1. Document and be absolutely certain of the "factual circumstances" when terminating an employee.
2. Do not allow anything in the employee's personnel file that cannot be substantiated.
3. Restrict information on the particulars of the termination to only those persons who absolutely need to know.
4. Do not make an example of a terminated employee as an indirect means of discouraging similar behavior in other employees. If it is absolutely necessary to make an example, be sure to know all the facts before making an announcement. Make sure the announcement contains only proven facts.
5. Do not give oral or written references to prospective employers without the written consent of the ex-employee.
6. In giving a reference, do not provide any information except dates of employment and position held.

In all cases, the employer should arrange for a trusted employee or colleague to be on the premises during the termination interview. For a small practice, this can be under the guise of being on hand to cover the telephones during the interview. The associate is not there to witness the interview, but to provide assistance in the rare but unfortunate instance when an interview gets out of control.

The employer must ensure that no employee is wrongfully discharged. Examples of wrongful discharge are: (a) calculated firing of an employee to avoid vesting and paying of benefits from a qualified retirement plan and (b) terminating an employee who was promised (orally or in writing) that he or she would not be terminated. However, the courts have ruled that employees who have received such promises can be terminated without just cause for economic reasons (e.g., an economic downturn that is beyond the employer's control).

SUMMARY

Advance planning will help the beginning practice identify staff requirements as early as the writing of the initial business plan. Identifying the skills the practice needs clarifies the screening and selection process.

In the areas of recruiting and selecting staff, audiology practices differ little from other businesses or industries. Using established search techniques, selection tools, and working with outside resources will assist the practice in efficiently addressing its staffing requirements.

Training new employees and associates provides the practice with an early opportunity to demonstrate its basic beliefs and operating philosophy. A successful training program removes ambiguity, relieves stress, and accelerates the contribution of new employees. A comprehensive and up-to-date Procedures Manual is essential.

Termination of employment is an unfortunate situation, the incidence of which can be significantly reduced by skilled hiring, training, and leadership. The owner/manager who assumes the responsibilities and obligations of leadership will successfully address the human resources aspects of the practice. This in turn will contribute to the long-term success of the practice. If termination must occur, it should be done decisively and performed in a manner that avoids potential defamation suits.

REFERENCES

Calabresi, M., Van Tassel, J., Riley, M., & Szczesny, J. R. (1993, November 22). Jobs in an age of insecurity. *Time Magazine*, pp. 31–39.

Chaney, D. (1994). *Overview of the closely-held business formation process.* Tucson: State Bar of Arizona.

Croghan, L. (1993, October 18). Theft by employees: A costly problem. *The Arizona Daily Star*, p. D1.

Desmond, A. (1994). Personnel management. In H. Hosford-Dunn, J. Baxter, A. Desmond, G. Jacobson, J. Johnson, P. Martin, & E. Cherow (Eds.), *Development and management of audiology practices* (chap 10, pp. 67–70). Rockville, MD: ASHA.

Drucker, P. (1992). *Managing for the future.* New York: Truman Talley Books/Plume.

Gardiner, G. (1990). *Tough-minded management.* New York: Fawcett Columbine.

Greco, S. (1992, July). The complete new-business survival guide. *Inc. Magazine*, pp. 49–66.

Jenkins, M. D. (1993). *Starting and operating a business in Arizona.* Grants Pass, OR: Oasis Press.

Kishel, G. F., & Kishel, P. G. (1993). *How to start, run, and stay in business.* New York: John Wiley.

Rizzo, S. R., Jr., & Frame, R. T. (1994). Foundations of leadership, management, and supervision. In S.R. Rizzo, Jr. & M.D. Trudeau (Eds.), *Clinical administration in audiology and speech-language pathology* (chap. 1, pp. 1–32). San Diego, CA: Singular Publishing Group.

Siropolis, N. (1990). *Small business management.* Boston: Houghton Mifflin.

Solomon, R. (1991). *Clinical practice management* (chap. 3). Gaithersburg, MD: Aspen.

Tway, P. (1992). *People, common sense and the small business.* Crozet, VA: Betterway.

Walberg, M. (1993, October 18). Applicant's bad credit may be due to job loss during recession. *The Arizona Daily Star,* p. D4.

Walton, M. (1986). *The Deming management method.* New York: Perigee Books.

Weiner, T. (1993, May 17). Mum's the word. *The Arizona Daily* Star, p. D8.

Welch, C., & Fowler, K. (1994). Human resource management. In S. R. Rizzo, Jr., & M. D. Trudeau (Eds.), *Clinical administration in audiology and speech-language pathology* (chap. 4, pp. 93–132). San Diego, CA: Singular Publishing Group.

Yate, M. J. (1987). *A manager's guide to effective interviewing.* Hanover, MA: Adams.

APPENDIX 11-A

Sample Job Description For An Audiologist At Cardinal Hearing Services, Inc.

TITLE: Senior Audiologist

JOB STATEMENT: Within the scope of audiology practice, determines patient's needs and provides patient care. This person has the skills, training, and professional manner necessary to operate patient care portions of the practice with minimal supervision. At all times, this person contributes to the marketing of quality by the practice by maintaining high standards of professional and personal conduct in all oral and written communications with patients, referral sources, and suppliers.

MAJOR DUTIES:
1. Arrives for work promptly and professionally attired.
2. Greets patients cheerfully and courteously, addressing their needs as first priority.
3. Performs diagnostic audiologic evaluations on adults and children, including tone and speech audiometry, PI functions, and acoustic immittance. Dates, signs, and completes all test forms, including identification of word lists, head phone type, labeling of acoustic reflex thresholds on the audiogram.
4. Performs hearing aid consultations, fittings, orientations, checks (electroacoustic, acoustic, and sound field), cleanings, and minor repairs. Takes ear impressions. Listens carefully to patients' comments about amplification. Is knowledgeable of new technology and appropriate applications, and provides concise summaries of amplification options to patients.
5. Prepares hearing aid orders (new and repair) and packages them correctly for Airborne pickup and delivery.
6. Prepares and sends formal reports to referral sources within 24 hours of evaluation. Reports are accurate, concise, and comprehensive. Less formal follow-up reports may be handwritten, but are also completed within 24 hours of encounter.
7. Documents all patient encounters in computerized patient chart notes, identifying date of encounter, provider's initials, and a brief summary of encounter.
8. Handles incoming patient or referral calls on an as-needed basis. Provides information in a courteous and complete manner (including fee and insurance billing information); schedules appropriately in terms of time and clinician assignment; answers general questions thoughtfully and respectfully.

MINOR DUTIES:
1. Removes cerumen when necessary and with the informed consent of the patient. Uses accepted procedures, extreme care, and antiseptic techniques.
2. Works on "team basis" with other staff, helping with testing, hearing aid checks, paperwork, cerumen management, and so on, on an as-needed basis.
3. Participates in training entry level audiologists and office staff by providing written instruction, observation, and commentary in a supportive manner.
4. Participates in ongoing chart analysis by reviewing computerized files, contacting patients for follow-up, correcting patient information in files (e.g., telephone number, change of address), and transferring inactive files to storage.

SHARED DUTIES:
5. Participates in performing office work as needed, including:
   a. places supply orders (e.g., batteries, ear impression materials, mailing boxes) on a timely basis, as needed.
   b. Prepares routine marketing projects (e.g., birthday card mailing list and labels; warranty notices) in a timely manner.
   c. Records financial transactions on daily production sheet, updating Accounts Receivable as payments are generated or received. Totals daily production sheet, completes daily deposit, and insures that they match.
   d. Chart preparation and reminder calls for scheduled patients; mail handling; matching of invoices to statements; filing of invoices; coffee table preparation; mailing labels; trash; recycling.
   e. Files charts accurately and in a timely fashion.
   f. Other duties as assigned.

RELATIONSHIPS: Reports to the office manager (i.e., owner). Provides supervision to other audiologist(s) and front office personnel at the direction of the office manager.

EDUCATION: Master's degree in Audiology, Certificate of Clinical Competence in Audiology (CCC-A)

EXPERIENCE: 3–5 years of significant clinical experience in audiology.

SKILLS: Must be able to operate test and repair equipment; operate computer equipment; use software for data bases, word processing, and scheduling; interact well with people.

APPENDIX 11-B

Sample Employment Application

Name_____ SSN:_____

Current Address_____

_____ # Yrs:_____

Previous Address_____

_____ # Yrs:_____

Telephone_____

May we contact your present and previous employers?_____

If yes, list any employers you do not wish us to contact: _____

Employment History (Last position first)

Company Name:_____From:_____To:_____

Address:_____#Hours/Wk:_____

_____Position:_____

Supervisor:_____

Reason for Leaving:_____

Company Name:_____From:_____To:_____

Address:_____#Hours/Wk:_____

_____Position:_____

Supervisor:_____

Reason for Leaving:_____

Company Name:_____From:_____To:_____

Address:_____#Hours/Wk:_____

_____Position:_____

Supervisor:_____

Reason for Leaving:_____

Education

Name/Address	Graduated?	Degree/Date

1._____

2._____

3._____

References

Name/Address	Telephone	Relationship
1.		
2.		

Remarks:_____

_____

_____

I understand that if I am employed and any statement is then found to be not true, I may be released immediately.

Signature_____Date_____

APPENDIX 11–C

Guidelines Regarding Discriminatory Questions

Acceptable Questions	Unacceptable Questions
Have you ever used another name?	What is your maiden name?
What is your place of residence?	Do you own or rent your home?
Can you show proof of age?	How old are you?
Are you over 18 years old?	What is your birthdate?
Can you provide verification of your right to work in the US?	Are you a US citizen? Where were you born?
What languages can you speak, read, or write?	What is your native tongue? Where were your parents born?
Can you perform the functions of this job with or without reasonable accommodation?	Do you have any physical disabilities?
How would you perform these functions?	Do you have a disability that would interfere with your ability to perform the job?
Can you meet the attendance requirements of this job?	How many days were you sick last year?
How many days of leave did you take last year?	Do you have AIDS? Do you have asthma?
Have you ever been convicted of a felony?	Have you ever been arrested?
What skills have you acquired through military service?	When did you serve in the military? How discharged?
What professional organizations do you belong to?	What organizations or clubs do you belong to?
	What is your height, weight?
	What race are you?
	What does your spouse do?
	How many children do you have?
	Their ages?

Source: Adapted from Kishel and Kishel, 1993, and Equal Employment Opportunity Commission (EEOC) employment guidelines

Note: For further information, the EEOC has recently published a document entitled *Enforcement Guidance on Preemployment Disability-Related Inquiries and Medical Examinations Under the Americans with Disabilities Act of 1990.*

APPENDIX 11-D

Sample Employment Agreement[1]

NOTE: This is a straightforward "at will" employment agreement suitable for a nonowner employee who is paid on an hourly basis. It is especially applicable for part-time employees. It contains various restrictions as to customer contact and protection of business information after termination as well as restriction on setting up a competing business. It could easily be revised to include other items discussed in the text of this chapter.

It is noted the compensation provision includes additional compensation ($25) intended to be consideration for being bound by the restrictive provisions which is consideration in addition to employment and payment of wages.

EMPLOYER: Cardinal Hearing Services, Inc.

EMPLOYEE: Mr. B

Position:_____

In consideration of employee's employment by Cardinal Hearing Services, Inc. (employer), employee agrees to all of the following terms and conditions including the restrictive provisions.

EMPLOYEE COMPENSATION: The employee shall be paid the following initial hourly rate for all hours of service on behalf of employer: $_____. It is acknowledged employer has not guaranteed employee any specific number of hours of work and pay per week or otherwise; however, it is agreed employer shall pay employee at the stated hourly rate and shall be responsible for withholdings and paying payroll taxes including the employer's share as well as worker's compensation on behalf of employee. Additional consideration to employee: employee acknowledges the receipt of a $25 check from employer upon execution of this agreement as additional consideration for entering into this agreement including being bound by the restrictive provisions of this agreement. Employee acknowledges he has had adequate time to review and understand this agreement and further states the restrictions are reasonable in time and space for the protection of employer's business and profitability and needed customer retention.

EMPLOYMENT AT WILL: Employee agrees employment at all times is "at will" meaning either the employer or the employee may terminate employment at any time with or without cause with employee to be immediately paid any due compensation. Employee acknowledges no statements, representations, or promises as to employment longevity have been made to employee whatsoever.

COVENANT NOT TO COMPETE: Employee agrees during the term of this employment and for a period of 1 year following termination not to engage as owner or investor in any or all portion of a business which directly or indirectly competes in_____ County in the same or similar audiology/hearing aid dispensing business as employer. The parties acknowledge this provision does not prohibit employee from being employed as an employee or contractor by a similar business and that employee, therefore, is not prohibited from using general skills learned while working for another employer.

NONSOLICITATION OF CUSTOMERS OF EMPLOYER: Employee agrees that during the term of employment and 1 year following termination that employee will not in the State

---

[1]Adapted from Chaney, 1994.

of _____, solicit, directly or indirectly, any customer of employer for services in any way related to audiology or hearing aid dispensing.

PROTECTION OF CONFIDENTIAL BUSINESS INFORMATION: Employee agrees upon termination to return all forms belonging to the employer as well as any other items related to the employer's method of business. Employee further agrees upon termination not to use any of said forms of items without obtaining written permission from the employer. Employee agrees not to use or divulge information from records of patients associated with the employer, or any information regarding those patients. Employee acknowledges that these files and information are confidential and are the sole property of the employer.

UTILIZATION OF EMPLOYER EQUIPMENT: Employee agrees at all times when any job whatsoever is done using the employer equipment that employee shall always represent that the job is being completed by Cardinal Hearing Services, Inc. All billings and fees for such jobs shall be tendered by employee to employer.

INJUNCTIVE RELIEF: Employee acknowledges violation of covenant not to compete and nonsolicitation obligations will cause employer irreparable harm and the remedy at law for such breach will be inadequate and damages flowing from such breaches is not readily susceptible to being measured in monetary terms. Therefore, employee agrees that employer is entitled to protection from such violations, including immediate protection by injunctive relief, in addition to all other remedies available under law.

MERGER: This agreement contains the complete agreement and understanding between employer and employee and this agreement may not be enlarged or modified except by writing executed by both parties.

RECOVERY OF EXPENSES: The parties agree in the event of breach of this contract, the breaching party will pay the other part costs and reasonable attorney fees incurred because of the breach whether a lawsuit is instituted or not.

SEVERABILITY: If any provision of this agreement is declared void and unenforceable, such provision shall be deemed severed from this agreement which shall otherwise remain in full force and effect. Further, if any such provision may be reduced and/or narrowed in scope or the like, such provision shall be reduced, narrowed, and/or the like, and so enforced. Additionally, in the event any term or provision of this agreement is declared to be illegal or invalid, because of the duration or geographic scope, such term or provision shall be reduced to the extent necessary to become enforceable, and shall be enforced as so reduced. The parties to this agreement acknowledge and agree the geographic scope and time period as to the respective restrictive covenant are reasonable and necessary for the protection of the business of employer including customer "base" and profitability.

WAIVER OF BREACH: Any failure by employer to insist upon strict adherence to any term(s) of this agreement on any occasion shall not be considered a waiver or deprive employer of the right thereafter to insist upon strict adherence to any term of this agreement.

EMPLOYEE ACKNOWLEDGEMENT AND UNDERSTANDING: By signature below employee acknowledges and signifies that employee has carefully read this entire agreement containing various restrictions against employee and has had time to consider the terms, including the opportunity to have it reviewed by independent counsel, and fully understands and agrees to all such provisions including the restrictive provisions.

Date of Execution: _____

_____
Dr. A, Owner, Cardinal Hearing Services, Inc.

_____
Mr. B, Employee, Cardinal Hearing Services, Inc.

APPENDIX 11–E

Sample Performance Evaluation

POSITION: Senior Audiologist

PERFORMANCE STANDARDS: This position is evaluated according to performance in three areas with the following weightings: <u>Operations (40%), Relationships (35%), and Administration (25%)</u>. While a person holding a senior position is expected to set an example in all areas, performance is weighted to reflect the time and importance associated with each area.

OPERATIONS: Performs diagnostic evaluations within the scope and standards of the audiology practice. This includes completing all records and forms as required in the job description. Prepares and sends formal reports to referral sources within 24 hours of encounter. Takes ear impressions, participates in hearing aid consultations, fittings, orientations, checks, cleanings, and minor repairs. Performs cerumen management in accordance with accepted procedures and techniques.

Comments:

Rating: Always   1   2   3   4   5   Almost Never

RELATIONSHIPS: Greets patients cheerfully and courteously, addressing their needs as first priority. Listens carefully to patients and provides them with knowledgeable, appropriate, and concise summaries of their hearing status and treatment options. Maintains a high standard of conduct in all communications with patients, referral sources and suppliers. Participates in training of entry level audiologists and office staff and works to maintain morale and teamwork.

Comments:

Rating: Always   1   2   3   4   5   Almost Never

ADMINISTRATION: Documents all patient encounters in computerized patient chart notes. Participates in on-going chart analysis and patient follow-up. Files charts accurately and in a timely manner. Performs office work as needed (e.g., ordering supplies, matching and filing invoices, patient warranty activities, minor bookkeeping, marketing efforts, and general housekeeping).

Comments:

Rating: Always   1   2   3   4   5   Almost Never

OVERALL: Reflects the weighted average of the above areas as well as any additional factors.

Comments:

Rating: Always   1   2   3   4   5   Almost Never

Signature Employee_____ Date_____

Signature Supervisor _____ Date_____

12

Managerial Accounting and Financial Analysis

> *Business in audiology is sometimes likened to unethical professional conduct. Thus, many audiologists disdain the "money end" of their practices. The consequence is a slipshod organization.*

Audiologists tend to categorize their activities into "professional" and "business" functions. Professional activities are those things that are taught in a traditional master's level graduate curriculum. They are grouped together under the rubric of "clinical services." On the other hand, *business activities are nonclinical requirements of audiology practices* that have rarely been included in professional training programs. Business activities are loosely grouped together under the rubric of "money." As money is the root of all evil, business enterprise in audiology is likened on occasion to unethical or shoddy professional conduct.[1] Thus, this categorization scheme establishes an artificial and adversarial relationship between the essential activities that autonomous audiologists must perform in order to maintain their practices. The unfortunate result is that many audiologists disdain the "money end" of their organizations, leaving accounting and financial analyses to their office managers, their accountants, administrators, and to chance. The consequence is a slipshod organization in which the ultimate losers are the patients and the audiologist.

---

[1] As an example: "We have always been driven by a purpose to educate our consumers and act in the spirit of public service, which differentiates us from the business section. For this reason, there will always be ethical conflicts between those strictly pursuing business interests and persons working in the professional spirit of public service" (Trace, 1993, p. 16).

The purpose of this chapter is not to instruct audiologists on how to get rich. Rather, it is to inform those in practice on how to use accounting and financial methods to maintain and improve their service delivery. These methods are a fundamental ingredient in becoming professionally autonomous, and at the time of this writing, these subjects are not included in the typical audiology curriculum.

This chapter focuses on the money aspects of basic audiology practices *as they relate to* clinical services.[2] It addresses a variety of topics such as bookkeeping, management accounting, and financial strategies. In business books, these topics usually have their own chapters (or entire books!) and typically are presented in a "logical" accounting order. Here, we have chosen to combine them because of our profession's traditional tendency to lump all things "business" or "money" together. Topics are introduced in an experiential rather than logical sequence, in an effort to simulate the order in which a newly independent practitioner might encounter principles associated with the handling of transactions.

BOOKKEEPING

Bookkeeping is the set of records describing the money coming into and money going out of a practice. Whitmyer, Rasberry, and Phillips (1989) state that it is the most important part of any business:

> Most people focus on marketing first, but this is a dangerous strategy . . . . Because almost anything you do to promote business will work. And the better you are at promotion the more business you can get. But without smoothly functioning financial and organizational systems in place, the increase in volume can swamp you and put you out of business overnight. *The worst possible response would be to provide lower-grade service or products because you are unable to keep up with the demand. So focus on your financial and organizational systems first.* (p. 17, italics added)

What are organizational systems? They are a group of procedures, forms, and source documents arranged by the audiology practice to allow record keeping, account management, and financial analyses. The procedures include estab-

Set up bookkeeping functions before initiating the practice

---

[2]Businesses operate under different types of legal formats. Long-term financial objectives and taxation planning are important factors that guide an owner's decision as to what structure the business should use. These considerations are addressed in Chapter 5.

lishing business bank accounts (checking and savings), depositing cash and check receipts on a daily basis, paying business expenses by company checks, keeping track of transactions chronologically and by type of transaction, and monthly reconciliation of bank statements. Forms include business checks, invoices, statements, stationery, business cards, and so on. Source documents are canceled checks and deposit slips; patient bills, statements, product contracts; supplier invoices and statements; insurance forms and explanation of benefits.

What are financial systems? They are a series of daily, weekly, monthly, quarterly, and annual journals, ledgers, and reports that are kept by the business to document money in and money out and describe the financial condition of the business at a point in time. They can be as simple as a drawer full of receipts and a list of bank deposits, but in most cases they should be elaborate enough to provide the necessary data for account management and financial analyses.

Nowadays, "doing the books" on the computer is faster than taking the drawer full of receipts to a bookkeeper or accountant. Many good software bookkeeping and accounting software packages are available that are easy to use and provide many different types of journals and reports.

Regardless of how the books are kept or who does them, the audiology practice must have records of: (a) sales, (b) cash receipts, (c) cash disbursements, (d) payroll, (e) accounts receivable, (f) accounts payable, and (g) fixed assets.

Accounting Terminology

All transactions must first be entered into *journals*. Journals document information about each transaction chronologically. At minimum, a journal entry must enter the date of the transaction, the amount of the transaction, a description of the transaction (e.g., check number, customer name), and some type of categorical description (e.g., "battery sale"). Each journal entry should be accompanied by the appropriate source document. Figure 12–1 is a simple example of an audiology practice cash receipts journal for tracking daily income.[3]

Journals are the first level of transaction analysis

One "does the books" by *posting* to a *ledger* in *single-* or *double-entry* form, based on a *cash* or an *accrual* method. Ledgers are the books, files, or computer records in which individual categories of transactions are maintained. Using

---

[3]A similar journal is needed for tracking expenses. This can be as simple as a checkbook ledger or may require drawing up a cash disbursements journal.

Date: January 1, 1995 CARDINAL HEARING SERVICES, INC.

PATIENT NAME	TYPE OF SERVICE	PROVIDER	TOTAL AMOUNT	AMOUNT PAID	CHECK OR CASH	BALANCE DUE
Miss X	battery	Dr. A	$ 6.96	$ 6.96	cash	$ 0.00
Mr. Y	dx test	Dr. A	100.00	0.00	——	100.00
Mrs. Z	cerumen	Mr. B	25.00	25.00	ck #396	0.00
TOTAL:			$131.96	$ 31.96		$100.00

Figure 12-1. Sample cash receipts journal.

the information shown in Figure 12–1, for example, one ledger category would be "Dx Tests," another would be "Battery Sales," another might be "Cerumen." In the ledger, such categories are referred to as account descriptions. Information from the journals is transferred into the individual ledger accounts (i.e., they are posted to the ledger). Thus, journals are the first level of transaction analysis, describing chronological events and arriving at across-the-board totals.

Ledgers are the second level of transaction analysis, separating data of the same kind from other journal entries and arriving at category totals. Ledgers are called books of secondary entry because of this two-stage process. In all cases, transactions are assigned to categories according to a *chart of accounts*.

Ledgers are the second level of transaction analysis

Chart of Accounts

A chart of accounts is a system of organizing transactions according to categories (e.g., "sales," "payroll") and/or account numbers. Figure 12–2 is a chart recommended by the American Institute of Certified Public Accountants.[4] In this system, a purchase of an audiometer would be posted to the ledger account "Machinery," with an account number assigned in the 201–250 range.

Charts of accounts should be tailored to the individual practice. It is important to set up the accounts correctly in

---

[4]These account numbers are not cast in stone. Different accountants use different numbers for accounts. Some computer accounting systems allow you to assign your own numbers when setting up the chart of acounts.

```
CHART OF ACCOUNTS              Account Numbers

      BALANCE SHEET                            001-500
ASSETS (the following are DEBIT ACCOUNTS)                    001-300
   Cash                                                      001-050
         Petty Cash
         Checking Accounts
         Savings Account
   Receivables                                                51-100
         Notes Receivable
         Accounts Receivable—Customers
         Accounts Receivable—Others
   Inventories                                               101-150
         Inventory—Goods for Sale
         Inventory—Supplies
   Prepaid Expenses                                          151-200
         Prepaid Advertising
         Prepaid Insurance
         Prepaid Interest
         Prepaid Rent
   Property and Equipment                                    201-250
         Land
         Buildings
         Buildings—Allowance for Depreciation
         Automobiles
         Automobiles—Allowance for Depreciation
         Furniture and Office Equipment
         Furniture and Office Equipment—Depreciation Allowance
         Machinery
         Machinery—Depreciation Allowance
         Leasehold Improvements (Rented Property)
         Leasehold Improvements (Amortization Allowance)
   Miscellaneous Assets                                      251-300
         Organization Expenses (Business Starting Costs)
         Deposits (Advance Payments)

LIABILITIES (the following are CREDIT ACCOUNTS)              301-450
   Notes & Amounts Payable to Others                         301-350
         Accounts Payable
         Sales Taxes Payable
         FICA Tax Withheld
         Federal Income Taxes Withheld
         State Income Taxes Withheld
         Expenses Owed to Others                             351-400
         Accrued Wages
         Accrued Commissions
         Accrued Interest
         Accrued Federal Unemployment Taxes
         Accrued State Unemployment Taxes
         Accrued Real Estate Taxes
         Accrued Federal Income Taxes
         Accrued State Income Taxes

                                                     (continued)
```

Figure 12–2. Sample chart of accounts.

Long-Term Obligations	401-450
Notes Payable—Long Term	
Mortgages Payable	

OWNER'S EQUITY (the following are *CREDIT ACCOUNTS*)	451-500
Capital Investment (for sole proprietors or partners)	
Capital Stock Issued (for corporations)	
Drawings to the Owner (for sole proprietors or partners)	
Retained Earnings (Profit Not Spent)	

<u>PROFIT OR LOSS STATEMENT</u>	501-999
REVENUES (the following are *CREDIT ACCOUNTS*)	501-550
Sales of Merchandise	
Sales Returns and Allowances	
Cash Discounts to Customers	
Service Charges	
Rental Income	
Cash Discounts from Suppliers	
Miscellaneous Income	

EXPENSE ACCOUNTS (the following are *DEBIT ACCOUNTS*)	551-600
Cost of Goods Sold	
Cost of Merchandise Sold	
Freight on Purchases	
Cost of Business Operations	601-700
Wages	
Labor from Agencies	
Supplies	
Tools	
Rental of Equipment	
Repairs to Equipment and Machinery	
Repairs to Vehicles Owned by the Business	
Vehicle Maintenance (gas and oil)	
Selling Expenses	701-750
Advertising	
Commissions	
Entertainment Expenses	
Travel Expenses	
Administrative Expenses (General Expenses)	751-800
Salaries	
Office Supplies	
Postage	
Telephones	
Dues and Subscriptions	
Insurance—Miscellaneous	
Group Insurance	
Workmen's Compensation Insurance	
Automobile Expense	
Professional Services	
Interest	
Miscellaneous Expenses	801-850

(continued)

Building Expenses	851-900
Rent	
Repairs to Building	
Utilities	
Depreciation	901-950
Buildings	
Automobiles	
Furniture and Office Equipment	
Machinery	
Amortization—Rented Property Improvements	
Taxes	951-999
FICA Taxes	
Unemployment Taxes	
Real Estate Taxes	
Miscellaneous Taxes	
Federal Income Taxes	
State Income Taxes	

Design chart of accounts to define activities of interest to the practice, to the government, and to other monitoring agencies

the beginning of the business, to monitor practice trends, easily access information in coming years, and facilitate compliance reporting (e.g., tax information for the government, sales figures for insurance audits).

The chart of accounts needs to be constructed with the help of a good accountant, with the audiologist communicating a comprehensive description of how the practice will be run. Not every practice will need every category shown in Figure 12–2. For example, many practices do not use outside sales people and therefore do not need some of the accounts in the Selling Expenses category. On the other hand, travel expenses may be an important and legitimate expense for audiologists attending training or association meetings. In that case, the chart of accounts for the practice should show Travel Expenses as an account, but not subcategorize it as a Selling Expense.

Another example of the tailoring process has to do with fees for diagnostic services, which is not shown in the sample Chart of Accounts. Audiologists need to add "Fees" in the Sales and Other Income Category. It is a good idea to subclassify fees according to types of tests (e.g., hearing screenings, diagnostic hearing tests, pediatric evaluation, acoustic immittance, electrophysiologic tests) and assign each an account number in the appropriate range. The same kind of subcategorizing can be applied to products (e.g., batteries, ear molds, hearing aids) and hearing aid services. For reporting and reimbursement purposes, many subcategories can be named according to procedure codes (e.g., CPT, HCPCS[5]).

---

[5]For information on procedural codes, see Chapter 15, "Reimbursement Issues."

Single-entry Bookkeeping

Single-entry bookkeeping is much like maintaining a check-book. It only looks at profit and loss and is not considered a complete accounting system. It is used only in the smallest businesses, where one person handles most of the funds and transactions. Only one entry is made per transaction, and there is no built-in system for error checking. Simple "write-it-once" systems for different kinds of businesses are available at office supply stores. The single-entry method usually includes three reports:

An incomplete accounting system

1. *Daily cash receipts journal.* This summarizes the day's cash sales activities, categorizing them according to total sales, sales by type of service or product, sales per employee, and so on.
2. *Monthly cash receipts summary.* Summarizes category totals from the daily cash receipts journal.
3. *Monthly cash disbursement report.* Itemizes payments for capital equipment, profit distributions, office supplies, debt payments, and so on.

Double-entry Bookkeeping

Double-entry bookkeeping is much more common in busi-nesses because it is a complete accounting system. It pro-vides a cross-check of all transactions because every trans-action must be entered twice to reflect money in and money out.[6] For example, if a patient purchases a hearing test for $100 and pays by check, the business checking account must be increased by $100 (money out to the bank) and the fees account must be increased by $100 as well (money into the practice). These double entries are called *debits* and *credits*, respectively.

A complete accounting system that "balances the books"

Contrary to common sense, a debit is not a subtraction and a credit is not an addition! In accounting terminology and consistent with the idea of a "double" entry, a debit is an entry on the left side of an account, whereas a credit is an entry on the right side of the account.[7] Thus, in the hear-ing test example, the checking account is debited and the fee account is credited. In every transaction, the same

[6]Assuming the chart of accounts has been carefully tailored for the busi-ness, the double entry system provides internal controls to ensure that all transactions are recorded. It not only reduces errors but provides an easy means of detecting errors as well as theft and embezzlement.

[7]This curious way of looking at things also prompts accountants to talk about accounts as "T Accounts." In a T Account, a line is drawn down the middle of the account with the name and type of account at the top (thus forming a "T"). Left sides are debits, right sides are credits.

Debit and credit accounts

amount must be simultaneously debited and credited, or an error occurs and the books cannot be *balanced.*

The hearing test example is not intuitive—after all, why should one account be debited and another credited when both are being increased? The answer has to do with the chart of accounts and the concept of balancing the books. Liability, revenue, and capital accounts are designated *credit accounts,* meaning that they are increased by entering a credit (right side). Asset and expense accounts are *debit accounts,* meaning they are increased by entering a debit (left side). In the hearing test example, the checking account is an asset, or debit account. It is increased by entering a $100 debit. The fees account is a revenue, or credit account. It is increased by entering a $100 credit. The accounts balance because $100 has been simultaneously credited and debited. This is illustrated in Figure 12–3.

There are many general ledger accounting software packages available on the market. Several are available for less than $100.00 that can meet all the bookkeeping needs of a small business. Most are easy to install and learn, but all should be set up in consultation with the practice's accountant.

Cash Versus Accrual Accounting

Accounting records are kept according to a cash or an accrual system. In cash accounting, income and expenses are reported

Example of a Debit Account

ACCOUNT: CHECKING   ACCOUNT NO. 21

Date	Item	Debits	Date	Item	Credits
1/1/95	Dx Test	$100.00			

Example of a Credit Account

ACCOUNT: FEES   ACCOUNT NO. 510

Date	Item	Debits	Date	Item	Credits
			1/1/95	Dx Test	$100.00

Figure 12–3. Example of double-entry bookkeeping by recording a fee transaction in debit and credit accounts.

at the time the money is exchanged. A practice works on a cash method if posting to revenue and expense accounts is done only when payments are made or when expenses are paid. In the example shown in Figure 12–1, the practice would post $31.96 in sales for January 1 if it is operating on a cash accounting basis.

In accrual accounting, income and expenses are reported at the time the obligation is made, regardless of when the money is actually received or paid out. In Figure 12–1, the practice would post $131.96 in sales for January 1 if it is operating on an accrual basis.

Cash accounting systems are easier to use than accrual systems and are probably used by most private practice audiologists for that reason. However, cash systems do not provide accurate information on true earnings and expenses for a given period and may distort the financial picture. For example, in a seasonal practice, payments may be high one month even though sales for the period are very low. Lacking knowledge of correct revenue for the month, the owner/manager may be too sanguine about the practice's financial health, make unsupported purchases, and encounter cash-flow problems later on.

The IRS requires any business with a physical inventory of products or parts to use the accrual system to keep track of inventory. Usually, if an audiology practice does not keep an inventory, it can choose either accounting method.[8] However, once a method is elected, the practice cannot change the method without filing a special application with the IRS for a change in accounting method prior to the change (IRS code section 446(e)). The election decision should be made after consulting with an accountant or tax consultant.

ACCOUNT MANAGEMENT

Aside from the IRS and other government regulators, what is the purpose of maintaining journals, source documents, and ledgers? Do they have intrinsic value? Yes they do! Their genuine value lies not in satisfying outside monitors, but in guiding the practice toward its financial and professional goals. In speaking of the importance of accounting systems, business books often use metaphors like road maps and air-

Use organizational systems to set and reach financial goals

---

[8]According to IRS code section 448(a), you must also elect the accrual method if you are a C corporation with average annual gross receipts greater than $5,000,000 for the three prior tax years.

plane radar systems: accurate books tell the practice where it has been, where it stands, and where it can go next. Accounting data provide current and correct feedback to anticipate and prevent potential problems and disasters.

An efficient accounting system is essential to make management decisions in the following areas:

- developing, implementing and evaluating marketing plans
- monitoring performance (e.g., profitability, staff production)
- setting and adjusting fees
- controlling accounts receivable
- negotiating contracts
- tracking expenses
- tracking depreciation
- predicting cash flow
- comparing performance to previous periods
- cost reduction
- staff planning
- adding or eliminating services/products
- identifying patients who warrant special attention
- identifying suppliers who provide the best discounts or the fastest service
- anticipating "tax events"
- identifying errors, theft, waste, or loss
- performing financial analyses (e.g., budgeting, forecasting, applying "financial health" formulas)

Good records are not just the bailiwick of private practitioners. It is equally important for clinic directors to have access to accurate accounting records in order to plan clinic growth, budget, market, protect clinic operations within health care infrastructures, and, in general, to ensure autonomy of practice. Unfortunately, not all clinic directors are provided with accurate accounting information. The only reasonable alternative in such cases is to construct an internal set of books and internal controls, and maintain them as religiously as one would in private practice.

Internal Accounting Controls

Use controls to avoid and detect financial abuses

Internal controls are common sense rules for handling transactions in ways that prevent errors, theft, and loss. In larger clinics, they are important because of the need to control the number of people who have access to the books. In smaller practices, they are important to avoid the potential for abuse when a single person handles too much of the record keeping. The following rules, adapted from Jenkins (1993), apply more or less depending on the number of people in the practice and their place in its organizational structure:

- The same person who handles the cash receipts should not also make the bank deposits.
- The person who writes checks should not also sign them or have the authority to sign checks.
- Whoever signs checks should sign them only when the bill that is being paid is presented at the same time. The check number should be written on the bill to avoid double payments or payments to a nonexistent vendor. No check should be written unless it is clear what the bill is for.
- Consider using some type of mechanical check imprinting equipment for all checks that are written, as a further means of preventing unauthorized payments.
- Use only prenumbered checks and keep all of the cancelled or voided checks on file.[9]
- Complete a monthly bank reconciliation or have an outside accountant do it. Never let the person who writes checks do the reconciliation.
- Deposit daily cash receipts in the bank each day. Do not comingle cash collections for one day with another day's collections.
- Use prenumbered sets of sales checks, invoices, and receipts to keep control of payments made and received.
- For cash on hand, write a check to petty cash, keep separate vouchers against expenditures to the petty cash fund, keep the cash in a locked box, count and reconcile the amount each day.

Scenario 12–1 analyzes a situation in which lax internal controls lead to problems.

---

[9]Accounting software packages often offer check writing capability, including numbered checks with automatically printed voucher slips and check "stubs." In addition to saving time, these features address internal control items 3, 4, and 5.

SCENARIO 12-1

Battery sales at CHS are handled through the petty cash box at the front desk. In fact, battery sales make up almost 90% of the petty cash activity. This unstructured arrangement has been convenient for drop-in patients as well as those who have a scheduled encounter. Lately, petty cash is dwindling and having to be replenished. Previously, petty cash had to be deposited once a week due to the amount of cash accumulated from battery sales. CHS battery orders have historically indicated an upward-trending sales volume, and there has been no change in this sales trend over the last few weeks. Where are the proceeds from the battery sales going?

ANALYSIS:

It is apparent that pilferage of petty cash or embezzlement has been occurring in recent weeks at CHS. It is important for Dr. A to determine as precisely as possible the time frame involved and the extent of the loss. Dr. A next needs to determine how to protect CHS's cash assets. This involves setting up safeguards, changing procedures, and identifying the source of the theft.

Questions and Management Suggestions for Dr. A

Question 1: Sales volume, based on battery orders from the manufacturer, is conforming to historical trends. When did the normal cash flow pattern change at CHS?

Suggested Answer: It's important for the Dr. A to determine as precisely as possible when the problem occurred. Any business needs to be able to accurately define all of its transactions. It is also important for Dr. A to determine if the problem is a theft, lost inventory, or sloppy bookkeeping.

Question 2: Assuming the approximate date for the change in the petty cash pattern can be established, what types of information can Dr. A obtain?

Suggested Answer: With the date roughly established, it is possible for the practice to go back through its daily encounters and determine who was seen and the nature of the visit. Patient records can also be checked for updates reflecting battery purchases. This is a good reason for using sign-in sheets for all direct patient encounters, which can then be used as cross-checks of encounters.

Question 3: Why is it important to establish the extent of the embezzlement, if that is what has been happening? What steps should the practice take in the future?

Suggested Answer: It is always essential for a business to accurately define its transactions. This definition can help in determining whether petty pilferage or more serious embezzlement has occurred. In the former situation the practice may be willing to take the loss. In the later, the practice may want to involve legal authorities.

An event like this is usually a signal to management that the practice has grown. That may seem like a trite statement but the people who own or manage businesses often are so busy running the business that they fail to step back from time to time and see just how much the practice has grown. This is mentioned because every good accounting system stresses a separation of duties. Separation of duties is used to protect against employee fraud or defalcation. When a practice first starts, duties cannot be divided much because the staff is small—often only the practitioner and perhaps a front office person. As the practice grows, staff is added but procedural changes are often overlooked. The practice becomes exposed to the unscrupulous employee. Procedures need to change as the practice changes.

Question 4: What other steps should the Dr. A consider in the scenario?

Suggested Answer: CHS can install new procedures that make pilfering or embezzlement more difficult. But what about the guilty party? If it is a small amount, perhaps it can be written off as an error. Do not dwell on it, but pay more attention on a daily basis to what is going on. If it is much more serious and obviously an ongoing situation, then Dr. A really needs to identify the thief. Weeding out the guilty party or parties may put a lot of stress on CHS and will probably require some outside assistance. But not resolving it will eat away at the fiber of the organization.

FINANCIAL ANALYSES

Financial analysis begins by always knowing the condition of the audiology practice's fiscal "health." For instance, a good owner/manager should know answers to questions such as:

- How profitable is the practice?
- What is the net income percentage to gross revenues?
- What is the cost of sales?
- How do these figures compare with previous periods in past years?
- What costs are a problem?
- What are the assets of the practice?
- How much have these assets been depreciated?
- How much is owed on what kinds of debts?
- How much is owed to the practice?
- Are budgetary goals being met?
- What are future goals for income and expense categories?
- Are there any cash-flow problems anticipated?

The answers to some of these questions are found in *financial statements* and *financial ratios* that are prepared and calculated from the original ledger data. Other questions are addressed by doing cash flow and pro forma predictions.

Financial Statements

The two major financial statements are the *balance sheet* and the *income statement*. These reports summarize activity for two different groups of accounts (see Figure 12–2): the balance sheet summarizes asset, liability, and owner's equity accounts, whereas the income statement summarizes income and expense accounts. Both statements are about a page long. Together, they summarize all the information contained in the detailed journals and ledgers of the business. Because they are drawn entirely from ledger records of the business, they should be very simple to create: the better the books, the easier financial analyses.

Balance Sheet

The balance sheet[10] is a summary of what the practice owns and owes at a particular point in time. It is a static descriptor, telling nothing about trends or changes in performance. For this reason, many accounting books liken it to a snapshot that freezes events in time.

As shown in Figures 12–2 and 12–4, the balance sheet has two main sections or sides, one listing assets of the practice and one listing the liabilities and owner's equity (also called *capital*)[11] of the practice. These two sides are simply two different ways of looking at the same business: the assets side tells what the business owns, the equities side tells who supplied the assets and how much they supplied. All assets in a business must be "owned" by someone—they are either owned outright by the practice (i.e., purchased with owner invested monies or with profits of the business) or they are supplied to the business by creditors. Therefore, in the balance sheet the two sides must always equate:

$$\text{ASSETS} = \text{LIABILITIES} + \text{OWNER'S EQUITY}$$

Perhaps a more intuitive way of looking at this equation from the owner's point of view is that the owner's share is everything left over after all debts are paid:

$$\text{OWNER'S EQUITY} = \text{ASSETS} - \text{LIABILITIES}$$

> The balance sheet shows the financial health of the practice at a fixed point in time

---

[10]Technically, this term is used in statements prepared on an accrual basis. Cash basis statements are more correctly called Statements of Assets and Liabilities (with or without owners' equity accounts).

[11]Liabilities and owner's equity are also called *equities*.

CARDINAL HEARING SERVICES, INC.
BALANCE SHEET
as of 12/31/95

Account	12/31/95 Balance

ASSETS

Current Assets

Cash and Bank Accounts		
Petty Cash	75.00	
Checking Balance	597.43	
Savings Balance	1,500.00	
Total Current Assets		2,172.43

Fixed Assets

Machinery and Equipment	25,000.00	
Furniture and Fixtures	5,000.00	
	30,000.00	
Less Accumulated Depreciation	(19,600.00)	
Total Fixed Assets		10,400.00

Other Assets

Refundable Deposits		140.00
TOTAL ASSETS		12,712.43

LIABILITIES AND EQUITY

Current Liabilities

Payroll Taxes Withheld	175.00	
FICA	132.57	
State Income Taxes	38.50	
	346.07	
		346.07
Sales Tax Payable		36.12
Total Current Liabilities		382.19

Stockholder's Equity

Common Stock, no par value:		
Authorized—10,000 shares		
Issued—1000 shares	45,564.60	
Retained Earnings (Deficit)	(33,234.36)	
		12,330.24
		12,712.43

Figure 12–4. Example of a Balance Sheet prepared for the start-up private practice described in Appendix 4-A in Chapter 4. This balance sheet indicates the status after one year of operation as a corporation. Note that accounts receivable & accounts payable are not shown because accounting is on a cash basis.

Assets

An asset is anything, physical or nonphysical, that has monetary value and is owned by the practice. Assets are listed on the balance sheet in order of their liquidity, with those that are easiest to convert to cash shown first. In this regard, assets fall into three categories:

1. *Current assets:* cash, accounts receivable, inventory
2. *Fixed assets:* Land, buildings, equipment, furniture and fixtures, vehicles
3. *Intangible assets*: Trademarks, copyrights, goodwill

According to the *cost principle* of accounting, assets are accounted for on the basis of what they cost to purchase. For example, the balance sheet may show a piece of land as an asset of the practice. The value of the asset is listed as the original purchase price, *not* the current value of the land.

It is important to remember that *balance sheets do not show how much a business is worth.* Because of the use of the cost basis for valuing assets on most balance sheets, the dollar amounts do not indicate the prices at which assets could be sold or at which they could be replaced. This is mainly because balance sheets are intended primarily to reflect the status of practices as continuing enterprises, not as final valuations for enterprises that are discontinuing because they are up for sale. Another reason is that original costs are factual information, whereas current market valuations are necessarily speculative and can fluctuate wildly from time to time.

Balance sheets can be constructed showing assets at current appraised values rather than at their historical cost. In selling an audiology practice, the owner may wish to consult an accountant about the wisdom of constructing this type of balance sheet.

Liabilities

These are all the debts owed by the practice, in the form of *current and long-term liabilities to creditors.* These are listed separately on the balance sheet, current liabilities first. Current liabilities include *accounts payable* (e.g., credit purchases such as hearing aids, supplies) and *accrued liabilities* (e.g., wages, interest, taxes, and deposits that are due but not yet paid). Long-term liabilities are debts or portions of debts that are not due in the next 12 months (e.g., mortgages, term loans).

Cost basis accounting has little effect on the valuation of liabilities on the balance sheet. This is because the amounts of liabilities are almost always fixed according to the original transactions with the creditors. Creditors have claims against the general assets of the business, rather than against individual assets. By law, creditors' claims have priority over the owner's claims: creditors must be paid even if it depletes these assets of the practice, in which case owner's equity is zero.

Owner's Equity

The owner is entitled to any residual assets that are left after all creditor's claims are paid. This residual is called *capital.* Capital includes the amount the owner invested in the company, as well as accumulated profits or losses. Capital is not always a positive amount.

In sole proprietorships and partnerships, capital investments and undistributed profits (i.e., income not taken as "draws") are listed in each owner's name. In corporations, owner investments for issued stock are listed as "capital stock" for the "par value" and additional paid-in capital for any additional amounts invested. Undistributed earnings to shareholders are listed as "retained earnings." In the example show in Figure 12–4, the start-up company has operated at a loss in its first year, so retained earnings is a deficit.

Income and Retained Earnings Statements

The income statement, or profit and loss statement (P&L), shows the sources and amounts of income, costs and expenses, and profits/losses for a specified time period (month, quarter, year). In contrast to the balance statement, the income statement does not address the overall financial state of the business, but focuses on whether the practice is profitable in a particular period. The income statement is likened to a motion picture because it provides a dynamic view of money in and money out over time.

There are two kinds of income statements. *Pro forma, or budgetary,* income statements estimate future profitability of a business by making educated guesses as to future sales and expenses. Accounting income statements are those generated for a given period, based on actual transactions entered in the practice's ledger. An example of a pro forma income statement is shown in Figure 12–5.

The income statement shows profitability in a window of time

	JAN–MAR 19--	APR–JUN 19--	JUL–SEP 19--	OCT–DEC 19--	TOTAL YEAR 1	TOTAL YEAR 2	TOTAL YEAR 3
INCOME							
Dx Fees	1,100.00	1,600.00	1,800.00	1,900.00	6,400.00	25,000.00	50,000.00
Batteries	120.00	228.00	360.00	516.00	1,224.00	1,744.00	2,320.00
Hearing Aids	12,100.00	19,300.00	22,900.00	30,900.00	85,200.00	151,200.00	216,000.00
TOTAL SALES	13,320.00	21,128.00	25,060.00	33,316.00	92,824.00	177,944.00	268,320.00
Returns/Discounts	800.00	1,135.00	1,395.00	1,630.00	4,960.00	12,130.00	20,900.00
NET SALES	12,520.00	19,993.00	23,665.00	31,686.00	87,864.00	165,814.00	247,420.00
Cost of Goods	4,872.00	6,856.00	8,856.00	11,069.00	31,653.00	55,006.40	78,392.00
GROSS PROFIT/LOSS	7,648.00	13,137.00	14,809.00	20,617.00	56,211.00	110,807.60	169,028.00
EXPENSES							
Accounting & Legal	1,000.00	250.00	250.00	250.00	1,750.00	1,500.00	1,500.00
Advertising/Promotion	1,300.00	325.00	1,000.00	325.00	2,950.00	1,800.00	1,800.00
Business Meals/Entertainment	186.00	86.00	86.00	286.00	644.00	644.00	200.00
Charitable Contributions	120.00	120.00	120.00	120.00	480.00	480.00	480.00
Depreciation	650.00	650.00	650.00	17,650.00	19,600.00	2,600.00	2,600.00
Dues & Subscriptions	400.00	0.00	0.00	0.00	400.00	400.00	600.00
Insurance							
Disability	300.00	300.00	300.00	300.00	1,200.00	1,200.00	1,200.00
Life	425.00	0.00	0.00	0.00	425.00	500.00	650.00
Malpractice	250.00	0.00	0.00	0.00	250.00	250.00	300.00
Office	300.00	0.00	0.00	0.00	300.00	300.00	350.00
Interest	0.00	0.00	0.00	0.00	0.00	0.00	0.00
Licenses	300.00	0.00	0.00	0.00	300.00	300.00	450.00
Office Expenses	1,300.00	300.00	300.00	300.00	2,200.00	2,000.00	2,000.00
Payroll Taxes	786.24	786.24	786.24	786.24	3,144.96	3,144.96	6,879.60
Pension Plan Contrib	0.00	0.00	0.00	0.00	0.00	6,240.00	13,650.00
Rent	3,000.00	3,000.00	3,000.00	3,000.00	12,000.00	12,000.00	12,000.00
Repairs & Maintenance	0.00	0.00	0.00	0.00	0.00	600.00	800.00
Salaries							
Officer	5,200.00	5,200.00	5,200.00	5,200.00	20,800.00	20,800.00	40,000.00
Other	5,200.00	5,200.00	5,200.00	5,200.00	20,800.00	21,800.00	51,000.00
Telephone	300.00	300.00	300.00	300.00	1,200.00	1,200.00	300.00
Travel/Education	0.00	0.00	0.00	0.00	0.00	1,200.00	2,500.00
Utilities	300.00	200.00	200.00	300.00	1,000.00	1,000.00	1,000.00
TOTAL EXPENSES	21,317.24	16,717.24	17,392.24	34,017.24	89,443.96	79,958.96	140,259.60
NET PROFIT/LOSS	(13,669.24)	(3,580.24)	(2,583.24)	(13,400.24)	(33,232.96)	30,848.64	28,768.40
RETAINED EARNINGS, BEGINNING	0.00	(13,669.24)	(17,249.48)	(19,832.72)	(33,232.96)	(33,232.96)	(2,384.32)
DIVIDENDS	0.00	0.00	0.00	0.00	0.00	0.00	25,000.00
RETAINED EARNINGS, ENDING	(13,669.24)	(17,249.48)	(19,832.72)	(33,232.96)	(33,232.96)	(2,384.32)	1,384.08

Figure 12-5. Projected profit/loss statement for the practice described in Appendix 4-A in Chapter 4 and the Balance Sheet in Figure 12–4.

Income and retained earnings statements are usually divided into sections:

- *Net sales*. For audiology practices, this includes total fees and sales of products for the time period, minus sales tax, discounts, and returns.
- *Cost of goods sold*: This is the total cost of products in the time period, less supplier discounts.
- *Gross profit/loss*: Net sales − Cost of goods sold
- *Operating expenses*: Selling expenses (i.e., advertising, commissions) and general and administrative expenses (i.e., rent, insurance, office supplies, payroll) for the specified time period
- *Net profit/loss*: Gross profit − Operating expenses
- *Dividends*: Distributed profits
- *Retained Earnings*: Accumulated[12] net profit − Dividends

Income statements should be prepared at least quarterly, and monthly if possible. Again, many software accounting packages are available that can quickly produce income statements for any time period specified.

Income statements are an important method of control for the practice manager. For start-up practices, pro forma (projected) income statements should be prepared for the first few years of operation and then compared to actual profit/loss statements for those periods. Existing practices should translate operating goals into dollars, form a budget, and project the budget out over a time frame in the form of a pro forma profit/loss statement. By comparing actual to projected income and expenses in both of these cases, businesses can quickly identify areas that need investigation (e.g., "Why were fees for diagnostic tests lower than expected in the third quarter?" "Why were hearing aid costs higher this year than last?").

How Income and Retained Earnings Statements Are Related to Balance Sheets

As we have seen, the balance sheet and the income statement present complementary analyses of the practice using information from separate accounting categories. The balance sheet is used to get a "snapshot" of what the practice

---

[12]This is not just net profits that have occurred in the present year. It also includes all undistributed profits since inception of the business.

owns and who it owes. The Income and Retained Earnings Statement is used to monitor profitability over time. But how do they relate to each other? Won't profitability (or losses) over time on the income statement eventually impact on the balance sheet?

The connection between the two reports is the way net profits and losses affect owner's equity. In the income and retained earnings statement, net profits may be taken as dividends. In that case, the impact on retained earnings is zero and the balance sheet is not affected. However, if net profits remain in the practice, they belong to the owner whether they are taken or not. In that case, retained earnings is increased by the amount of the net profit, which now shows up on the balance sheet as *retained earnings* in the owner's equity. It is this essential connection between profitability and equities that underscores the oft repeated admonition to "heed the bottom line!"

Cash Flow Projections and Budgeting

Almost anyone who has run a successful audiology practice for any length of time has encountered the paradoxical situation where the profits promised by the income statement do not materialize as cash in the bank! This is because neither the balance sheet nor the profit/loss statement measures cash flow. Seasonal fluctuations in sales, inventory, and slow paying accounts receivable are all variables that can compromise cash flow, even in the midst of rising profits. Depreciation can also confuse the cash flow picture (Siropolis, 1990). Depreciation[13] is a noncash expense in the income statement.

For these reasons, it is important to prepare reports of cash flow projections based on predicted income and budgeted estimates of expenses. An example of a cash budget is shown in Figure 12–6.

---

[13]Actual depreciation expenses for audiology assets are not described in this book. The new rules set forth in the Tax Reform Act of 1986 make it essential that an accountant be consulted for the proper way to depreciated assets in individual practices. Under the modified accelerated cost recovery system (MACRS), assets are depreciated according to asset depreciation ranges (ADRs) that vary from industry to industry (IRS code, subsection 168). Under certain conditions, the MACRS allows up to $17,500 of depreciable items purchased in a fiscal year to be fully deducted in that year (e.g., see Figures 12–4 and 12–5).

CARDINAL HEARING SERVICES, INC.
CASH FLOW ANALYSIS
FIRST 12 MONTHS, 19--

	JAN–MAR	APR–JUN	JUL–SEP	OCT–DEC	YEAR
INCOME					
Dx Fees	1,100.00	1,600.00	1,800.00	1,900.00	6,400.00
Batteries	120.00	228.00	360.00	516.00	1,224.00
Hearing Aids	12,100.00	19,300.00	22,900.00	30,900.00	85,200.00
TOTAL SALES	13,320.00	21,128.00	25,060.00	33,316.00	92,824.00
Returns/Discounts	350.00	940.00	1,275.00	1,535.00	4,100.00
NET PROFIT/LOSS	12,970.00	20,188.00	23,785.00	31,781.00	88,724.00
Cost of Goods	3,282.29	6,216.80	8,216.00	10,429.60	28,144.69
CASH INFLOWS	9,687.71	13,971.20	15,569.00	21,351.40	60,579.31
EXPENSES					
Accounting & Legal	1,000.00	250.00	250.00	250.00	1,750.00
Advertising/Promotion	1,300.00	325.00	1,000.00	325.00	2,950.00
Business Meals/Entertainment	186.00	86.00	86.00	286.00	644.00
Charitable Contributions	120.00	120.00	120.00	120.00	480.00
Dues & Subscriptions	400.00	0.00	0.00	0.00	400.00
Insurance					
Disability	300.00	300.00	300.00	300.00	1,200.00
Life	425.00	0.00	0.00	0.00	425.00
Malpractice	250.00	0.00	0.00	0.00	250.00
Office	300.00	0.00	0.00	0.00	300.00
Licenses	300.00	0.00	0.00	0.00	300.00
Office Expenses	1,300.00	300.00	300.00	300.00	2,200.00
Payroll Taxes	524.16	786.24	786.24	786.24	2,882.88
Rent	3,000.00	3,000.00	3,000.00	3,000.00	12,000.00
Repairs & Maintenance	0.00	0.00	0.00	0.00	0.00
Salaries					
Officers	5,200.00	5,200.00	5,200.00	5,200.00	20,800.00
Other	5,200.00	5,200.00	5,200.00	5,200.00	20,800.00
Telephone	300.00	300.00	300.00	300.00	1,100.00
Utilities	200.00	300.00	200.00	300.00	1,000.00
CASH OUTFLOWS	20,205.16	16,167.24	16,742.24	16,367.24	69,481.88
CASH GAIN OR LOSS	(10,517.45)	(2,196.04)	(1,173.24)	4,984.16	(8,902.57)
BEGINNING CASH	11,000.00	482.55	(1,713.49)	(2,886.73)	(11,000.00)
ENDING CASH	482.55	(1,713.49)	(2,886.73)	2,097.43	2,097.43

Figure 12–6. Projected cash flow analysis for the first year of operation for the private practice corporation described in Appendix 4-A in Chapter 4 and in the Balance Sheet and Pro Forma Profit statement shown in Figures 12–4 and 12–5.

Comparative Financial Statements

Any of the reports described above can be compared with other similar reports. It is wise to compare overall trends as well as individual accounting items by comparing like data from different periods.

There are two types of comparisons. *Horizontal analysis* compares the same category at different times, year to year, season to season, and so on. This type of analysis can identify trends that are helpful in predicting cash flow, making staffing decision, and ordering supplies.

Vertical analysis looks at individual categories in a report, comparing them to some single base (usually revenues). For instance, income may be up but profit may be down. A vertical analysis may show that the percentage of cost of goods to hearing aid sales is 35%. A horizontal analysis of this same statistic shows that it is up from 25% last year. Further investigation leads to the conclusion that increased sales of programmable instruments are raising income but costing more to purchase from the manufacturers.

Financial Ratios

The comparative analyses discussed in the previous section are simple examples of financial ratios used to interpret data in the financial reports. There are other less intuitive ratios that are used routinely to pinpoint strengths and weaknesses of businesses. *Liquidity and profitability* ratios are easy to calculate and are often included in financial software packages (Kishel & Kishel, 1993). Freeman (1990) discussed the application of these ratios to audiology practices.

Liquidity Ratios

The following equations measure the practice's ability to convert assets to cash and meet its obligations:

Current Ratio

The most commonly used ratio, it determines the practices ability to meet its obligations within the next 12 months. It's good to have a ratio of at least 2:1.

$$\text{CURRENT RATIO} = \frac{\text{CURRENT ASSETS}}{\text{CURRENT LIABILITIES}}$$

Acid-test Ratio or Quick Ratio

Asks whether obligations can be met if income declines suddenly. A ratio of 1:1 is acceptable if accounts receivable are being collected appropriately.

$$\text{ACID-TEST RATIO} = \frac{\text{CASH} + \text{ACCOUNTS RECEIVABLE}}{\text{CURRENT LIABILITIES}}$$

Working Capital Ratio

Looks at the practice's ability to pay unforeseen expenses and handle financial setbacks. A subtraction and not a ratio, it should always be a positive number. Lenders will often set a minimum level for working capital.

$$\text{WORKING CAPITAL} = \text{CURRENT ASSETS} - \text{CURRENT LIABILITIES}$$

Average Collection Period

A two-step process that assesses the practice's ability to convert accounts receivable to cash. The rule of thumb is that the average collection period should not be more than 1.3 times the credit terms (i.e., $1.3 \times 30 = 40$ days for a 30-day credit policy).

Step 1

$$\text{AVERAGE DAY'S SALES} = \frac{\text{NET INCOME}}{365 \text{ DAYS}}$$

Step 2

$$\text{AVERAGE COLLECTION PERIOD} = \frac{\text{ACCOUNTS RECEIVABLE}}{\text{AVERAGE DAY'S SALES}}$$

Profitability Ratios

These ratios look at the "bottom line" in terms of total sales or total assets. Essentially, they indicate how hard the business is working or how much money it is taking to turn a profit.

Net Profit on Sales

Determines the percentage of sales that are net profit.

$$\text{NET PROFIT ON SALES} = \frac{\text{NET PROFIT}}{\text{NET SALES}} \times 100$$

Excluding compensation to the owner as an operating expense, 50% net profit is very good. For example, a practice has $100,000 in revenues, $30,000 in cost of goods, and $60,000 in operating expenses (including $30,000 salary to the owner). The calculation is as follows:

Net Sales	$100,000
Cost of Goods	−30,000
Gross Profit	70,000
Expenses (excluding Owner compensation)	−30,000
Net Profit	40,000

$$\text{Net profit on sales} = \frac{40,000}{100,000} = 40\%$$

Thus, in this example, the practice realizes a 40% profit, the bulk of which goes to the owner in the form of draws or salary.

Return on Investment

This ratio looks at the practice as an investment. To determine whether putting resources into the practice was a good investment, compare the ROI to figures from comparable businesses, or to the outcome if the money had been put into mutual funds or some other investment vehicle.

$$\text{RETURN ON INVESTMENT} = \frac{\text{NET PROFIT}}{\text{TOTAL ASSETS}}$$

LIMITATIONS OF ACCOUNTING AND FINANCIAL ANALYSIS

Financial reports alone cannot set the value of a practice

Accounting data, reports, and analyses rely on dollar values. For this reason, accounting and financial information cannot yield a full picture of a practice. Reputation in the community, technical skills and knowledge, staff teamwork, years of experience, and personal dedication are examples of vital, nonfinancial factors that may describe a practice much more adequately than its financial statements.

Even in dollars, accounting information cannot measure the actual worth of a practice. This is because assets are valued by their original cost, as discussed earlier in this chapter. In addition, the purchasing power of the dollar is less than it used to be, but assets are recorded according to their original cost without adjustments for price inflation.

SUMMARY

Bookkeeping, management accounting, and financial analysis are interlocking parts of financial systems set up by practices to monitor and analyze the flow of money in and money out of a practice. Basic bookkeeping and accounting starts with journal entries for every transaction. These entries are then posted to individual ledger accounts, according to a chart of accounts that is tailored to the practice. The ledger accounts are subsequently analyzed and summarized into financial statements. The main financial statements are the Balance Sheet, which states what is owned and what is owed by the practice at a given time, and the Income Statement, which shows income, expenses, and profitability for a period of time. Pro Forma Income Statements and Cash Flow Budgets are predictive reports used to estimate profitability and cash on hand. Finally, financial ratios are applied to the data in these reports to determine the liquidity and profitability of the practice.

Accounting and financial systems are essential for making short- and long-term management decisions in any audiology practice. This is true even in multi-clinic settings where actual financial control is exercised remotely by nonaudiology administrators. Good financial systems minimize errors, waste, theft, and loss, promote profitability, and help secure a practice's autonomy.

REFERENCES

Freeman, B. A. (1990, July/August). Private practice. *Audiology Today*, p. 17.

Jenkins, M. D. (1993). *Starting and operating a business in Arizona.* Grants Pass, OR: Oasis Press.

Kishel, G. F., & Kishel, P. G. (1993). *How to start, run, and stay in business.* New York: John Wiley.

Siropolis, N. C. (1990). *Small business management* (4th ed.). Princeton: Houghton Mifflin.

Trace, R. (1993, November 8). Doing the right thing. *Advance Magazine for Speech-Language Pathologists and Audiologists*, pp. 16–20.

Whitmyer, C., Rasberry, S., & Phillips, M. (1989). *Running a one-person business.* Berkeley, CA: Ten-Speed Press.

Marketing

Elements of Marketing

- *Sociology*
- *Psychology*
- *Education*
- *Human Engineering*
- *Product Engineering*
- *Public Relations*
- *Cost Analysis*
- *Management*

This chapter discusses the cornerstones of marketing as they apply to emerging, technologically dynamic fields like hearing health care. Whenever possible, marketing principles and marketing strategies are illustrated and discussed using specific examples from audiology and hearing aid dispensing.

Marketing is a fascinating field that incorporates elements of sociology, psychology, education, human engineering, product engineering, public relations, cost analysis, and management. The simplest marketing "chain" begins with identifying a need and ends with satisfying that need through marketing exchange. The connecting links of the chain include products, pricing, market analysis, and marketing strategies. A multitude of good marketing books are available that address some or all of these marketing subfunctions. It is impossible to do justice to all of these sources in a single chapter. Instead, we have leaned heavily on the integrative and innovative works of two marketing experts with divergent backgrounds. Kotler (1991), one of the world's leading academic authorities on marketing, provides a scholarly and comprehensive discussion of marketing and marketing management. McKenna (1986), a successful marketing consultant in Silicon Valley, has written a step-by-step approach to developing marketing strategy in technology-based industries. With few exceptions, the theoretical concepts discussed in this chapter are taken from Kotler and are illustrated with

A simple marketing chain includes products, pricing, analysis, and strategies

"how-to's" from McKenna. Rather than reference them at every instance, readers are encouraged to refer to these sources for further information on marketing.

The chapter begins with broad definitions and applications, then narrows to discussions of individual links in the marketing chain. Having identified the marketing links, the discussion progresses to a consideration of marketing strategies for "positioning" products and practices in the hearing health care market place. The market is analyzed in terms of its *infrastructure:* all of the people, industries, programs, and regulations between the audiologist and the consumer that have an influence on the buying process.

The chapter culminates with a discussion of Continuous Quality Improvement (CQI) as the premiere marketing strategy. It is not by accident that this book lacks a chapter on Quality Improvement. This chapter takes the position that the most successful (and appropriate) way to market audiology services and expertise is to establish the credibility of our "products" and our credibility as providers within the health care (and hearing health care) industries. CQI, in its best and broadest interpretation, is an ideal way to establish our credibility in the hearing health care infrastructure.

The chapter concludes with Appendix 13-A, which discusses elements of a marketing plan for a small dispensing audiology practice.

OUR ATTITUDES TOWARD MARKETING: THE MARKETING OF AUDIOLOGISTS

According to Kotler (1991),

Marketing is:

the creation and delivery of a standard of living. (p. 4)

Marketing Management is:

the process of planning and executing the conception, pricing, promotion, and distribution of ideas, goods, and services to create exchanges that satisfy individual and organizational objectives. (p. 11)

Societal Marketing is the process of determining:

the needs, wants, and interests of target markets and delivering the desired satisfactions more effectively and efficiently than competitors in a way that preserves or enhances the consumer's and the society's well-being. (p. 26)

These definitions of marketing may seem foreign or contrived to some audiologists. Like other novices, people in our field often confuse marketing with advertising or sales, when in fact the latter are just two links in the long chain of thoughts and events that define marketing processes. Our ignorance and prejudice toward marketing has its roots in three areas. The first root is our training: few, if any, graduate programs include marketing in their curricula; only in the last few years has the ASHA recognized "marketing" as a topic worthy of inclusion in its calendar of professional programs for continuing education. The second root has to do with professional attitudes that promulgate fear of marketing. As Kotler (1991) points out:

Think positively about marketing

> The resistance [to marketing] is especially strong in industries where marketing is being introduced or proposed for the first time, for instance, in law offices, colleges, hospitals, or government agencies. Colleges have to face the hostility of professors, and hospitals have to face the hostility of doctors, because each group thinks that "marketing" their services would be degrading. (p. 24)

The third root lies with hearing aids. Until the late 1970s, audiologists violated their own professional code and lost their professional status if they sold hearing aids. There was some basis for this position. At that time, and even today, the traditional marketing approach of hearing aid manufacturers and hearing aid "dealers" emphasized sales and advertising rather than education, quality improvement, and ethical conduct.

Ironically, the ASHA's draconian measures designed to differentiate audiologists from persons and products associated with the hearing aid industry by positioning them as professionals rather than sales people or technicians, is a straightforward example of *"product positioning"*—one of the first and most fundamental steps in marketing strategy (McKenna, 1986). Product positioning (of audiologists) continues today as our scope of practice is defined and refined to differentiate hearing loss and communication disorders from ear disease (Beck, 1994), as quality improvement measures are adopted, the professional doctorate in audiology becomes a reality, and the American Academy of Audiology (AAA) becomes a reckoning body.

Audiologists have to position themselves in the marketplace

Currently, the AAA and ASHA are working at establishing *"market positioning"* for audiologists by consumer education and advertising efforts and also by testimonials and position papers to governing bodies like the FDA and Senate Committee on Aging. *"Corporate positioning"* of AAA and perhaps ASHA lies largely in the future and will depend on how successful these organizations are in establishing productive affiliations with government agencies, technological leaders, and other health care professions.

All three types of positioning—product, market, and corporate—are interactive. Each is necessary to sustain the long-term success of audiologists. The same can be said on the microcosmic level of individual audiology practices, as we will examine in later parts of this chapter.

THE MARKETING CHAIN

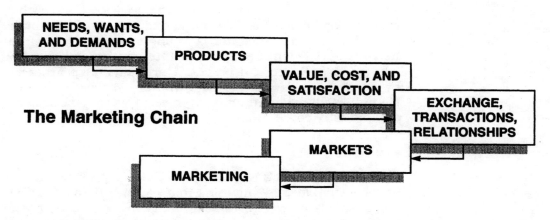

Figure 13–1. The marketing chain. (Adapted from Kotler, 1991.)

Needs, Wants, and Demands

Human *needs* are requirements, not creations, of society (e.g., food, shelter, hearing). Needs are a precondition for a market, they are not created by marketing. The beginning of the first link in the marketing chain, then, is to identify a need. Congenital hearing loss, noise-induced hearing loss, balance disorders, and tinnitus are examples of human conditions that present needs in our society. As such, they represent potential markets.

Human *wants* are desires for specific means to satisfy needs (e.g., designer label clothing, programmable hearing aids). Wants are created and shaped by social and institutional forces in the environment (e.g., families, schools, workplaces, clubs, government, corporations, research and development), as well as by marketing efforts. Once a need is identified, typically several wants are associated with it. Thus, congenital hearing loss prompts a want for early identification and a want for early intervention, once the public is made aware of the consequences of congenital hearing loss and the steps required to minimize those effects. This type of public education is an example of what audiologists are trained and expected to do, and it expands the first link in the marketing chain by creating or expanding a market for our services.

Marketing works by influencing demand

A want becomes a *demand* when it is accompanied by the ability and willingness to purchase. Marketing attempts to influence demand by finding ways to make the product or service as attractive, affordable, and accessible as possible, thereby completing the first marketing link. As an example, not every community can or is willing to support a comprehensive early identification and intervention program for hearing loss. Successful programs are usually spearheaded by hearing health professionals who are actively marketing via public education, funding agencies, government liaisons, and industry connections.

Products

The second marketing link is to create a product. Kotler defines a *product* as "anything that can be offered to someone to satisfy a need or want" (p. 5). People get hearing tests to find out if they have a hearing problem. They purchase hearing aids to satisfy their need to hear, not because they like hearing aids. *It is incumbent on audiologists to remember that the product we market is always hearing care, not a new test or treatment technology.*

Audiologists' product is hearing care

Value, Cost, and Satisfaction

The third link in the marketing chain is to assign a cost to the product that is consistent with its perceived value. Kotler defines *value* as the "consumer's estimate of the product's overall capacity to satisfy his or her needs" (p. 6). An adult with acquired hearing loss may have a "need set" consisting of obtaining a hearing examination at a reasonable cost and in a reasonable time period from a nearby practitioner who can recommend a treatment plan. Thus, cost, time, accessibility, and outcome are factors that determine value in this example. The consumer may find that the hearing examination is covered by HMO insurance, but the only provider is located at a hospital across town and has no appointments available till next month. On the other hand, an appointment is available tomorrow with a nearby audiologist who is highly recommended by friends who wear hearing aids, but the test fee will have to be out-of-pocket. The consumer's choice in this example will reflect the "product" (i.e., hearing evaluation) that produces the most perceived value per dollar.

Exchange, Transactions, and Relationships

The fourth marketing link has to do with what we usually think of as selling, but is more rightly called exchange. *Exchange* involves satisfying a demand for a product by offering something in return (it need not be money). Kotler identifies five requirements for a satisfactory exchange:

1. There are at least two parties.
2. Each party has something that might be of value to the other party.
3. Each party is capable of communication and delivery.
4. Each party is free to accept or reject the offer.
5. Each party believes it is appropriate or desirable to deal with the other party. (p. 7)

In an audiology practice, exchange occurs whenever there is a fee for service, whether it is for a tangible (e.g., batteries, hearing aids) or intangible (e.g., tympanogram) product. The audiologist's purview includes all products available for exchange in the practice, not just intangibles. The only difference between "selling" batteries and "providing" diagnostic hearing evaluations is the fee (and value) assigned to each exchange.

The bill, check, or receipt represents the *transaction* that occurs when an exchange occurs. A transaction itemizes the two things of value (product and money), the date, and the place of service.

In the previous section, a consumer assigned value to a future exchange based on an audiologist's reputation in the community, in addition to other factors such as product cost. This is an example of *relationship marketing*. In relationship marketing, exchanges between a company and its markets are mutually satisfactory to the point that exchanges cease to be one-time transactions and become routine

Use relationship marketing to build marketing networks

arrangements as long-term trusts are established. Relationship marketing reduces the costs and time of transactions and maximizes benefits to both parties. In audiology practices, *marketing networks* based on relationships need to be established not only with patients, but also with suppliers and referral sources.

Markets, Marketing, and Marketers

From the preceding discussion of marketing links, it is clear that a *market* is all the people sharing a need or want for a product who may be willing and able to obtain it through exchange. Targeting these markets is the fifth link in the marketing chain. Markets can be defined broadly (e.g., all people with hearing loss) or very narrowly (e.g., all males over 55 years old with noise-induced hearing loss and annual incomes greater than $100,000 who live in the Central City area).

The final link is marketing. Marketing is the effort by marketers to maximize the likelihood of exchange by identifying a need, creating a demand, and offering a product that satisfies that demand at the best value. ASHA and AAA representatives are marketing when they state to the FDA that consumers' best interests are served by having comprehensive audiology examinations prior to obtaining hearing aids. *Audiologists are marketers whenever they put forth their services as high quality and professional.* In short, we are always marketing if we are doing a good job, which takes us back to the definition of societal marketing, modified for an audiology practice:

> *The process of determining the needs, wants, and interests of people with auditory (or vestibular) disorders and delivering the desired diagnostic evaluations, treatments, and tangible products more effectively and efficiently than other hearing health providers in a way that preserves or enhances the consumer's and the society's well-being.*

POSITIONING STRATEGIES

Central to all marketing strategies is the concept of "positioning." All links in the marketing chain relate to positioning. It is futile to attempt to provide services or sell products if they are not right for the market, if they are priced incorrectly, if the practice is not known to the market, or if the practice lacks a credible image.

The vast array of material available to consumers has made information a disposable commodity in our society. This means that traditional marketing approaches (e.g., advertising, public relations) have limited value and must be exquisitely timed. Both Kotler and McKenna advocate relationship marketing strategies based on: (a) long-term alliances, (b) educational efforts, and (c) high-quality products. Strategic relationships should be established with suppliers, investors, and patients. Relationship marketing not only reduces the cost of doing business, but it can also provide the intuitive knowledge, flexibility, and solid operating base that are necessary to survive in industries like hearing health care where rapid improvements in technology are transforming the profession.

In technical fields like audiology and hearing aid manufacturing, the complexity and diversity of information and products confuses and intimidates many consumers. In marketing parlance, they *want* to know more about their hearing problem and about hearing aids before they can decide how best to *satisfy* their *hearing needs*. The best strategy in such cases is to use marketing as an educational process that informs the consumer and, in the case of tangible products, provides reassurances regarding performance and warranties.

Marketing is an ongoing educational process

McKenna identifies three key steps every business needs to take when developing marketing strategies:

1. Know where you are going. As part of the business plan, and at intervals thereafter, identify strengths, weaknesses, and goals of the practice. The practice's mission statement should be posted and its goals need to be discussed periodically with employees. Use internal audits to find out if everyone in the practice is going in the same direction and if the practice has developed a coherent identity. Failure in these regards can result in missed opportunities, infighting, and inertia.

Adopt and use a mission statement

2. Know what business you are in. The famous management expert Peter Drucker has observed that the only way to know what business you are in is to look at it from the outside, from the point of view of the customer and the market. Listen to patients' desires and frustrations. Only by listening carefully to patients and understanding their attitudes and perceptions can management know the market environment and develop an intuitive knowledge of what will and will not work. Spend time in the marketplace and look for patterns and trends outside and within the practice. Maintain a fresh and unbiased view of the marketplace by "thinking small": make sure everyone in the practice interacts and listens to customers and suppliers on a regular basis.

View the practice through the eyes of the consumers

3. Decide on a positioning strategy. Use the information from steps 1 and 2 to define concrete steps the practice will take to identify its products and its image. These steps are, of course, unique to each practice, but there are some underlying basic concepts.

The Four Ps

The Four Ps of Marketing
- *Product*
- *Price*
- *Place*
- *Promotion*

In modern marketing theory, positioning is a functional marketing strategy designed to optimize profitable sales to target markets through design and implementation of "marketing mixes." The marketing mix refers to the type and combination of marketing tools that are used to pursue the objective. Staab and Jelonek (1994) give a concise summary of practical applications of different marketing mixes for hearing health professionals.

One well-known classification of marketing mix tools is the "four Ps:" *product, price, place,* and *promotion* (McCarthy, 1981). For audiologists, these components are represented as follows:

1. Product (or service). This is the most basic of the marketing mix tools, encompassing all goods and services the practice offers to consumers. It addresses topics including what services to emphasize, which are most profitable, what images they project, and what consumer needs do they meet (Pearce & Robinson, 1991). For hearing aids, the product component portion of the strategy will address brand names, variety, quality, design, features, size, service, warranties, and returns.

2. Price. Pricing strategies may be cost-oriented (wholesale cost plus markup), market-oriented (based on demand), competition-oriented (discounting), or a combination of these strategies. Pricing must be consistent with perceived value and must also generate a gross profit margin. For audiologic tests and services, the pricing component addresses third party reimbursement levels within the community, time to perform the services, cost of equipment used, and staff costs. For hearing aids, the pricing component addresses wholesale cost of goods, manufacturers' discounts and payment plans, discounts to patients and patient payment plans, cost of warranties, and cost of returns.

3. Place. This marketing mix tool asks where, when, and by whom products and services are offered? Are products/services easily accessible and available? An audiology practice invokes this marketing tool when selecting its location. It may emphasize this tool heavily when competing for contracts (e.g., assigning an audiologist with portable equipment to cover nursing homes or hospital nurseries) or obtaining new patients (e.g., mobile test vans, screenings at retirement enclaves).

4. Promotion. This last marketing mix tool is the most familiar, incorporating decisions regarding advertising, media, sales promotion, public relations, and direct marketing. Different audiology practices' marketing strategies rely more or less strongly on this tool in their marketing mix, using some variety of the following: yellow page column listing or display ads; direct mail pieces (often in a co-op arrangement with a hearing aid manufacturer); newsletters[1] (written by the practice or purchased from a national distributor); business cards, maps, and brochures; biographical sketches of staff audiologists; letters to referrals and patients; letters to or meetings with potential referral sources; television or radio talk show appearances; published or broadcast interviews or articles; newspaper advertisements or announcements; professional speaking engagements; logos and/or announcements appearing on anything from plastic magazine covers to billboards; coupon book advertisements; hand-outs (e.g., stickers, bags, pencils, etc.); product/referral packages for physicians (e.g., Hear Pens).

---

[1]In addition to their promotional utility, newsletters and other direct-mail literature that are sent, bulk mail can serve a secondary function of purging and updating patient records. Simply have the words "Address Correction Requested" printed in the upper left hand corner of the mailer below the return address. All items with incorrect addresses will be returned to sender with corrected information, for a minimal cost.

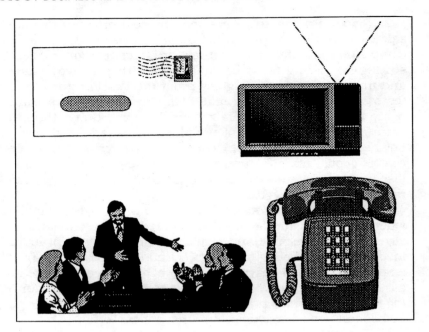

Dynamic Positioning

All positioning is competitive because consumers use hierarchical comparisons to evaluate products and services of different companies and different professionals (e.g., "This was a much more thorough test than I received at Audiologists Unlimited").[2] It is extremely important to establish a positive position at the outset. Once an image is set in the public's mind, it is very hard to change. "Creating an image" amounts to the aggregate of all the things the practice does in the marketplace.

McKenna makes the distinction between "marketing-driven" strategies (based on advertising and promotion) versus "market-driven" strategies (developing strong products and relationships with others in the marketplace). Avoid focussing too much marketing effort on tangible products, technologies, advertisements, or promotions. New technologies

---

[2]Always exercise extreme caution if comparing professions negatively in advertisements, brochures, etc. For example, the FDA (Davids, 1994, p. 1) specifically warns audiologists against using the following statements:

"the average hearing aid dealer is not always qualified to do all the tests and evaluation central to a person's hearing."

"[FDA] found that fewer than 50% of the people who bought hearing aids were adequately tested and evaluated."

"[FDA] advises you to consult an audiologist . . . before purchasing a hearing aid."

"success with hearing aids is 13 times greater when they are provided by an audiologist."

can quickly undermine a marketing position that is based on a particular piece of hardware (e.g., ABR) or technology (e.g., "noise suppression" circuitry). Consumers are deluged with so much promotional material nowadays that they tend to cast a jaundiced eye on advertising efforts. This "discount factor" prevents advertising and promotion from being image builders—they can reinforce an image but they cannot build one.

McKenna describes three progressive stages of "dynamic positioning" that evolve as a business matures: product positioning, market positioning, and corporate positioning. These positions were briefly touched on at the beginning of the chapter and will now be described as they apply to individual audiology practices.

Product Positioning

Product positioning asks the question *"How does what I do fit into the present marketing environment?"* It is answered by identifying product(s), differentiating them according to market trends, and targeting specific audiences. The products an audiology practice can offer are: screening, testing, rehabilitation services, hearing conservation programs, hearing aids, assistive listening devices, and supplies. The first four are intangibles, the last three are tangibles. *All seven fall under the general product, which is hearing care.*

Product positioning requires that the practice establish a unique position for these product(s) by *differentiation*. Differentiation in an audiology practice can be done in a variety of ways, and some ways are better than others at contributing to a positive image:

- *Technology.* Does the practice use state-of-the-art diagnostic applications? Real-ear measurements? Programmable instruments?
- *Price.* One of the most obvious and overused methods is to undercut competitors on pricing of hearing aids or to offer "free hearing tests."
- *Application.* As examples, a practice might imprint the idea with local neurologists that hearing evaluations are an important part of balance assessments; write educational articles for the public on why hearing tests are important for everyone, not just seniors.
- *Quality.* Stress the importance of quality service delivery to referral sources and staff by discussing it, posting quality goals, and constantly trying to improve quality. Imprint the image of quality at every patient encounter by ensuring that all staff

interactions with each other, with patients, and with their referral sources live up to that quality image.

■ *Distribution channels.* Hearing aid dispensers and some audiologists have traditionally offered home visits to patients—a custom that certainly has its pluses and minuses, depending on locale. Another example of differentiation along this dimension would be to offer audiology and hearing aid services through a health maintenance organization (HMO), or managed care network, where a practice achieves some degree of exclusive access to enrolled patients by virtue of its preferred provider status.

■ *Target audiences.* This is discussed below as the "third golden rule."

■ *Qualifications.* Do employees in the practice have any unique skills? Do they have stronger educational backgrounds, better credentials, or more experience than competitors?

How should one decide which of these avenues to choose for distinguishing the products of the practice? McKenna (1986) identifies four "golden rules" for product positioning.

Four Golden Rules for Product Positioning

- *Understand market trends*

- *Focus on intangible positioning factors having to do with quality*

- *Focus on a specific audience and serve it better than anyone else*

- *Experiment and pay attention to market reaction*

Golden Rule #1. McKenna's first rule is to *understand market trends.* Product differentiation is useless if it is along dimensions that do not interest the market, hence the adage that *the market actually positions products.* Identical products can be perceived quite differently by the market, depending on how they are presented. As examples:

A patient may receive duplicate hearing evaluations in two audiology practices but assign a much higher value to one than the other, depending on how the history was taken, the audiologist's credentials, how the equipment looked, how cordial the staff was, and how quickly results were communicated to a physician.

The same brand and model hearing aid can be dispensed in two practices, yet be perceived as completely different by the patient, depending on whether it is marketed as part of a hearing health care program or as an expensive piece of technology.

Marketing trends are dynamic, hence another adage that "timing is everything." Knowing what is available, what to say about it, and when to say it constitutes the marketers' proverbial window of opportunity. Two timely examples:

National discussions on regulation of hearing aid sales have placed emphasis on the word "comprehensive," lending new meaning (and probably value) to the product dubbed "comprehensive audiologic evaluation." It is a good idea to recognize the market trend and start using these words. An even better idea is to improve diagnostic services (e.g., start doing speech roll-over testing on every patient; design a better history form) in response to market demand.

Due to massive advertising and technological development in the personal computer industry, the words "programmable," "computerized," "digital," and "user-friendly" have acquired new meaning (and value) to most Americans. The advent of sophisticated hearing aid circuits in the same period has allowed the hearing care industry to usurp those words to describe hearing aids. Thus, hearing aids can piggyback on a high-tech market trend, with the result that consumers are responsive to the concept of "computerized" hearing aids and place added value on such instruments.

Golden Rule #2. McKenna's second golden rule is to *focus on intangible positioning factors having to do with quality.*

New technologies can fade away

McKenna bases this rule on the observations that tangible products often move quickly from leading edge to obsolescence and also that consumers are more interested in quality, service, and support than they are in narrow technical differences between products. He cautions against positioning through "specmanship" (e.g., "Our ABR equipment has a sampling rate of 50 Khz, much better than the 20 Khz machine used at Audiologists Unlimited"), since few consumers base their buying decisions on objective standards.

The concept of quality improvement underlies good marketing practices

What *does* motivate consumers to purchase is the perception that a business is a technological leader that consistently offers services of the highest quality, products of the highest technology, and provides total support for all products. Once again, the concept of Quality Improvement underlies good marketing. Dispensing audiology practices that focus on all aspects of quality in service delivery are positioning their product(s) as high quality and low risk to the patient. This type of positioning establishes an aura of trust and confidence with their patients, irrespective of the brands and types of hearing aids the practice may choose to recommend.

Golden Rule #3. McKenna's third golden rule is to *focus on a specific audience (market niche) and serve it better than anyone else*. Markets can be targeted many ways, including geographically, by age, by income, by profession, or "psychographically" (e.g., see discussion of psychological mapping in Chapter 6). It is not wise to try to be all things to all people—doing so puts the practice in competition with everyone else and reduces the overall quality of the product. It is also not necessary. The hearing health care industries (audiology and hearing aids) are both in the early stages of their development, and there is more than enough room for everyone in the marketplace.

In addition to maintaining market share, look for new markets

What *is* necessary is to decide what market niche the practice will service and then proceed to position the audiology products to meet the demands of that niche group. For example, a practice that announces free hearing tests and "$50 off all hearing aids" is targeting a niche group that values cost over quality and service. The mirror image of that niche group—those who value quality and service over cost—will probably seek services through a practice that markets through physician contacts and community lectures.

What *is* wise is to identify new types of markets and expand the practice not by taking market share away from competitors, but by increasing the overall market. Depending on the locale, there are various examples of opening new markets including:

Pediatric audiology came into its own in recent years as physicians and parents learned to appreciate the complexities of pediatric audiologic evaluation, interpretation and management strategies and the importance of early intervention.

There is now a market for recreational use of ear protection and electronic noise reduction devices, thanks to technological improvements and product positioning.

Recently published research on auditory sensory deprivation has created a whole new group of binaurally aided individuals.

Successful application of hearing aids to persons with precipitous high-frequency hearing loss often caused by noise exposure requires special knowledge and experience with amplification.

Golden Rule #4. McKenna's last golden rule for product positioning is to *experiment and pay attention to market reaction.* This is not to say that patients are treated as guinea pigs. New techniques and new technologies may or may not have a place in a practice, but that is difficult to know until they are tried. For example, in the early 1980s, impedance testing (now know as acoustic immittance) was slow to be accepted in some circles as part of a "comprehensive" audiologic evaluation. Not infrequently, it was taught and implemented only as a test of middle ear function (and still is in some graduate programs!). Fortunately, some audiologists and researchers were quick to add the technique to the standard test battery and just as quick to discover that it was a robust test of retrocochlear integrity. At that point, the product positioning of impedance testing changed dramatically (including its name), much to the benefit of the profession and patients.

Market Positioning

Market positioning asks the question *"How do I get my products recognized and establish credibility with my target audiences?"* It is answered by a slow building process based on *inference, reference, and evidence.* Achieving good market positioning takes time, patience, and consistently high-quality performance. A practice must develop solid marketing networks with reputable professionals within and outside of the profession (inference) and with patients and referral sources who are satisfied and willing to tell others (reference). Success in these regards breeds success (evidence), to the point where the practice and its products eventually gain credibility in the marketplace. McKenna identifies five methods for establishing market position by building credibility. They are described in the following sections.

Five Methods for Establishing Market Position

- *Word of mouth*
- *Develop the infrastructure*
- *Form strategic relationships*
- *Buy from the right suppliers and sell to the right customers*
- *Know how to deal with the media*

Word of Mouth

Everyone knows about word of mouth, but few businesses set up a plan to direct it. The first step is to decide what message to spread. As discussed in product positioning, the message should most likely focus on intangibles such as quality (e.g., complete and accurate diagnostic testing; hearing aids dispensed as part of an aural rehabilitation "package") or efficiency (e.g., one-day turnaround on reports) rather than on hearing aids or a particular technology.

The next step is to decide who is to receive the message. In the example where "quality" is the message, the impression of quality should be apparent to everyone who comes in contact with the business, for example:

■ Customers know that they received complete and accurate services by qualified professionals who listened carefully to their concerns and took appropriate steps to address those concerns;

■ Sales and customer representatives know that staff members were respectful, open, knowledgeable, and interested in learning about new products and services (regardless of whether the office made purchases);

■ Physicians' offices know that their patients will be thoroughly evaluated and that treatment recommendations will be based solely on the patients' needs; in every case, physicians know that they will receive appropriate and timely communications from the audiologists regarding results and recommendations;

■ Community people (delivery people, people being interviewed, people who wander into the practice looking for directions, people calling for information). People who come in contact with the practice know that they were treated with respect and helped to the best of the staff's ability.

The next step is to decide who gives the message. In the "quality" example above, it is obvious that the answer must be "Everyone in the practice!"

The final step is to find out if the message is being received. This should be done formally, on a regular basis, through the use of surveys for patients (cf., Welch, 1994). ASHA sells a customer survey form for office use (see sample in Appendix A, Section C, at the end of the book). This step should also be performed informally on a daily basis by asking patients how they feel about the personal treatment, services, and equipment that they have received in the office.

How important is word of mouth? According to surveys done by the Technical Assistance Research Programs Institute in Washington, D.C., it is very important, especially if the message is bad (Boyett & Conn, 1991). Those surveys yielded the following information:

■ Consumers were five times more likely to stop doing business with a company for poor service than for poor product quality or high cost.

■ 96% of a company's dissatisfied customers never complained to the company, but 90% quit doing business with the company.

■ The average dissatisfied customer complains about the company to nine other people. Thirteen percent complain to at least 20 people!
■ The cost of losing a customer is five times the annual value of the customer's account.

In contrast, the research shows that a reputation for good service and high quality pays off in many ways (Boyett & Conn, 1991):

■ An undifferentiated product accompanied by outstanding service may command up to a 10% price premium.
■ A customer who is pleased with a company will tell five other people about the company. Many of these people become customers of the company.
■ Almost all customers (95%) with a complaint will stay with a company if their complaint is resolved quickly.
■ Improving quality of service is much more cost-effective than other promotional efforts: it costs five times as much to obtain a customer than to keep one.

Develop the Infrastructure

To paraphrase McKenna, the infrastructure is all those people between the product and the customer who have an influence on the buying process. These people give credibility to the product and the company. Without the support of the infrastructure, the product and company are sure to fail. McKenna pictures infrastructures as inverted pyramids, with the company or product at the narrow tip, consumers at the wide base, and layers of related groups in between. Information about the product and company percolates up to consumers through these layers, primarily by word of mouth, and each layer influences other layers, especially those above it. McKenna (1986) explains the rationale for the inverted pyramid by describing the communication within an industry's infrastructure:

> The spreading enthusiasm [about a product, a service, an audiologist, or a practice] bounces up and down the infrastructures.... Eventually, the word reaches the top of the pyramid and the customers begin buying. It's like a massive game of whispering down the lane, with more and more people involved at each level. Each part of the infrastructure validates the others. (p. 65)

Infrastructures can be drawn up for the hearing aid industry, the audiology profession, and for individual audiology practices.

Figure 13–2 is an infrastructure for an autonomous audiology practice,[3] showing hearing services as the product. Let's look at how the infrastructure begins with a closely defined, small group of people and expands "outward and upward" as more and more people with different backgrounds and interests become involved.

The hearing care "product" is born in our university training programs and shaped for delivery to consumers by government regulations and by technological changes. It is defined within our scope of practice by our national organizations, which work to achieve good positioning for the profession and its products by third party carriers and other agencies. It is further defined by the hearing aid manufacturers, with constant changes in the way hearing losses are treated. All of these influences on the product of hearing care are discussed in our professional journals and in other media by "luminaries" in the profession (e.g., Mead Killion's letter to the Food and Drug Administration [Killion, 1994]), by important opinion makers (e.g., former Surgeon General Everett Koop), and at our professional meetings. Audiologists relate the results of these discussions to other professionals (physicians, speech pathologists, industrial health directors). Portions of discussions in the infrastructure are picked up by the media as newsworthy (e.g., FDA censorship of hearing aid manufacturers) and read by consumers, who then complete the infrastructure by talking with other consumers.

McKenna points out that infrastructures are most critical when confusion in the marketplace is greatest. Marketplace confusion over hearing care has been high in the 1990s as the nation debated managed health care, the FDA examined hearing aid regulations, and consumer protection groups testified about unethical behavior by hearing aid dispensers. It is a good idea for individual audiology practices to construct and cultivate their own infrastructures. Use the infrastructure to identify key members and delineate hierarchies of influence. Develop relationships with key members and others throughout the infrastructure. An infrastructure that is fully developed in this way is one of the best means of establishing and maintaining a practice's position in a volatile marketplace.

---

[3]The degree of automony influences the layers near the "point" of the infrastructure. The illustration is for a stand-alone practice. An infrastructure for a practice that is part of an otolaryngology practice would have ENTs near the bottom of the inverted triangle, rather than near the top as portrayed in Figure 13–2.

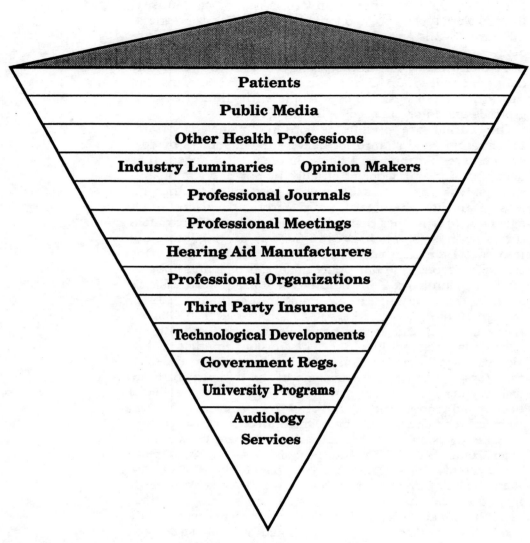

Figure 13-2. The infrastructure of audiology services.

Form Strategic Relationships

Credibility for small companies increases when they make alliances with large, reputable companies and respected groups in the community. For audiology practices, examples include but are not limited to: (a) associating with managed care networks, (b) obtaining hospital privileges, (c) affiliating with university training programs, and (d) perhaps teaching courses at the university or community college. More peripherally, it means volunteering to sit on the board of one or more community groups and participating in service clubs.

Strategic relationships must be mutually beneficial. A small practice must avoid becoming overly dependent or controlled by its more powerful affiliates. When the practice loses its autonomy, the relationship is no longer strategic and credibility suffers.

Buy from the Right Suppliers and Sell to the Right Customers

As tempting as they make it, hearing aid manufacturers that offer deep discounting, enchanting cruises, and great customer service are not always the best suppliers for an audiology practice. In searching for the right suppliers, audiologists should bear in mind their role as "customers." They need to interview each supplier, inquiring about the company's philosophy, goals, training, technical orientation, pricing, and customer support policies. The "right" supplier is one who consistently offers excellent hearing aids with cutting-edge technology at reasonable costs, sends them on time and supports them with a top-notch repair staff. A practice that accepts less than this as a customer will in turn erode its own credibility with its patients.

Market analysis divides customers into four groups according to their responsiveness to change: (a) *Innovators* are those who are willing to try something in its developmental stage. They account for only 2.5% of all consumers, but exercise greater influence over the (b) *early adopters* (13.5%), (c) *majority* (68%), and (d) *laggards* (16%). Practices should cultivate relationships with innovators to gain early insight into new products and how they should (or should not) be positioned.

There are four types of customers

Deal with the Media

It is not always easy to get the attention of the local press, but information about hearing care should be sent to specific persons in the media on a periodic basis. Newspaper articles and radio or television interviews are perceived by the public as more objective than advertisements. They also afford an opportunity to provide more information. Toward that end, articles and interviews should be informative and educational rather than promotional. Save advertising for

Aim to educate, not commercialize

last and use it to reinforce an image in the community, not create the image.

Corporate Positioning

> # Benefits of Corporate Positioning
>
> - *Lower cost of borrowing money*
> - *Lower cost of sales*
> - *Patient loyalty*
> - *Better recruiting and staff loyalty*
> - *Better sales*

Corporate positioning asks the question: *"How does my company compare with others in the health care profession?"* Corporate positioning can occur only after product and market positioning have succeeded. It is based on only one variable: financial success. McKenna recommends mixing basics with "silver bullets": relying on standard services (e.g., diagnostic audiometry, hearing aid repairs and sales) to supply practice revenues, while actively promoting a few outstanding services (e.g., otoacoustic emissions, new technology hearing aids) to maintain and build on the practice image. Once a practice achieves a reputation as a respected and prosperous business, it will benefit in the following ways:

■ *Lower cost of borrowing money.* A practice with a proven track record in the community and a good set of tax returns has leverage when it approaches banking institutions. In tight times, it can get a loan when others cannot; in freer times, it can get a loan or a line of credit at rates that are close to prime.

- *Lower cost of sales due to less advertising and bigger discounts from suppliers.* In the hypothetical practice described in the appendices of Chapters 4 and 12, early operating costs were higher because of the need to use direct mail and newspaper advertisements. Projected operating costs in later years were lower as the practice gained product, market, and corporate positioning in the community. Along the way, suppliers would begin to offer the practice larger discounts on hearing aids, more lenient payment terms, and capital equipment purchase opportunities.
- *Patient loyalty.* Repeat patients are the best part of any practice. Fixed costs are all paid and the patient is pleased to return for unsolicited services. It is a profitable encounter for all concerned.
- *Better recruiting and staff loyalty.* Maintaining and improving the quality of services cannot happen unless the staffing is consistent and of the highest quality. People like to work for a financially solid and reputable business that has positioned itself as a leader.
- *Higher volume.* Physicians do not like to commit their patients and customers do not like to commit financially to a marginal practice.

QUALITY IMPROVEMENT—THE BEST MARKETING STRATEGY OF ALL

A practice that has achieved successful product, market, and corporate positioning has only one question left to answer: *"How do we continue to improve our positioning?"* The answer lies in Continuous Quality Improvement.

Much has been written in our field and in the health care generally about Continuous Quality Improvement (CQI) (aka Quality Assurance [QA] or Total Quality Management [TQM]). CQI is discussed in terms of improving "structure," "evaluation," "process," "outcome," "functional assessment," "documentation," "customer satisfaction," and accreditation standards. In short, CQI is discussed in every aspect of what we do *except* "marketing." In fact, CQI represents the very ideal of marketing. CQI strives to clearly delineate needs ("evaluation") and address them as efficiently ("structure," "process," "documentation") and well as possible ("outcomes," "functional assessment"). In doing so, CQI aims to achieve good product and market positioning ("customer satisfaction," meeting accreditation standards). By achieving these goals, CQI enables good corporate positioning for audiology in the marketplace (cf. Harrison, 1994).

The concept of quality has been discussed in many and varied examples in this chapter. These examples are meant to illustrate that quality and marketing are integrally entwined—describable only in terms of continuous efforts, not single or limited events. It is just as nonsensical to talk about a "quality hearing test" as it is to ask "How much time should be spent on marketing?" Marketing is the sum of all of a practice's endeavors and quality is the descriptor of the success of the marketing effort.

Deming says doing your best is not good enough

W. Edwards Deming has described management steps that are necessary for the promulgation of quality improvement. He points out that "doing your best" is not good enough. Quality improvement requires that everyone in the group must first know what to do and then do their best. In marketing parlance, this parallels McKenna's three key steps for developing marketing strategies (Know Where You're Going, Know What Business You are In, Decide on a Positioning Strategy). We will conclude this chapter by summarizing Deming's Fourteen Points (Reisberg & Frattali, 1990; Walton, 1986), because they are so essential to the success of any marketing plan and any practice.

1. *Create constancy of purpose for improvement of product and services.* The marketing goal of the practice is not to make money, the goal is to stay in business and provide jobs through innovation, research, constant improvement, and maintenance.
2. *Adopt the new philosophy.* Mistakes and negativism are unacceptable.
3. *Cease dependence on inspection to improve quality.* Quality comes from improving the process, not from inspection of what is already done. Properly instructed workers can contribute to this improvement.
4. *End the practice of awarding business on price tag alone.* Price has no meaning without consideration of quality (as perceived by the practitioner as well as the consumer).
5. *Improve constantly and forever the system of production and service.* Again, quality is not a one-time event. Always strive to improve quality and productivity, thereby reducing costs.
6. *Institute training on the job.*

7. *Institute leadership.* Help employees do a better job and identify those who need individual help.
8. *Drive out fear.* Everyone in the practice needs to feel secure in order to do their best and ask enough questions to be sure they "know where they are going."
9. *Break down barriers between staff areas.* Make sure everyone in the practice works together as a team.
10. *Eliminate slogans, exhortations, and targets for the workforce* (e.g., "THINK" doesn't help!!).
11. *Eliminate numerical quotas.* Selling on commission or doing X number of audiograms per day is antithetical to the marketing of quality.
12. *Remove barriers to pride of workmanship.* Be sure the practice is properly equipped and that everyone is encouraged for doing their best.
13. *Institute a vigorous program of education and retraining.*
14. *Put everyone in the practice to work to accomplish these steps.*

SUMMARY

Marketing is not advertising. Marketing is a chain of events that begins with identifying a need and ends with satisfying that need through exchange. The best marketers are those who use a "marketing mix" to plan and implement marketing strategies that efficiently and effectively yield the highest quality satisfaction to consumers.

In the case of audiology, hearing and vestibular problems are needs that can be satisfied by the products of hearing health care. Whether or not a consumer visits an audiologist depends on the cost and accessibility of services, the value the consumer assigns to hearing care, and the audiologist's image as a care provider. Successful audiology practices must make their hearing services valuable to consumers and establish relationships with those consumers. They must also establish good working relationships with other groups in the infrastructure of hearing health care. They must achieve and maintain profitability. These efforts compose marketing strategies.

Marketing strategies encompass education, alliances, technological applications, research, listening, public relations, and advertising. Intentionally or not, everything that is done in and by an audiology practice contributes to the marketing of the practice, either positively or negatively. For this reason, it is important for everyone in the practice to understand the mission and goals of the practice. Practice goals are reached by *product positioning* (identifying and providing services and goods for which there is a need and a want); *market positioning* (distinguishing a practice from competitors through inference, reference, and evidence); and *corporate positioning* (achieving financial stability).

Quality is the measure of success for marketing strategies. Quality reflects the efficiency, effectiveness, and satisfaction associated with a practice's goods and services, as perceived by others in the infrastructure. The best long-term marketing strategy is Continuous Quality Improvement (CQI). CQI is the means by which a successful practice continues to build on its success, as manifest in Deming's 14 points for constant improvement.

REFERENCES

Beck, L. B. (1994). 1994 presidential address. Healthcare and audiology: Qualified quality providers. *Audiology Today, 6*(4), 4–6.

Boyett, J. H., & Conn, H. P. (1991). *Workplace 2000.* New York: Plume.

Davis, J. (1994). Letter from the Department of Health and Human Services to Frederick Spahr, Executive Director of the American Speech-Language-Hearing Association. Rockville, MD: Food and Drug Administration.

Harrison, M. (Ed.). (1994). Total quality management: Application to audiology. *Seminars in Hearing, 15*(4), 259–330.

Killion, M. C. (1994, March 31). *Open letter to Hearing Aid Regulation Division of the Food and Drug Administration.* Elk Grove Village, IL: Author.

Kotler, P. (1991). *Marketing management. Analysis, planning, implementation, and control* (7th ed.). Englewood Cliffs, NJ: Prentice-Hall.

McCarthy, E. J. (1981). *Basic marketing: A managerial approach* (9th ed.). Boston: Richard D. Irwin.

McKenna, R. (1986). *The Regis touch. New marketing strategies for uncertain times.* New York: Addison-Wesley.

Pearce, J. A., & Robinson, R. B., Jr. (1991). *Formulation, implementation, and control of competitive strategy* (4th ed.). Boston: Irwin.

Reisberg, M., & Frattali, C. (1990, October). Toward total quality management. *Quality Assurance Digest,* pp. 1–5.

Staab, W., & Jelonek, S. (1994). Are you finding your competitive advantage? *Hearing Instruments, 45*(7), 20–21.

Walton, M. (1986). *The Deming management method.* New York: Perigee/Putnam.

Welch, D. S. (1994). How do you know if your customers are satisfied? *Hearing Instruments, 45*(4), 17–19.

SUGGESTED READING

Harrison, M. (Ed.). (1994). Total quality management: Application to audiology. *Seminars in Hearing, 15*(4), 259–330.

APPENDIX 13-A

Elements of a Marketing Plan

Marketing plans spell out strategies and marketing-mix programs for achieving objectives. They can be very formal and have a number of sections, but this depends on their readership and the reasons for their preparation. The following is a brief outline of basic aspects of a marketing plan, some of which have been further illustrated in the Sample Business Plan contained in Appendix 4-A of Chapter 4.

I. <u>Executive Summary</u>
A very brief overview of the plan.

II. <u>Current Marketing Situation</u>
Provides data on the target market(s), products, competition, distribution (e.g., how many hearing aids sold nationally last year), and broad societal trends. (See Appendix 4-A in Chapter 4 for an example of this section.)

III. <u>SWOT Analysis</u>
(Strengths/Weaknesses, Opportunities/Threats). Strengths and weaknesses are factors within the company. Widespread and reputable name recognition is an example of a strength. Inexperienced staff is a weakness. Opportunities and threats are factors outside the company. An emphasis by the FDA on hearing testing prior to hearing aid fitting is an opportunity; a perception of otolaryngologists as the entry level for hearing health care is a threat.
SWOT factors are written along with possible actions that could be taken. They are ranked according to importance.

IV. <u>Issues Analysis</u>
SWOT factors are used to define the main issues the plan will address (e.g., Should the practice hire another experienced audiologist? Should the practice affiliate with an otolaryngology practice?).

V. <u>Financial Objectives</u>
Based on the issues, goals are set for net profits, cash flow, rate of return on investment, etc. (see Chapter 12 for an explanation of financial terms). For example, the practice might set a financial objective to increase net profits by 10% in the next year.

VI. <u>Marketing Objectives</u>
The financial objectives must be translated into marketing efforts. These objectives need to be stated in a measureable form for a stated period. They should be internally consistent and attainable. They should be stated in order of importance. In the example financial objective given above, the marketing objectives might be:

1. Increase revenues from comprehensive audiologic evaluations by 30% over last year.
2. Therefore, increase the number of diagnostic tests by 20% over last year.
3. Increase the number of primary care physicians (PCPs) that refer to Cardinal Hearing Services, Inc.(CHS) by an average of two per month.

4. Increase the number of referrals from established PCP referral sources by an average of one patient per month.
5. Aim for an average reimbursement of $___ per comprehensive diagnostic hearing evaluation.

VII. Marketing Strategy
In paragraph or list form, broadly state the manner in which marketing tools will be used to reach objectives. For example in the marketing objectives above:
"Cardinal Hearing Services, Inc. (CHS)'s basic strategy for increasing diagnostic revenues is to target primary care physicians (PCPs), particularly those with gerontology certification. Our comprehensive diagnostic evaluation will be expanded, at little cost to the patient. We will take steps to guarantee efficiency in communicating results to PCPs and in performing third-party billing. A new and intensified promotional campaign will be developed to increase PCP awareness of auditory communication disorders in seniors and augment their perception of CHS's expertise and efficiency. Finally, we will put more funds into test equipment."

VIII. Action Programs
Given the broad objectives of the strategy, action programs now describe the "who, what, when, where, and how" elements of the program. Continuing the above example:

January. Incorporate a central processing screening with speech materials into comprehensive hearing evaluations on adults over 65 years of age; also, automated loudness-growth functions at four frequencies in cases of sensorineural hearing loss. Additional fees for these services amount to $25, in line with Medicare reimbursement rates. Dr. A will arrange for purchase of equipment for loudness growth testing, at planned cost of $1,000.

Mail patient reports and results to the PCP on the same day as the evaluation. Do electronic Medicare patient billing at the time of service. Mr. B will handle this at no projected cost.

Monthly. Schedule brief meetings with four PCPs in their offices, one per week. Bring in lunch if possible. Provide hearing screening devices to the physicians and/or staff. Dr. A and Mr. B will handle this, at a planned cost of $1,500.

Quarterly. Mail a quarterly physicians' newsletter to all PCPs in the Central City area, introducing an individual staff member in each issue and featuring one of the following topics:

1. Communication handicap and hearing loss
2. Central processing problems in the elderly
3. Level-dependent compression circuitry for accelerated loudness growth functions
4. Assistive listening devices

Dr. A and Mr. B will handle this, at a planned cost of $400.

June. Purchase a small, used sound booth and install it in the second consultation room, to accommodate increased diagnostic test scheduling. Equip it with the portable 1.5 channel audiometer already owned by CHS. Mr. B will handle this, at a planned cost of $3,500.

IX. Projected Profit-and-Loss Statement
This is a budget in which the number of projected tests and the average fees are shown on the revenue side. The costs of marketing, equipment, and staffing are

shown on the expense side. The difference in expenses to revenues is the projected profit or loss.

X. <u>Controls</u>

Steps are outlined for monitoring the action programs (e.g., monthly production reports, new patient reports, referral analysis reports). Contingency plans may be stated (e.g., "If printing costs sky-rocket, we will move to desktop publishing").

Pricing

Pricing is only one of the "four Ps" of marketing discussed in Chapter 13, but it is so important that it deserves separate discussion. If the **Price** is unacceptable to customers,[1] then there is no point in putting efforts into the other three Ps (**Product**—technology, expertise; **Place**—office location, service delivery; and **Promotion**—advertising, publicity). Of the five deadly business sins identified by Drucker (1993), three of them have to do with pricing![2]

Even though price is one of the four Ps in the marketing mix, it is rarely considered a strong marketing tool. Yet, as Mondello (1992) observes:

> for many companies (particularly start-ups or small, growing businesses) there is no other marketing or sales decision that more immediately affects customer acceptance or rejection of what you sell, your cash flow, and perhaps even your overall success or failure. (p. 80)

But is this true in the "business" of hearing health care? After all, our diagnostic fees are set to a large extent by federal, state, and HMO reimbursement schedules. Our competitors dictate what we can charge for hearing aids and other tangible products. Why think about pricing when we cannot use it as a marketing tool? The answer is that in-depth thinking about pricing forces the audiologist to consider costs, productivity, quality, and competition. Pricing that carefully addresses these and other marketing management issues is of paramount importance to hearing health care providers as they learn to compete in the era of health care reform.

> The ASHA (1994a) sums it up without pulling any punches: In the new system of health care delivery and reimbursement, cost of services will be of primary importance. Purchasers want to know our estimated costs for serving populations . . . and they want to know those costs up-front, before they buy our services. Like any prudent buyer, they want the best value for the least cost . . . . How will you respond? Do you know your average costs for providing services to individuals . . . ? (p. 17)

---

[1]"Customers" is the word of choice in this chapter for two reasons: (1) pricing is a marketing activity and (2) customers are not only patients, they may also be hospitals, insurance organizations (HMOs or private insurers), nursing homes, physicians, industrial groups, and so on etc.

[2]These three are: (1) The worship of high profit margins and of "premium pricing," (2) Mispricing a new product by charging "what the market will bear," and (3) Cost-driven pricing.

THE CONCEPT OF PRICING

Pricing is the point where marketing theory and economic theory join forces to produce a practical result. In combination, they give providers the means to set fees for hearing health care fees that (a) correspond to the value consumers assign to the products, (b) cover all costs, and (c) give the maximum return to the provider.

Arriving at optimum pricing for an individual practice requires three steps by the owner/manager (see Figure 14–1). First, decide which *pricing objective* best meets the marketing objectives developed in the business plan. Is the practice most interested in maximizing profits, the number of sales, or maintaining the status quo? Second, select a *target measure*. Depending on the pricing objective, the target measure may be profits, sales, market share, competitive comparisons, and so on. Finally, implement a *pricing method*. Pricing methods are formulas that use the target measure as the independent variable. For example, the Return on Investment pricing method sets a percentage of profit as the target measure and calculates what prices must be to meet that goal.

All of this makes pricing sound tedious and academic. Why not just calculate costs and markup? This approach gains validity from articles in hearing health care journals that describe principles and steps for setting prices that consist of plugging numbers into expense/income formulas (Kamara, 1988; Navarro & Klodd, 1989). In all likelihood, most audiology fees, regardless of setting are set in this fashion. Costs and formulas are certainly an integral step in the price setting process, but they should be the *last* step in the process. Putting them first or using them alone limits the audiology practice. Like putting the proverbial cart before the horse, the revenues begin to dictate what the practice does, rather than the practice using revenues to further its long-term goals.

Pricing is more than costs and formulas

The following sections follow the outline presented in Figure 14–1, considering pricing objectives and pricing targets first, then relating pricing methods to pricing objectives. The chapter ends with a discussion of pricing strategies.

PRICING OBJECTIVES AND TARGET MEASURES

Figure 14–1 identifies three types of pricing objectives, each with its corresponding target measures and pricing methods:

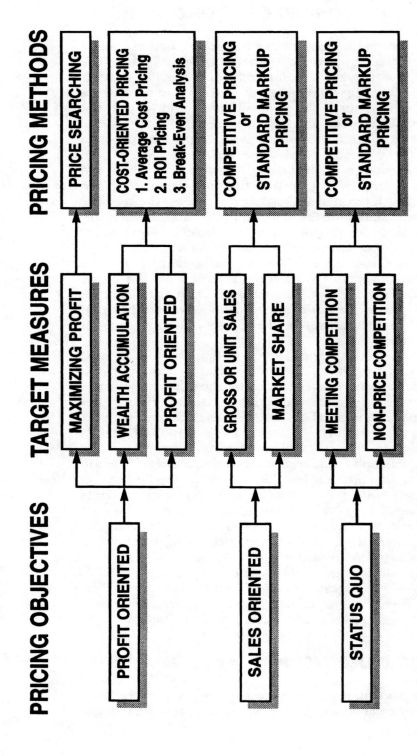

Figure14-1. Steps for determining optimum pricing.

1. Profit-oriented
2. Sales-oriented
3. Status-quo oriented

Pricing objectives dictate how compatible the practice's fees and charges are with everything else the practice is trying to achieve. The owner/manager should make this important decision by getting out the business plan, reviewing the company's written goals and marketing objectives, and selecting the pricing objective(s) that reflects the philosophy and furthers the goals of the business. Is the practice committed to increasing market share? maximizing cash flow or profit? establishing a particular image? deterring competition? increasing sales? holding on until retirement?

To ensure compatibility, the pricing objective should be *put in writing and explained to staff members*. It is the framework for the pricing methods and pricing policies that follow.

Profit-oriented Pricing

These objectives set some measure of money as their target measure. Objectives may be stated in terms of numerical *target returns,* such as a set percentage of profit, return on investment, or increase in profit over some previous period.

In many cases, the objectives are stated not by a numerical target, but in terms of "comfort" targets. Examples would be practices in which the goal is to: (a) make "some" amount of profit (e.g., the bottom line is positive), (b) support a certain work style (e.g., enough income to support lavish staff without going in the red), or (c) provide a comfortable life style (e.g., high owner income).

Profit maximization is a target that seeks not just some profit, but *as much profit as possible.* On the face of it, this seems reprehensible and socially irresponsible. In fact, profit maximization is often the best and most socially responsible objective that autonomous audiologists can select, for two reasons:

1. Competition drives down price. Hearing health care operates in what economists call *monopolistic competition.* In such environments, demand increases as price decreases, every business has several close competitors, and no business is able to prevent other competitors from entering the market unless they lower prices to equal costs, thereby denying profitability to anyone (Mulligan, 1989). Competitive environments foster lower prices by encouraging competitors to offer higher quality services/goods at lower prices to spur demand. Therefore, a *profit maximization target aims to maximize profits by lowering prices and costs.*

2. Elasticity drives down price. Elasticity refers to how much the demand for a product fluctuates with price. Demand for necessities is inelastic because need supersedes price. Price increases translate to more profit because demand does not drop. For example, a patient with an ear infection does not wait for medicine to go on sale before purchasing a prescription. In contrast, luxury and high technology items are elastic products because relatively small changes in price drive demand up or down. Hearing care is a good example of an elastic product. One has only to look at the number of consumers who respond to a free hearing screening versus the number who elect to schedule hearing tests. *For elastic products, a profit-maximization target aims to lower prices to a point where increased volume produces optimal profit.*

Sales-oriented Pricing

In contrast to profit-oriented pricing objectives, sales-oriented pricing looks at target measures (e.g., revenues, number of sales, market share) without regard to profit. The pitfall for audiology practices that adopt sales-oriented objectives is "profitless success." Such practices may do very high volumes, bring in lots of revenue, have large market shares, and operate at a loss.

Avoid profitless success

Why would any practice adopt sales-oriented pricing objectives? First, it is much easier to count sales than it is to try to maximize profits. Second, some high-volume products like hearing aid batteries lend themselves to this approach. Third, some practices pay commission based on number of sales. Fourth, it seems to be inherent in our professional culture. What clinic director exists who does not characterize his or her operation in terms of number of patient visits per year, per clinician, and so on? What hearing aid manufacturer or practice broker exists who does not categorize dispensing audiologists according to the number of hearing aids they sell per month?

Status-quo Pricing

This type of objective may be chosen by practices whose owners are happy with the way things are going and do not feel competitive pressures. In stable environments, status quo pricing objectives are a means of avoiding price competition, but they also discourage creative thinking on the part of management. Status-quo pricing objectives can also be part of a marketing plan aimed at nonprice competition. Here, prices are left unchanged while one or more of the other three Ps are enhanced. For example, quality of diagnostic services is improved (Product), a new office is opened (Place), or a series of lectures is offered at local retirement centers (Place and Promotion).

PRICING METHODS

Competitive Pricing

This is the simplest and most deceptively simple-minded pricing method. It is employed to satisfy status quo or sales-oriented pricing objectives. Service fees and product charges are set at or below those of competitors, *without regard to profitability*. An obvious example of this method is the "price war" in which hearing aids are advertised at low prices designed to undercut the competition. A less obvious example is in managed competition when hospitals or managed care organizations award services to the lowest bidder.

No skill is required to set prices the same as or lower than competitors, but a good deal of skill is required to ensure profitability. Thus, *competitive pricing is an inadequate pricing method because it does not take market demand and profits into account.* What if prices are set below profitability? Is there a break-even point? If there is, how long until it is predicted to occur? What assumptions are being made about future costs and number of services/sales? To answer these questions, the owner/manager of the audiology practice must do a complete financial analysis of all fixed and variable costs associated with the service or product and estimate how many of each service or product will be provided. *If costs exceed predicted revenues, expenses must be forced to conform by reducing overhead or wholesale costs. This is known as "demand-backward pricing."*

In highly competitive markets, there is little choice but to use the competitive pricing method. In hearing health care, this may be especially true for audiologists who offer diagnostic services or even hearing aids in managed care environments. In such cases, the audiologist is cautioned to do demand-backward price analyses based on third party reimbursement rates, or before committing to contractual pricing agreements (see Chapter 15).

Sometimes this is the only method of choice

Standard Markup Pricing

This is another very simple approach used to meet status quo or sales-oriented pricing objectives. Markup is the dollar amount added to the cost of products or services to get the selling price. It is usually described as a *percent value.*

The simplest application of markup pricing is *keystone markup,* in which the cost of each item is simply doubled to arrive at its selling price. This is a common approach for pricing of hearing aid batteries and other inventory-type items. More often, a business will apply different standard markups for each type of sales category (e.g., hearing aids, diagnostic audiometry, ABR).

Batteries lend themselves to this method

Typically, markup means the percentage of selling price that is added to the cost. A hearing screening that costs the practice $15 and generates a charge of $30 has a 50%, or $15 markup.[3] The formula for calculating markup in percent for a particular price is:

$$\text{MARKUP} = \frac{\text{SELLING PRICE} - \text{COST OF SERVICE OR GOODS}}{\text{SELLING PRICE}} \times 100$$

The formula for calculating price for a given markup in percent is:

$$\text{SELLING PRICE} = \frac{\text{COST OF SERVICE OR GOODS}}{100 - \text{MARKUP}} \times 100$$

It is very important to include all overhead expenses in the cost calculation. A hearing aid with a wholesale cost of $500 and a sale price of $1500 has a markup of 66.6% over its invoice cost, but this does not reflect dispensing costs. If those service costs amount to $700, the total cost to the audiology practice is $1200, so the markup is only 20%. If the sale price includes maintenance and follow-up services that amount to $200 (total cost to dispenser of $1400), the true markup associated with dispensing and maintaining the hearing aid is only 6.6%.

Markups do not always translate into profits. Incomplete analysis of the cost of service delivery can result in inadequate markups that convert into losses rather than profits. Even if cost analysis is correct, markups may be too high to generate adequate sales. The result is low profits or even losses.

Cost-oriented Pricing

This is a more complex and accurate pricing method than competitive or standard markup pricing. It is used when the business selects profit-oriented pricing objectives. Cost-oriented

---

[3]The reason markup is calculated as a percentage of sale price rather than cost is to reflect actual earnings.

pricing methods are most applicable to businesses that offer specialized services and customized goods, such as dispensing audiology practices. Prices are set individually, based on the cost of goods sold, cost of services, fixed expenses, and profit margin. Depending on the target measure, there are various ways of implementing a cost-oriented pricing method.

Return on Investment (ROI) Pricing

This is one type of cost-oriented pricing. Here, the price is based on the amount of profit desired from original investment dollars. This method requires accurate estimates of fixed and variable expenses for a given time, as well as a good estimate of the number of sales for that period and the cost of those sales.

The formula for ROI Pricing is:

$$\text{SELLING PRICE} = \frac{[(100 + \%\text{ROI})/100] \times (\text{EXPENSES} + \text{COST OF GOODS SOLD})}{\text{NUMBER OF SERVICES OR GOODS SOLD}}$$

For example, Cardinal Hearing Services, Inc. (CHS), expects to perform 20 otoacoustic emittance screenings in the intensive care nursery each month, at a cost of $50 each. Therefore, expenses will total $50 × 20 × 12 = $12,000 for the year. There is no cost of goods. The number of services will total 240 for the year. CHS wants a profit margin of 10% for the year. Plugging these numbers into the formula, the charge for each test must be: (1.1 × 12,000)/240 = $55.

In another example using a tangible good, CHS expects to dispense 10 programmable hearing aids per month over the next year. From past experience, they predict an average cost of goods of $650/aid, or $78,000 annually. Average expenses associated with dispensing and maintaining programmable instruments are estimated at $900 per hearing aid, yielding annual expenses of $900 × 10 × 12 = $108,000. CHS desires a profit margin of 12%. Again, plugging these values into the formula yields a selling price of:

[1.12 × (108,000 + 78,000)]/120 = $1736 per hearing aid

Average-Cost Pricing

ROI is just a specialized version of average-cost pricing, which is the most common kind of cost-oriented pricing. In this general method, previous records or predicted costs are used to estimate total and average costs:

- *Total fixed cost.* Total fixed cost is the sum of all costs that are fixed, regardless of sales. These include rent, depreciation, owner/manager salaries, property taxes, insurance. Divide total fixed cost by the number of goods sold, or services provided, to obtain the average fixed cost.
- *Total variable cost.* Total variable cost is the sum of all expenses that vary with production. These include cost of goods, wages, and selling costs (e.g., commissions, packaging, forms, shipping). Divide total variable cost by the number of goods sold or services provided to obtain average variable cost.
- *Average cost per unit* is the sum of total fixed and variable costs divided by the number of goods sold or services provided.

Setting Fees Based on Average Cost Analysis

Professional fee setting in audiology practices is often based on average-cost pricing formulas. For example, assume that a practice has total fixed costs of $75,000 per year and does 1000 diagnostic audiometric evaluations annually. Total variable costs associated with performing those tests are $25,000 per year. The practice wants to make a "reasonable profit" of 10%. Calculate the planned profit as follows:

$$
\begin{array}{lll}
\text{Total Fixed Costs} & = & \$\,75{,}000 \\
\text{Total Variable Costs} & = & 25{,}000 \\
\hline
\text{Total Costs} & = & 100{,}000 \\
\text{"Reasonable" profit} & = & 10{,}000 \\
\hline
\text{Total Costs + Profit} & = & 110{,}000
\end{array}
$$

Calculate the fee for the diagnostic tests as follows:

$$
\frac{\text{Total Costs + Profit}}{\text{Number of Tests}} = \frac{110{,}000}{1000} = \$110.00
$$

These calculations are only as good as the estimates on which they are based. The most common pitfalls in estimating fees for services are: (a) *underestimating* total expenses and (b) *overestimating* productivity. Whitmyer, Rasberry, and Phillips (1989) offer the worksheet shown in Figure 14–2 as a method for calculating professional fees.

Worksheet for calculating fees

1	Yearly Salary	_____ *(Supply the salary you wish to earn.)*
2a	Days worked per month	_____ *(Supply the number of days you wish to work.)*
2b	Days worked per year	_____ Multiply 12 months by number of days you wish to work per month
3	Desired percent profit	_____ *(Supply the percent of profit you want.)*

4 EXPENSES (Fill in the lines below for your expenses.)
   Operating Overhead Office Expenses

Rent	_____	x 12 = _____
Office Help	_____	x 12 = _____
Postage	_____	x 12 = _____
Telephone	_____	x 12 = _____
Utilities	_____	x 12 = _____
Other	_____	x 12 = _____
Subtotal	_____	_____

Support Services

Insurance	_____	x 12 = _____
Marketing	_____	x 12 = _____
Legal & Accounting	_____	x 12 = _____
Promotion	_____	x 12 = _____
Other	_____	x 12 = _____
Subtotal	_____	_____

Additional Expenses

Automobile	_____	x 12 = _____
Entertainment	_____	x 12 = _____
Travel	_____	x 12 = _____
Vacation	_____	x 12 = _____
Miscellaneous	_____	x 12 = _____
Subtotal	_____	_____

5 Total expenses (Add the expense figures and put total here.) _____

6	Daily Overhead	_____ *(Divide total yearly expenses by number of days worked per year.)*
7	Daily Salary	_____ *(Divide total yearly expenses by number of days worked per year.)*
8	Revenue Requirement	_____ *(Sum of Daily Overhead (6) and Daily Salary (7).)*
9	Daily Profit	_____ *(Multiply Desired Percent Profit (3) by Revenue Requirement (8) and divide by 100.)*

10	Required Billing Rate	_____ *(As Daily Overhead (6), Daily Salary (7), and Daily Profit (8).)*
11	Equivalent Hourly Rate	_____ *(Divide Required Billing Rate by the number of billable hours worked per day.)*

Figure 14-2. "Worksheet for calculating fees" from *Running a One-Person Business*, Copyright ©1989 By C. Whitmeyer, S. Rasberry, and M. Phillips, with permission by Ten Speed Press, P.O. Box 7123, Berkely, CA 94707.

Break-even Analysis

This is a way of calculating whether pricing will cover costs by identifying the break-even point (BEP) where costs equal revenues. Figure 14–3 is a graphic example of BEP analysis.

BEP can also be computed as follows:

$$\text{BEP (in units)} = \frac{\text{Total fixed cost}}{\text{Fixed cost contribution per unit}}$$

Fixed cost contribution per unit is the sale price minus the variable cost of the unit. This formula is more intuitive than it looks: fixed costs have to be covered in order to break even. This is accomplished by taking the revenue from each unit (after subtracting variable costs) and calculating how many units must be sold before those revenues equal fixed costs.

For example, assume total fixed costs for a practice are $100,000 annually. The practice objective is to have diagnostic procedures cover all fixed costs. If the average diagnostic fee is $100 and variable costs are $15 per procedure, then the BEP is $100,000/85 = 1176. The practice must perform 1176 diagnostic tests per year, or an average of 4.5 tests per day just to cover fixed costs.

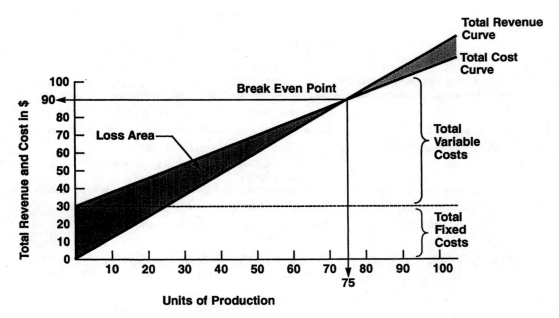

Figure14–3. Break even analysis graph.

Weaknesses of Cost-oriented Pricing

Average-cost pricing can be risky if expenses change unexpectedly. In audiology practices this can happen if rent increases, suppliers are changed, or staffing requirements increase. The result may still be profits, but not maximum profits.

The other weakness with any kind of cost-oriented pricing is that demand is not considered as a variable. Thus, *cost-oriented pricing, like competitive pricing and standard markup pricing, is an inadequate pricing method because it fails to incorporate predictions of future demand.* Pricing that is too high may drive down demand and result in a loss. Pricing that is too low may spur demand but not cover costs, resulting in a loss. Curiously, the most profitable situations will be those in which neither the highest or the lowest prices are employed.

Average cost pricing works best in stable markets. When it works it produces profit, but not usually maximum profits. A better way to maximize profits is to include the customer in the formula by estimating product demand.

Average cost pricing works best in stable markets

Price Searching

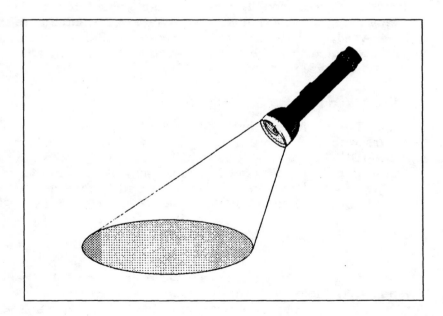

This approach, traditionally called *demand-oriented pricing*, comes from economic analysis of supply and demand. By forecasting demand and linking that variable to cost-oriented measures, price searching comes closest to identifying ranges of profitability (Heyne, 1992).

Although cost-oriented pricing strives to achieve *some* profit, demand-oriented pricing aims to maximize profits. But, why "go for the gold?" Aren't there more important objectives for a practice than maximizing profit? In most cases, yes, but an owner/manager who knows the best way to make the highest profit is in the best position to decide what other objectives to pursue and at what loss of profit.

Use demand estimates to maximize profit

Margin Analysis

Margin analysis is a demand-oriented pricing method that searches for the best price and also identifies a range of profitability. It asks the question: "Is it always better to try to sell as many units as possible?" For audiology practices, this translates to questions such as: "Is there ever a time when performing and billing for 50 audiometric tests is more profitable than performing and billing for 100 tests?"

Margin analysis is a more technical approach to price setting than previously discussed methods, but it is easy and fun to implement in a computer spreadsheet, once a few basics are understood. These basics are defined in the following paragraphs and illustrated in Table 14–1 and Figure 14–4, which tabulate and graph the costs, profits, and margins associated with the sale of programmable hearing aids in a hypothetical practice.

Downward Demand Curve

Demand and price are inversely related. Increasing demand occurs with decreasing price, as shown by the demand curve (DC) in Figure 14–4. In this example, demand is assumed to decline to zero when programmable hearing aids are priced at 4000 units each. Demand is forecast to increase by one aid for every decrease of 500 units in price.

Marginal Revenue

If unit price is reduced just enough to sell one more unit, what change will that single sale make in revenue? In the example in Table 14–1, the question is answered by scanning down the number of programmable hearing aids sold and looking at the corresponding change in the marginal revenue (MR) column.

In competitive markets, the marginal revenue curve is always below the demand curve, as shown in Figure 14–4.

Table 14–1. Example of marginal analysis for pricing programmable hearing aids.

Quantity Q	Price P	Total Revenue TR=Q×P	Total Cost[a] TC	Marginal Profit (TR−TC)	Marginal Revenue[b] MR	Marginal Cost[c] MC	Profit M=MR−MC
0	4000	0	500	− 500	——	——	——
1	3500	3500	1800	1700	3500	1300	1200
2	3000	6000	3100	2900	2500	1300	1200
3	2500	7500	4400	3100	1500	1300	200[d]
4	2000	8000	5700	2300	500	1300	− 800
5	1500	7500[e]	7500	0	− 500	1800	− 2300

[a]Assumes hypothetical fixed costs of 500/day, wholesale hearing aid costs of 500/aid, and variable costs of 800/aid. .
[b]The change in total revenue that results from the sale of one more programmable hearing aid.
[c]The change in total cost that results from selling one more programmable hearing aid.
[d]For this example, this is the point of maximum profit.
[e]Assumes fixed costs will rise to 1000/day, due to need to bring in an additional full-time employee and move to larger quarters to accommodate increased sales activity!

Note that there comes a point where price is so low that the sale of additional units yields negative marginal revenues, although total revenues may remain positive. In Table 14–1, this point occurs somewhere between four and five hearing aid sales, where marginal revenue for the fifth aid sold drops to −500, even though total revenue is 7500.

Marginal Cost

How much does total cost change when one more unit is sold? In a dispensing practice, fixed costs are the same whether one or two hearing aids are sold. But total cost goes up by the wholesale cost of the second aid and the cost of dispensing the instrument. That increase is the marginal cost of selling one more unit. In Table 14–1, the marginal cost is 1300 per aid (500 wholesale cost + 800 dispensing cost), so the marginal cost curve (MC) in Figure 14–4 is a horizontal line at 1300.

But, at some point on the downward demand curve, the volume of hearing aids sold becomes so large that the practice must hire more staff and perhaps expand into larger quarters. Marginal cost increases at this point. For purposes of illustration, Table 14–1 shows this cost increase occurring

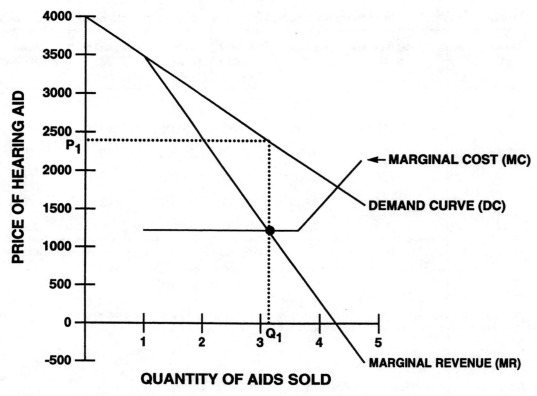

Figure14–4. Graph of demand curve, marginal revenue, and cost for selling programmable hearing aids. Q_1 is the profit maximizing output and P_1 is the point of maximum profit.

with the sale of the fifth hearing aid. The increase in marginal cost (MC) is shown in Figure 14–4.[4]

Marginal Profit

This is the extra profit achieved by selling one more hearing aid. It is the difference between marginal revenue (which decreases with demand) and marginal cost (which eventually increases with demand). At some price point, the increased revenues from selling one more aid are just about offset by the cost of selling that unit. *The price where marginal cost cancels out marginal revenue is the price where marginal profit is near zero and, paradoxically, this is also the price*

[4]Note that the MC curve continues to rise theoretically after staff expansion occurs. This is because management time is proportional to staff size. It is always faster (and cheaper) to manage oneself than it is to manage a large staff.

that produces maximum profits! In the same data of Table 14–1, marginal profit is barely positive when the price is 2500. This is the best price to maximize profits from programmable hearing aids in this practice.

This point is better illustrated by examining the curves in Figure 14–4. The intersection of the marginal revenue (MR) and marginal cost (MC) curves is the point where the two are equal and marginal profit is zero. Q_1 represents the "profit-maximizing output"—slightly more than three hearing aid sales. P_1 is the corresponding price for Q_1 hearing aid sales. Thus, the point of maximum profit, P_1, is just under 2500 per aid.

Finding the Range of Profitability

Marginal analysis, then, consists of searching for the best price by creating a demand curve and then calculating the marginal profit associated with each price/demand combination. In graphic terms, this is the point of intersection of the marginal cost and marginal revenue curves. But what if the real world does not follow the graph? As Table 14–1 shows, there is a range of profitability surrounding the ideal point. In fact, for these data there is some profit to be made whenever one to four hearing aids are sold. Knowing the limits of profitability[5] marked by this range is of more value than the ideal point.

To perform a marginal analysis, simply construct a table with the headings shown in Table 14–1 and fill in the data required for the desired analysis. Demand forecasts in the first and second columns should be based on marketing analysis data; also on previous history if the practice is ongoing.

But what if the demand curve is wrong? Like the point of maximum profit, the demand curve is also an ideal, based on the owner/manager's knowledge of market conditions. Demand curves can change with increasing competition (i.e., shift downward, indicating lower demand at each price level). It is a good idea to construct marginal analysis data from a family of demand curves to appreciate the full extent of pricing effects. As McCarthy and Perreault (1987) observe:

> The major difficulty with demand-oriented pricing is estimating the demand curve. But experienced managers—aided perhaps by marketing research—can estimate the nature of demand for their products. Such estimates are useful—even if

---

[5]Or in bad economic times, the range that is the *least unprofitable.*

they aren't exact. They get you thinking in the right "ball-park." Sometimes, when all you need is a decision about raising or lowering price, even "rough" demand estimates can be very revealing . . . . when managers are setting a price, they have to consider what customers will be willing to pay. This isn't always easy. But it's nice to know that there is a profit range around the "best" price. Therefore, even "guesstimates" about what potential customers will buy at various prices will probably lead to a better price than mechanical use of traditional markups or cost-oriented formulas. (p. 511)

A Caveat on Pricing Methods

Other factors affect pricing success

Pricing methods cannot be used in a vacuum. Various formulas have been discussed for setting price, but they must be implemented in an environmental framework that takes other, uncontrollable variables into account. Even price searching is restricted if demand forecasts are based solely on past experience of the practice, or on wishful thinking in a start-up venture.

Pricing must be sensitive to and consistent with the prevailing business climate. That climate is determined by the competitive environment, economic environment, technological environment, political and legal environment, cultural and social environment, and the company environment (McCarthy & Perreault, 1987). Pricing in this framework requires pricing strategies.

PRICING STRATEGIES

Societal Dictates

Pricing strategies must be *legal and ethical* to succeed in the long run. But what does this mean? When a strategy is unlawful, is it unethical? When a strategy is legal, is it ethical? By whose ethics?[6]

Our professional codes of ethics are relatively silent on the subject of pricing. They simply state that audiologists:

shall not charge for services not rendered, nor shall [we] misrepresent, in any fashion, services rendered or products dispensed (ASHA, 1994b);

---

[6]No attempt is made to answer this larger question. The reader is referred to Resnick (1993) for a thoughtful consideration of ethical questions in hearing health care.

shall charge only for services rendered (American Academy of Audiology, 1991).

ASHA guidelines say that published fees should declare fixed prices or a range of prices for specific services and indicate when additional charges may be incurred. The listing should not be misleading. For example, "one level of service (diagnostic) may not be offered at a specified fee, when in fact a lower level of service (screening) is provided for that fee" (ASHA, 1992). ASHA guidelines also comment that there is no basis for setting fees at a different level than normal when services are performed by students in training under the supervision of certified audiologists (ASHA, 1994c).

In contrast, state and federal laws on pricing are numerous and complicated. It is not necessarily clear whether control of pricing strategies is designed to protect consumers or to protect businesses from the rigors of competitive life (Heyne, 1992). The following are the laws associated with pricing, with occasional commentary that is intended to stimulate and titillate, *not* instruct!

■ *It is illegal in many states to sell below cost.* Unfair trade practice acts in these states require at least a minimum markup. It is *not* illegal to charge very high prices (although it may be ruinous in the long run).

   Comment. The laws were developed to control companies that might use "predatory pricing" strategies to run competitors with fewer resources out of business. By this reasoning, are "free" hearing tests illegal? Is it illegal for otolaryngologists to negotiate HMO contracts by offering audiology services below cost? Are not-for-profit institutions with low fees guilty of predatory pricing? Or, are such laws just a means of sheltering businesses from aggressive competition?

■ *It is illegal to lie about prices.* The Wheeler Lea Amendment bans "unfair or deceptive acts in commerce," such as use of phony "list" prices[7] (McCarthy & Perreault, 1987).

   Comment. Is it lying, and therefore illegal, for an audiologist to post a hearing aid fee schedule, but mark off a 10% discount on every hearing aid sale?

---

[7]Hearing aid manufacturers supply a suggested retail price schedule for hearing aids and accessories. These are not phoney list prices, but are valid because (a) that price is what patients pay who go directly to the manufacturer to obtain their hearing aids and (b) some hearing aid dispensers charge the suggested retail price.

■ *Price fixing is illegal.* When the marketing mix boils down to price as the only arbiter of success, competitors may be tempted to make agreements on pricing. According to the Sherman Act and the Federal Trade Commission Act, this is conspiracy and it is illegal. It is *not* illegal to request a competitor's fee schedule, but it *is* illegal to arrive at similar prices by agreement.

■ *Price discrimination is illegal . . . sometimes.* By the Robinson-Patman Act, the same service or merchandise cannot be sold to different customers at different prices if it injures competition. It is *not* illegal to sell the same product at different prices if there is a cost difference or if there is a need to meet competition.

Comment. Price discrimination seems unethical even if it is *not* illegal. But what about Senior Discounts, sliding fee scales, or accepting insurance assignment for some (but not all) patients? These are examples of legal and ethical price discrimination: the strategy seeks to provide goods and services to as many people as possible, according to some estimate of their ability to pay. Does price discrimination "exploit" those who can afford to pay, or does it benefit those who otherwise could not afford the product?

What about "price lining" strategies in which identical products (e.g., two hearing aids from the same manufacturer, one with a "prestige" label, the other with a "budget" label), are sold at different prices? Illegal but ethical or vice versa—or neither?

In the end, how is one to proceed in devising pricing strategies that are legal, ethical, and maximize profits? One strategy is to de-emphasize price in the marketing mix and offer the same cost-oriented prices to all customers. In many practices, this may be the best approach to setting fees for diagnostic tests. The strategy is consistent with the ASHA guidelines for ethical practice. Just as importantly, it acknowledges price "bars" set by Medicare, Medicaid, private third party payers, and HMOs. Here, the strategy involves setting prices above the reimbursement "bar," which periodically moves up or down depending on the economy and the political climate. The strategy must avoid two types of barriers in order to avoid penalties:

1. Prices must not exceed upper barriers set by some insurers (e.g., Medicare[8]), and
2. fees for the same services must not be priced differently according to the patient's insurance. For example, Medicare does not look kindly on being billed more for a service just because its reimbursement bar is set higher than that of another insurer!

At the other extreme, creative pricing strategy premiers pricing as an imaginative and effective marketing tool. Creative pricing strategies usually work best with merchandise or special programs (e.g., speech reading programs).

Regardless of where one ends up on the tactical continuum, the pricing strategy should be consistent with Principle 1 of the AAA Code of Ethics:

> Members shall provide professional services with honesty and compassion and shall respect the dignity, worth and rights of those served. (AAA, 1991)

Creative Pricing Strategies

Mondello (1992) suggests a rule for thinking creatively and proactively about pricing: "Forget absolutely everything you know about 'how it's done in my business,' and start looking at how it's done in other businesses" (p. 83). While agreeing with Mondello that assimilation, flexibility, and brainstorming are important attributes of successful pricing strategies, we would add two equally important corollaries:

1. Do not forget *anything* you know about laws and ethics.
2. Use strategies only if they are consistent with the professional image we must create and maintain to position ourselves in the health care marketplace.

With these caveats in mind, it is safe to ask "How *is* it done in other businesses?" Kishel and Kishel (1993) list the following:

■ *Skimming:* Set prices high for new, high-technology products, to quickly sell to the "innovators" at the top of the demand curve. "Step down" the demand curve

---

[8]For more discussion of Medicare and other third-party insurer's reimbursement schedules, see Chapters 15 and 16.

by lowering price over time as the product becomes more widely accepted and competition increases.

■ *Penetration:* Set prices low and keep them low in order to gain a large market share in very competitive markets. Use this strategy for low-cost, high-volume merchandise (e.g., batteries).

■ *Price-lining:* Categorize merchandise and set prices in several ranges (high, medium, low) to accommodate what customers are willing to spend.

■ *Promotional pricing:* Set prices artificially low for introductory offers or for special occasions (e.g., infrared listening systems as "stocking stuffers" at Christmas). Raise prices as soon as the special is over.

■ *Price bundling:* Put separate but related products/services together and price as a "bundle" to sell more of them (e.g., hearing aids sold with three-year warranties).

■ *Time period pricing:* Raise prices in high seasons, lower them in low seasons to maintain demand.

■ *Value-added pricing:* Offer an additional service or gift when a customer buys a product (e.g., a year's supply of batteries with the purchase of a hearing aid).

■ *Captive pricing:* Set a low price for one product, then sell other products that go with it (e.g., free hearing test, which results in purchase of hearing aids).

Figure 14–5 is adapted from Mondello's (1992) "Creative Pricing Primer," in which he presents pricing approaches gleaned from consumer products, services, and business-to-business situations. He recommends going "through the primer, and for every approach presented, jot down in the space provided some way your company might be able to use that type of pricing" (p. 83).

We have listed possibilities that we have seen used in various dispensing practices, and have left additional room for the reader's ideas. This is a brainstorming exercise, designed to acknowledge "what is out there," and prompt you to think creatively about pricing. The exercise is not designed to sanction or denounce the various pricing strategies. However, keep our two corollaries in mind and think critically as well as creatively. Just because we have observed these applications (and therefore included them in the list), does not mean that we chose to use some of them in our own practices! Applications must fit into an overall, quality-oriented, marketing plan that keeps patient satisfaction primary. Haphazard and cavalier use of many of these applications amounts to no more than gimmickry. Gimmickry has long-term deleterious effects on a practice and on our profession.

PRICING APPROACH	HOW IT WORKS	EXAMPLE	HOW IT MIGHT APPLY TO AUDIOLOGISTS
Bundling or unbundling	Sell products or services together as packages or break them apart, priced accordingly.	Season tickets; stereo equipment; car rentals charging for air conditioning.	Combining air, bone, and speech testing, billing as a "comprehensive" evaluation.
Time-period pricing	Adjust price up or down during specific times to spur or acknowledge changes in demand.	Off-season travel fares to build demand; peak-period fees on bank ATMs (to shift demand).	Free hearing screening during "May is Better Speech and Hearing Month."
Trial pricing	Make it easy and lower the risk for a customer to try out what you sell.	Three month health club starter memberships; low, nonrefundable "preview fees" on training videos.	One-week programmable hearing aid trial for only the cost of an ear mold.
Image pricing	Sometimes the customer *wants* to pay more, so price accordingly.	Most expensive hotel room in town; private-label vitamins raising price to signal quality.	Completely-in-the-Canal (CIC) hearing aids at prestige pricing.
Value-added price packages	Include free services to appeal to bargain shoppers, without lowering price.	A magazine's offering advertisers free merchandising tie-ins when they buy ad space.	Free batteries with hearing aid purchase.
Pay-one-price	Unlimited use or unlimited amount of a service or product for one set fee.	Amusement parks; office copier contracts; salad bars.	Free follow-up for lifetime of hearing aid.
Constant promotional pricing	Although a "regular" price exists, no one ever pays it.	Consumer electronics retailers always matching "lowest price in town"; always offering one pizza free with one purchased at regular price.	Discount on all hearing aid sales.
Change the standard	Rather than adjust price, adjust the standard to make your price seem different and better.	A magazine clearinghouse's selling a $20 subscription for "four payments for only $4.99."	Selling a $1500 hearing aid for three payments of $499 each.
Variable pricing tied to a creative variable	Set up a "price per" pricing schedule tied to a related variable.	Children's haircuts at 10 cents per inch of a child's height; marina space billed at $25 per foot of boat.	Seniority discount tied to age.
Different names for different price segments	Sell essentially the same product under different names, to appeal to different price segments.	Separate model numbers or variations of the same TV for discounters, department stores, and electronic stores.	Order the same type of hearing aid from two different manufacturers with different pricing structures.
Captive pricing	Lock in your customer by selling the system cheap, and the profit by selling high-margin items.	The classic example; selling razors at cost, with all the margin made on razor blade sales.	Free hearing tests to prompt hearing aid sales.
Product-line	Establish a range of price points within your line. Structure the prices to encourage customers to buy your highest-profit product.	Luxury-car lines (high-end models enhance prestige of entire line but are priced to encourage sale of more profitable low end).	Programmable hearing aid prices set as high-end, priced to encourage purchase of mid-range priced compression aids.
Differential pricing	Charge each customer segment what each will pay.	In new-car sales, a deal for every buyer; Colorado lift tickets sold locally at a dis-	Different prices for different industrial or managed care contracts

Figure 14–5. Creative Pricing Primer. (Adapted from Mondello, M.D. (1992, July). Naming your price. *INC.*, pp 80–83.) *(continued)*

PRICING APPROACH	HOW IT WORKS	EXAMPLE	HOW IT MIGHT APPLY TO AUDIOLOGISTS
Quality discount	Set up a standard pricing practice, which can be done several ways.	Per-unit discount on all units, as with article reprints; discounts only on the units above a certain level, as with record clubs.	Battery clubs.
Fixed, then variable pricing	Institute an introductory charge, followed by a variable charge.	Taxi fares, phone services tied to usage.	Basic hearing evaluation charge, with acoustic immittance and ABR charges added if needed.
"Don't break that price point"	Price just below important thresholds for the buyer, to give a perception of lower price.	Charging $499 for a suit; $195,000 instead of $200,000 for a design project.	$69 for a basic hearing evaluation; $1490 instead of $1500 for biaural hearing aids.

Figure 14–5. *(continued)*

SUMMARY

Audiologists should view pricing as a strong marketing tool for competing in the era of health care reform. Successful practices in the 1990s must set fees that cover all costs, spur demand, and maximize profit. This is accomplished by identifying pricing objectives that are compatible with the practice's goals, setting measurable targets to meet those objectives, and "running the numbers" through appropriate pricing method formulas. The pricing methods are: competitive pricing, standard markup, averaged cost analysis, break-even analysis, and price searching. The only pricing method that includes consumer demand in its formula is price searching.

Pricing objectives, targets, and formulas may differ within a practice, depending on the product. Examples include (a) inexpensive, inelastic products like batteries priced with a standard markup to meet a sales-oriented objective; (b) diagnostic fees set according to competitive pricing; (c) high technology products such as programmable hearing aids priced by margin analysis to maximize profit.

Pricing strategies are marketing efforts to sell products at particular prices. They can be routine or creative, stabilizing or predatory, uniform or discriminating. Like pricing objectives, pricing strategies should be compatible with the audiology practice's business philosophy. They should be consistent with the prevailing business climate. Above all, they should be lawful and ethical.

REFERENCES

American Academy of Audiology. (1991). *Code of ethics.* Houston, TX: Author.

American Speech-Language-Hearing Association. (1992). Public announcements and public statements. *Asha, 34*(Suppl. 9), 13–14.

American Speech-Language-Hearing Association. (1994a). How will health care reform affect our professional practices? *Asha, 36*(2), 17–18.

American Speech-Language-Hearing Association. (1994b). Code of Ethics. *Asha, 36*(Suppl. 13), 1–2.

American Speech-Language-Hearing Association. (1994c). Fees for clinical service provided by students. *Asha, 36*(Suppl. 13), 26.

Drucker, P. F. (1993, October). The five deadly business sins. *The Wall Street Journal,* p. A18.

Heyne, P. (1992). *The economic way of thinking* (6th ed.). New York: Macmillan.

Kamara, C. A. (1988). Determining fees in private practice. *Asha, 30*(1), 37–39.

Kishel, G. F., & Kishel, P. G. (1993). *How to start, run, and stay in business.* New York: John Wiley.

McCarthy, J. E., & Perreault, W. D., Jr. (1987). *Basic marketing* (9th ed.). Homewood, Il: Irwin.

Mondello, M. D. (1992, July). Naming your price. *INC.,* pp. 80–83.

Mulligan, J. G. (1989). *Managerial economics. Strategy for profit.* Boston: Allyn & Bacon.

Navarro, M. R., & Klodd, D. A. (1989). Sound principles for pricing. *Hearing Journal, 42*(7), 24–27.

Resnick, D. M. (1993). *Professional ethics for audiologists and speech-language pathologists.* San Diego, CA: Singular Publishing Group.

Whitmyer, C., Rasberry, S., & Phillips, M. (1989). *Running a one-person business.* Berkeley, CA: Ten Speed Press.

15

Reimbursement

*Although the issues
are complex, the goal
is simple: maintain
positive cash flow*

Audiologists face a perplexing variety of reimbursement issues in today's health care market. Simplistically, all of the reimbursement issues can be boiled down to one concern— how to maintain positive cash flow. Unfortunately, most audiology practices lack complete control of reimbursements, so decisions to promote cash flow vary according to the reimbursement issue. For purposes of discussion in this chapter, the various reimbursement issues are divided into two groups, those that are *external* and those that are *internal* in origin.

Foremost among the externally generated issues is professional recognition of audiologists as hearing care providers. Traditional third party insurers do not always acknowledge audiologists as providers, nor do managed care plans necessarily admit audiologists to their ranks. A related external issue, then, is how to integrate audiology services into managed care.

Beyond that, audiologists who qualify as providers must make their way through the thicket of distinct reimbursement rules for each health care plan, carefully monitor their provider appointments and contracts, and stay abreast of reimbursement coding systems. These are all externally generated issues.

In addition to external reimbursement issues that are dictated by insurance companies and health plans, fee for service patients present the practice with wholly different, internal reimbursement issues. The practice must develop its own billing and collection policies for services and products that are purchased directly by patients. It must generate procedures and forms that are consistent with those policies and review them periodically.

Traditionally, diagnostic tests are likely to be covered by third party reimbursement, but hearing aids are not. Therefore, audiologists deal with externally generated reimbursement issues for tests and with internally generated reimbursement issues for hearing aids.

This chapter is organized to discuss internal reimbursement issues first for two reasons: (1) fee for service has been around longer and is a more familiar model to most independent practices and (2) hearing aid income is such an important part of cash flow for most audiology practices. Following a discussion of fee for service, the chapter addresses external reimbursement issues. It concludes with comments on changes in reimbursement issues as managed competition emerges in the health care market place.

FEE FOR SERVICE REIMBURSEMENT

The Paradox and the Solution

Like marketing and pricing, fee collection is viewed by many audiologists as a nonprofessional, demeaning activity—a necessary evil that the business world forces on service professions. Audiologists with this perception tend to set up practices in which billing and collection are left to a front office person who develops credit and collection "policies" as questions arise. Strangely, the same audiologists who disdain discussing money with patients may have no difficulty fighting tooth and nail with agencies and third party insurers to maximize their reimbursements!

The difference is mainly in perception. Both cases involve transactions in which hearing "products" are traded for money. But, in the first instance the transaction is direct whereas in the second instance the transaction is through an intermediary. The resulting misperception, broadly stated, is that asking for payment is legitimate so long as it is not from the person receiving the service.

The misperception is buttressed by emotional factors. What if the patient does not make the promised payments or makes a scene? Quite naturally, audiologists fear these events because they can create ill will and tarnish their image as caring providers. In particularly unpleasant cases, the audiologist may get emotionally involved and take a patient's comments personally.

Paradoxically, the audiologists who suffer from these misperceptions and emotional responses are the ones most likely to experience billing and collection problems. This is because they skirt the issues and fail to set up fair and reasonable credit and collection policies in advance. Formulating such policies is the solution to the paradox. The idea of policies is to avoid reimbursement problems through preven-

Set up fair and reasonable credit and collection policies in advance

tive measures that preserve the dignity of all parties and maintain the professional decorum of the practice. Like the mission statement, practice philosophy, and many other management tools discussed in this book, the credit and collection policies need to be thought out before the practice commences. They need to be written down, discussed with all staff members, posted prominently for the benefit of patients and employees, and reviewed on a regular basis to make changes that reflect current market conditions.

Credit Policy

Some credit is needed in all practices to avoid lost sales

Credit exists whenever a transaction is not totally covered by cash at the time of purchase. Some credit is needed in all practices to avoid lost sales, but each practice must decide how much credit to extend. Coordinate the credit policy with sales goals. Apply it consistently to avoid the old cliche "You set the price; I'll set the terms" (Scott, 1990, p. 14). Answer basic questions such as: How much down payment is required? What are the billing terms? Are there discounts for early payments? Are there late charges? If so, when do they start?

The following are a few rules of thumb that are helpful in deciding what credit policies are best for an individual practice.

- *Economic situation.* In good economic times, extend more credit. In economic down-turns, adopt a more conservative credit policy.
- *Market demands.* The wealthier the target market, the more credit they expect and the more they can handle. Be prepared to extend more credit in high-end practices, but remember that there is a potential downside:

  > The rich are used to getting the finest products and services, and they can be very demanding, even finicky. Thus, a business catering to the wealthy can have more problems with returns, and more disputes over services, than other businesses. (Scott, 1990, p. 19)

- *Size of transaction.* The larger the transaction, the more likely the need for credit.
- *Competition.* Credit policies need to be competitive.
- *Repeat customers.* The more likely a customer is to return, the more likely that credit is extended.
- *Cash flow.* The stronger the practice's own financial situation, the more credit it can afford to offer.

Types of Credit

Each practice must make decisions about what forms of credit it will use. The following are some comments about basic types of credit. Many of the comments in this section and the following section on contracts address worst-case scenarios. It is highly unlikely that a well-run dispensing audiology practice will encounter these scenarios except on rare occasions. However, it bears repeating that part of being a well-run practice is anticipating rare and undesirable events by developing policies and procedures to defuse them.

Credit
- *Checks*
- *Credit Cards*
- *Finance Companies*

Checks

Checks are often thought of as cash, but they are really a form of credit until they clear the bank. Several things can happen that keep a check from turning into cash. The most obvious is a bad check. This can happen if there are insufficient funds in the account, the check is not filled out properly, or if the bank account is closed. Bad checks are a problem for several reasons: (a) authorities rarely will get involved, especially if inadequate information was collected at the time of writing; and (b) to prosecute, the practice must show that the customer had intent *not* to pay, which is very difficult to prove.

Even if the check is good, payment can be stopped. It is legal for a patient to put a stop payment on a check if he or she feels there is a "good" reason (e.g., thinks the price is too high, decides to return merchandise). Finally, checks can be lost by the practice or by the bank.

The remedies for these situations involve careful documentation at the time of transaction. As a minimum, be sure to verify the address on the check with another piece of identifi-

Document all checks

cation (e.g., driver's license). The driver's license number is useful for finding people who move. Unless there are legal rulings against it in your state, request a major credit card and write down the credit card number. A valid card is a basis for assuming the person has good credit. It may be uncomfortable for you to ask for this documentation, but much of it is required by authorities before they will even consider action against the writer. Explain to the patient that the documentation is a formality of the credit policy—which, indeed, it is in all cases but bad checks.

Make copies of checks or keep a check deposit record that chronicles account numbers and notations on the checks. These are useful if it is necessary to contact the bank, or if a check is lost.

If there is any doubt about the customer's credit on large checks, call the bank to verify that the checking account is open and that there are sufficient funds. If necessary, deposit such checks on the same day, hold merchandise until the check clears, or simply do not enter into a transaction.

Another preventive measure is to have patients sign agreement forms (e.g., a hearing aid purchase agreement, or an acknowledgement of office policies on fees and collections). Along those lines, it is a good idea to suggest that patients annotate their checks (e.g., "hearing aid payment"; "payment on account").

Credit Cards

Credit cards are like checks with a built-in discount. Your bank charges a "merchant discount" that ranges from 2.5 to 5.5% of the charged amount on each transaction.[1] This is in addition to set-up fees, monthly fees, and equipment purchases. However, these charges are partially offset by the bank and credit card company doing credit checks, collection, and establishing policy decisions.

Credit cards do not guarantee payment. Credit cards can be invalid, credit lines may be exceeded, or charges can be disputed, resulting in "charge-backs" to the practice. Preventative steps when handling credit card transactions are: (1) check the list of invalid cards provided by the credit card company or call the company to check the card and (2) have patients sign agreement forms.

---

[1]It is illegal to charge a reduced fee (equivalent to the discount rate) for cash purchases to discourage credit card use.

Finance Companies

Recently, a few banking associations have begun to offer financing services to audiologists and hearing aid dispensers. These companies purchase "Professional Service Contracts" from an audiology or hearing aid practice. Professional services include any services or goods provided by the practice to a customer. The purchase price for the contract covers the total amount billed, minus down payments and portions covered by insurance.

The finance company takes over all billing and collection on the account, often paying the practice up-front for the amount due. The amount due to the practice is the purchase price of the contract, less an agreed-on discount percentage of the financed amount (typically 5%). The practice also pays an initial set-up fee.

This type of service encourages sales by offering monthly payment options to patients who might not otherwise be able to afford to purchase hearing aids. The advantages to the audiologist/dispenser, besides more sales, are timely payment and no collection costs beyond the discount percentage (which must be factored into the pricing structure). A possible disadvantage is that the professional loses some control over patient care. However, this concern would only arise if the customer or the finance company abused the relationship. In the latter case, the professional can avoid further problems by terminating the contract, usually with 30 days notice.

Contracts

Once the practice decides how much credit to offer, to whom, and in what form, the next step is to decide what contractual forms are needed.[2] An effective contract does at least six things:

1. designates the services and merchandise that are provided,
2. assigns the price for each service or good,
3. specifies payment amounts, due dates, and charges for late payments,
4. describes customers' remedies,
5. provides proof of full disclosure to the customer,

---

[2]For an example of a service and hearing aid contract, refer to Appendix I at the end of this book.

6. provides proof of what the customer has agreed to in terms of accepting services and goods, payments, collections, and remedies.

In many states, the precise wording of hearing aid contracts is mandated by law. *The contract should be composed and printed before the first hearing aid is sold.* Contracts should contain "protective clauses" to cover nonpayment. In addition to describing the services and merchandise, the amount of payment, and the due date, customer remedies need to be fully described. A hearing aid purchase agreement should explain how the customer can act if he or she has a complaint about the hearing aid or associated service. As an example, the clause might contain the following wording (with bracketed portions filled in appropriately): *"30-day trial period with full refund on merchandise, if returned in original condition, and [partial] refund on services; otherwise, it is assumed [the customer] has received the merchandise in satisfactory condition."*

The practice may also have patients sign release forms for hearing aids and other devices, stating that the customer is satisfied with the purchase and agrees to the stated procedures for collecting disputed funds. This helps prevent stops on checks and charge-backs in credit card disputes.

Contracts may contain a protective clause that states that the debtor is responsible for collection costs if the debt is not paid when due. This is necessary if the practice plans to charge interest or overdue charges. Scott (1990) provides a sample clause:

> If the amount due in this agreement is not paid by the date indicated, and it is necessary to take steps to collect on this debt, then the customer agrees to pay all reasonable collections costs, including attorney fees, that are necessary to collect the debt. (p 36)

All of these protective clauses make the process of fitting and selling a hearing aid seem more like practicing law than audiology. Indeed, when contemplating how to get everything on the form and not scare the patient away, one begins to appreciate the meaning of the term "fine print." The audiologist can reassure the patient that the clauses are only formalities, implying that this is so because the patient will certainly be paying on time. Explain that their inclusion is only to protect the practice in the very rare event that there is a collection problem. In the equally rare event that a patient refuses to sign the agreement, this is a good sign that you have headed off a bad debt and avoided the expense and discomfort of trying to collect.

Collection Procedures

Even the best of practices will have an occasional collection problem. These problems take a financial, emotional, and professional toll on those in the practice and can even get the practice in trouble. The following are a few do's and don'ts of collection.

DO:
- Install a good billing system, with bills reflecting all transactions (including insurance and other payments) that are mailed at regular monthly intervals (Colan, 1994);
- Get the patient to acknowledge and accept the debt
- Get a post-dated check or hold merchandise, if possible
- Find out the reason for nonpayment
- Use legal and dignified methods to motivate the patient to pay the debt
- Maintain good will

Assume that the patient is responsible and honest, but does not understand the bill, has forgotten the payment, or has problems that are preventing payment. In the latter case, be sympathetic and offer to work out a revised payment schedule. If the patient is disputing the bill because he feels he has a valid grievance, listen carefully to the grievance. Try to get payment for nondisputed portions of the debt and make adjustments to the remainder, if appropriate.

Steps in the collection process vary according to the situation and the practice's collection policies, but some standard steps are:

- *Stamped reminder.* Simply mail a second copy of the bill with a red-inked stamped message (e.g., "Past Due," "Your account is over due," "A friendly reminder!").
- *Letter or telephone call.* Either call the patient or send him or her a courteous and tactful letter. Firmly but politely request payment by a specified date. Ask the patient to contact the office if there are reasons why the bill cannot be promptly paid.
- *Reminder call or letter.* If there is no response to Step 2 within the specified time frame, contact the

patient one more time (e.g., "You did not respond to our last letter..."). Explain the consequences of non-payment (e.g., collection agency) and remind the patient of the signed commitment to pay.

■ *Further reminders, collection agency, attorney, small claims court, or write off.* These are the alternatives if there is no response to Step 3. Further reminders and Small Claims Court actions take time and may not result in payment. Attorneys will not accept cases for small debts and *their* fees make collection on large debts a bit prohibitive. This leaves the options of using the collection agency or writing the debt off, depending on circumstances and business policies. The advantages of using collection agencies are that they are trained in debt collection procedures and use a systematic approach, they can locate missing debtors, and they are taken more seriously by the debtor. The disadvantage of the collection agencies is that they retain as much as 50% of whatever they collect. Not all collection agencies are equal. Exercise caution when choosing an agency and be sure that their reputation and business policies are compatible with your practice.

DON'T:
■ Use deception or misreption or misrepresentation
■ Harassment
■ Charge excessive interest (usury)
■ Malign the patient's reputation

Exercise caution when "notifying" patients

It is illegal[3] to send out collection notices that look like court documents, or to state that the account will be turned over to the practice's "legal department for collection" (unless the practice has such a department). It is also illegal to threaten to turn an account over to collection or to file a lawsuit unless that really is the next step. Threatening to tell the debtor's friends or employer or notify other creditors about the debt may constitute extortion.

It is illegal to make repeated telephone calls or let the telephone ring nonstop. Only one call per day is allowed and that call cannot be to the debtor's work place if he or she has asked that you not call there. Although you can visit debtors in their homes, you cannot refuse to leave when asked.

---

[3]Refer to the Fair Debt Collection Practices Act (Public Law 95-109) of 1977 for further information.

Slander or libel charges may be brought if the debt is discussed with another person or if defamatory statements about the debtor are heard or read by a third party (e.g., "I don't think he's truthful"). You cannot "publicize" the debt by sending the debtor a postcard that mentions the debt, or even a letter in a sealed envelope if it is likely that someone else will open the letter. Always mark such envelopes as "PERSONAL AND CONFIDENTIAL."

Summary of Fee For Service Reimbursement Policies

Develop credit and collection policies and procedures before initiating transactions in the practice. Apply the policies uniformly and fairly. Review the policies frequently, taking into account economic environment, sales goals, competitors' policies, target markets, and financial status of the practice. Use signed agreements with protective clauses to avert collection problems and billing disputes. Approach delinquent debtors legally and respectfully, accommodating them when possible. Maintain good will and professional dignity. Never become emotionally involved with nonpayors. Never resort to threats and never discuss nonpayors with third parties.

INSURANCE REIMBURSEMENT

Insurance reimbursements for audiology and hearing aid services are of two general types: (1) traditional indemnity policies and (2) managed care plans. By mid-1993, managed care plans enrolled 18.5% of the total population in the United States. With enrollments growing at a rate of 6.5% in the first half of 1993, managed care plans are quickly assuming dominance in health care (Marion Merrell Dow, 1993). This is happening much more rapidly in some markets than others: by the beginning of 1993, more than half of the people in Minnesota were receiving their health services through an HMO (Johnson & Anderson, 1994).

Glossary of Health Insurance Terms

The proliferation of patients, services, providers, policies, and plans has prompted a virtual family of health care acronyms. Their definitions are necessary in order to follow even the simple discussion of insurance reimbursement issues provided in this chapter. The following is a glossary of health care terms.

AMA. American Medical Association.

CPT. Current Procedural Terminology. Developed by the AMA, it assigns a five-digit code to each service or procedure. "These procedure codes have become the standard adopted by third party payers for identifying services (procedures) rendered. Their use by nonphysicians may be inappropriate or inaccurate, but often no recognized substitute codes are available" (American Speech-Language-Hearing Association [ASHA], 1992). The 1995 edition of the CPT code book is available at most medical book stores, or can be ordered from the AMA (hard copy) or government offices (hard copy or tape).[4] All CPT codes, descriptions, and 2-digit modifiers are under copyright by the American Medical Association.

HCFA: Health Care Financing Administration. Developed HCFA/1500 standardized health insurance claim forms. Address is: HCFA, US Department of Health and Human Services, 6325 Security Blvd., Baltimore, MD 21207.

HCPCS. HCFA Common Procedure Coding System. There are three levels of HCPCS. Level 1 HCPCS codes are the same as CPT codes, assigned by the American Medical Association. Level 2 codes are alphanumeric (A0000-V9999), describing services not included in CPT codes that are assigned and maintained by HCFA. Most Level 2 HCPCS codes are not included in the current Medicare reimbursement structure (White & Kander, 1992). Level 3 codes are also alphanumeric (W0000-Z9999), describing services and supplies that are assigned and maintained by a local carrier and not contained in the CPT code book. Audiology HCPCS codes, and proposed codes, are shown in Appendix 15-A.

HMO and HSMO. Health Maintained Organization, more correctly called a Health Service Maintenance Organization. A form of managed care.

HPPC/HIPC-HA: Health Plan Purchasing Cooperative/ Health Insurance Purchasing Cooperative-Health Alliance. In managed competition, these are purchasing pools that negotiate and purchase plans for employee health care.

---

[4]Ordering addresses for hard copy are: AMA, Order Department, PO Box 109050, Chicago, IL 60610 (1-800-621-8335); or Superintendent of Documents, U.S. Government Printing Office, Washington, D.C. 20402, 202-512-1800. Order address for the tape version of the CPT manual is: National Technical Information Service, U.S. Department of Commerce, 5285 Port Royal Rd., Springfield, VA 22161 (703-487-4650).

HSMO/Insurance. Health Maintenance Organization that also has a license with the state to provide insurance. A response to market demand, this type of organization offers clients health care choices ranging from HSMO, to POS, PPO, and Indemnity policies.

ICD-9-CM. International Classification of Diseases-9th Edition-Clinical Modification. Lists principal medical diagnoses. Created for research and statistical tracking of epidemics, it also serves as a means of deciding on payment for services. Updated ICD-9 codes went into effect October 1, 1994.[5]

IPA. Independent Physicians Association. A group of independent physicians (as opposed to a clinic, for example) formed to negotiate agreements and provide services as an entity.

Managed Care. Refers to organizations that control health care costs by using methods such as putting selected physicians on salary, contracting with some specialists, specifying how illnesses are treated, limiting specialist referrals, requiring preauthorization for hospitalization, and so on. The Health Insurance Association of America defines managed care as "systems that integrate the financing and delivery of appropriate health care services to covered individuals by means of the following basic elements: arrangements with selected providers, standards of selection of providers, formal quality assurance and utilization management and financial incentives for membership." (Breske, 1994, p. 9)

Managed Competition. A type of health care reform, using governmental regulation of insurers.

PHO. Physician Hospital Organization.

POS. Point of Service. A marketing product offered by some HSMOs that combines HSMO and indemnity coverage. Members chose the level of benefits at the point of service, moving freely between HSMO services for some purposes and indemnity benefits for other purposes.

PPO. Preferred Provider Organization. A marketing product offered by some HSMOs in which members can chose from a list of independent providers who agree to provide services to members at discounted fees.

RBRVS. Resource-Based Relative Value Scale. Designed to gradually replace the CPT charges in the Medicare system

---

[5]At the time of writing [1994] copies of the ICD-9 codes are available through: Practice Management Information (PMI), 2001 Butterfield Rd., Downers Grove, IL 60515 (1-800-633-7467) or the American Medical Association (AMA), PO Box 109050, Chicago, IL 60610 (1-800-621-8335).

by 1996. RBRVS assigns a value to every CPT procedure, based on three components: (1) a work, or "professional" component that takes into account time, technical skill, judgment, physical effort, and stress; (2) a "technical" component based on the amount of overhead required to perform the service; and (3) malpractice cost associated with the service of procedure. Currently, Medicare does not recognize a professional component for services performed by independent audiologists. True RBRVS values have been developed for some health care professions but not others, including audiology.[6]

UPIN: Unique Physician Identification Number. A national number assigned to a physician Medicare provider to identify the physician ordering or referring services. A UPIN is required on Medicare claims for the following services: laboratory, consultations, durable medical equipment, prosthetics and orthotics, radiology, diagnostic tests.

Indemnity Insurance

Indemnity insurance is designed to restore the policy holder to a similar financial condition as was enjoyed before a health condition arose. Thus, if a procedure or test costs $100, an indemnity policy traditionally reimburses most of that amount to the patient. A secondary indemnity policy often reimburses most of the remainder.

So-called "80-20" plans are what usually comes to mind when discussing indemnity insurance. Large, private insurance companies such as Blue Cross/Blue Shield or Aetna issue such indemnity policies to individual policyholders, ensuring 80% coverage of the *approved amount*[7] for the test or procedure. The remaining 20% is paid either out of pocket by the policy holder or by a secondary indemnity policy he or she has purchased.

Changes in Collection Procedures

Originally, providers treated indemnity insurance like fee for service, collecting the total fee from the patient at the time of service, and leaving the responsibility for reimbursement to the patient. More and more, market forces are making this model obsolete. Independent audiology practices frequently

---

[6]As of this writing (1994), ASHA has used RBRVS methodology to develop relative work values for audiology (*American Journal of Audiology*, in press).

[7]The approved amount is usually based on a "usual and customary" fee schedule developed by the carrier for providers in a given region.

submit the insurance forms for patients. In some cases (i.e., Medicare), they are required to do so by law.[8] Audiology practices often wait to collect anything from the patient until insurance reimbursements are received. In many cases, audiologists "accept assignment," by which they agree to accept the approved amount as payment in full.

These changes in insurance reimbursement procedures have significant ramifications for *all* audiology practices. First, they create a sizable accounts receivable that is often weighted heavily with aging accounts. This is because insurance payors are often slow and because claims with even minor errors are often rejected and must be resubmitted.

The second ramification is that excellent (sometimes obsessive) and timely record keeping is necessary to ensure that claims are submitted and reimbursed correctly and promptly. This requirement is desirable from a quality standpoint, but undesirable financially. Practices must increase capital expenditures (e.g., more computer strength) and operating expenses (e.g., more nonprofessional staff) in the face of reduced cash flow and gross income.

The third ramification is that managers and staff members must be well informed and continuously updated on the policies and procedures of many different insurance carriers.[9] This adds considerably to the audiologist's knowledge base requirements, which in turn increases the practice's overhead expenses. Graduate programs in audiology do not provide knowledge about insurance. Audiology practices must assume the role of preparing employees by allocating a significant amount of staff time to non-income-producing educational training.

Insurance reimbursement can be a time-consuming and slow process

Basic Information and Procedures

Whenever possible, practice managers should contact insurance carriers prior to encountering their policy holders as patients. Find a contact person in the insurance organization, get a billing address or phone number for automatic billing,

---

[8]See Chapter 16 for a discussion of allowable billing by audiologists working in a practice that is owned wholly or in part by a referring physician.

[9]Insurance carriers sometimes initiate policy and procedural changes with little or no notification to providers, who learn of the changes only when they receive payment explanations on claims submitted several months earlier. In such cases, it is quite possible that 2 to 3 months of claims may be submitted incorrectly before the provider is even aware that a problem exists. To avoid this scenario, carefully read all information that insurance carriers send out to providers, but do not rely passively on the carriers to provide all information. Develop contacts at each insurance company and arrange for office staff members to communicate on a regular basis with these key people.

and put that information in hard copy and computer files. For each indemnity insurance carrier, a practice manager must:

■ determine whether the carrier recognizes audiologists as providers,
■ make sure that the practice and/or the individual audiologists in the practice are properly registered with the carrier,
■ find out the carrier's reimbursement rates and decide on a collection procedure for nonreimbursed balances,
■ obtain special forms or software (if any) that are used by the carrier for submitting or disputing claims,
■ educate professional and nonprofession staff about the carrier's policies and the practice's collection procedures,
■ review and update steps 1–5 at least annually.

When scheduling patients or at patient encounters, staff members must be prepared to verify:

■ enrollment status
■ eligibility for audiology services
■ coverage and deductible amount
■ whether a physician referral is required

If necessary and feasible, acquire this information by copying the patient's insurance card and calling the carrier for verification. Submit charges on appropriate forms, along with supporting documents, if required (e.g., physician referral). Have patients sign and date their forms. Note the date of submission and make a copy for the office. When submitting electronically, generate a hardcopy for the patient to sign.

Medicare: A Government Indemnity Plan[10]

Medicare is a federally funded indemnity insurance program, primarily for people 65 and over. Those covered by Medicare are called beneficiaries. Medicare is an "80-20" plan for outpatient care. Audiologists may chose to accept assignment or not. Medicare's scope of coverage for audiology services is

---

[10]Medicare is only one example of a government plan. There are others that cover hearing services (e.g., Medicaid, Medi-Cal, Vocational Rehabilitation, Childrens' Rehabilitation Services). For a discussion of these plans and a more detailed description of the Medicare system for audiology services, see "Sources and Methods of Reimbursement," in *Developing and Managing Audiology Practices* (Kander, Martin, & Hosford-Dunn, 1994). For specifics on state plans (e.g., Medi-Cal and Medicaid), consult the appropriate state office.

very simple: "Audiology services are covered when a physician orders testing to help determine if medical or surgical treatment is appropriate for a hearing deficit or a related medical problem" (Kander, Martin, & Hosford-Dunn, 1994). *Hearing aids are not covered.*

Medicare is complex because the government contracts with different private insurance companies to handle and pay claims for two kinds of care. *Part A* covers inpatient care in hospitals and skilled nursing facilities (SNFs) and also home health and hospice care. Inpatient audiology services are covered if they are performed by audiologists who are employed by the hospital or under arrangements with the hospital (e.g., contract, staff privileges). The hospital, not the audiologist, is paid by Medicare under the *Prospective Payment System using Diagnosis Related Groups (DRGs).*[11] A Medicare *fiscal intermediary* reviews the claim and makes payment. Audiologists cannot bill Medicare directly for inpatient services.

Part B is a supplemental medical insurance to which Part A participants can subscribe by paying a monthly premium. Outpatient audiology services are Part B benefits. Audiologists bill directly and receive direct reimbursement for Part B services. Audiologists may sign a contract each year with Medicare to accept assignment on all claims, thereby becoming *participating providers.* Claims are submitted to *Medicare carriers.*

Information for Submitting Part B Medicare Claims

Be sure to ask patients whether they belong to an HSMO. Many patients who belong to HSMOs but pay for Part B supplements are under the mistaken belief that they can still choose any provider they want, as in an indemnity plan.

Always make a copy of a patient's Medicare card before submitting a claim to Medicare. This gives the patient's name as it is registered with Medicare, as well as the Medicare number. Medicare numbers are nine digits (some "Railroad Medicare" numbers are only six digits), corresponding to the social security number of the wage earner. All Medicare numbers have a Health Insurance Claim (HIC) suffix code, usually at the end, which indicates the manner in which the beneficiary is collecting social security benefits. Railroad

---

[11]Under the Prospective Payments System, hospitals are reimbursed by Medicare based primarily on the principle diagnosis of the inpatient. Prospective payment levels are set annually for each of the clusters of principal diagnoses that form Diagnosis Related Groups (DRGs).

Medicare numbers are readily identified because they always *begin* with a HIC suffix code. All other Medicare numbers *end* with a suffix code. The most common codes are:

A: beneficiary is collecting social security benefits on wages earned by the beneficiary;

B: wife is beneficiary, collecting social security benefits on wages earned by the husband;

B1: husband is beneficiary, collecting social security benefits on wages earned by wife;

D: spouse is beneficiary, collecting social security benefits on wages earned by deceased spouse.

Medicare contracts with different carriers in different states, so claims procedures vary on a state-by-state basis.[12] There are a few universal rules, however. Paper claims are submitted on HCFA 1500 forms. The patient must sign and date the form, or their signature must be on file. Claims are filed in the state where services are incurred, except for patients with "Railroad Medicare," in which case the claims are submitted to regional centers.[13]

Things to Know About Medicare and Audiologists

The following is a potpourri of Medicare information, some of it essential, some simply interesting:

■ Audiologists are recognized as nonphysician providers by Medicare, but we technically did not exist until 1994! The original Medicare statute references speech therapy and speech treatment, but there was no reference to audiology. Efforts to amend the Medicare statute to include audiology and define audiology services did not meet with success until the Social Security Amendment of 1994 was signed into law on October 31, 1994.[14]

---

[12]For example, the availability, sophistication, and cost of computerized billing to Medicare varies dramatically from one carrier to another, as of this writing (1994).

[13]At the time of writing (1994), for the 25 states west of the Mississippi River, the Medicare carrier is: Travelers Railroad Medicare, P.O. Box 30050, Salt Lake City, UT 84130-0050 (801-364-0548). For the states east of the Mississippi, the Medicare carrier is: Travelers Railroad Medicare, P.O. Box 10066, Augusta, GA 30999 (706-855-1386).

[14]Public Law 103-436 amends the Social Security Act to define "qualified audiologists" and "audiology services."

■ The Medicare reimbursement concept of "billable time"[15] does not apply to audiologists. Audiology services billed to Medicare are payed on an "inclusive procedure basis" that does not recognize nondirect time spent on patient care.

■ Audiologists must obtain a provider number from their state's Medicare carrier before providing services for which claims will be submitted.

■ Effective September 1, 1992, providers are required by law to submit all eligible Part B claims for Medicare beneficiaries.

■ Accepting Medicare assignment is a *legal* agreement that carries specific terms that the provider should read carefully. The provider agrees to accept the Medicare allowable as payment in full on all claims. Once *assignment* is made, a participating provider cannot cancel the assignment, even if a patient gives his or her consent. Under Public Law 95-142, a provider in violation of the assignment agreement may be charged with a misdemeanor. If convicted, he or she is suspended from the Medicare and Medicaid programs and penalized further by fines and possible imprisonment.

■ Effective January 1, 1994, nonparticipating audiologists (those who do not accept assignment on all claims) cannot bill more than 115% of the Medicare fee schedule rate. If they bill the patient for more than the Medicare allowable rate, they should notify the patient in writing at the time of the service.

■ Medicare claims are submitted on the HCFA 1500 claim form. A sample HCFA 1500 is included in Appendix I at the end of this book. Alternatively, claims can be submitted electronically via telephone modem.

■ Some carriers require that audiology claims be accompanied by the written physician referral. Other carriers take the position that, under the Physicians Paperwork Reform Act, evidence that a referral was made must be documented in the chart (Aetna, 1992; author's [HHD] personal communication with Aetna, March, 1994).

---

[15]"Billable time is related to activity involved in implementing a plan of care. It is appropriate to include in the cost of a visit the time spent in face-to-face contact as well as the client-specific yet nondirect time. Nondirect client services include such activities as documentation, development of care plans, and meetings or phone conversations with other care givers" (Asha, 1993b, p. 23).

■ Regarding routine audiologic testing (i.e., annual follow-up evaluations), the official interpretation of the Health Care Financing Administration is that the Medicare statute ". . . is clear in prohibiting payment for all routine physical checkups and testing and this would obviously include routine audiologic testing."[16]

Disputing Insurance Claim Denials

Private Indemnity Claim Denials

If an insurance company refuses to pay a claim or pays at a reduced rate, it is appropriate to dispute the decision if you feel it is unfair. The following steps are recommended (Thompson, 1993):

1. *Call the carrier.* Say the problem is complicated and ask to speak to the supervisor of the claims department (not a service representative).
2. *Ask the supervisor for a detailed explanation* of why the payment was denied or reduced. Take notes, including full names of everyone with whom you speak.
3. *Get the supervisor to agree to review the claim again.* State why you feel the claim was handled incorrectly.
4. *Send a written appeal.* If the supervisor still says the claim was handled correctly, state your disagreement and find out where to send a written appeal that will be reviewed by an "impartial" party—not the same supervisor who denied the claim.
5. *Write a clear and concise appeal letter,* stating all the reasons why the claim should be paid. Include a statement from the referring physician. If appropriate, point out cost-effectiveness. Reference definitions in the policy to show that the service falls within the coverage limits. Ask for specific reasons if the appeal is denied.

Medicare Denials

Medicare appeal rights are spelled out in laws and regulations. Audiologists may appeal under Part B if they accepted assignment. They may also appeal if they did not accept

---

[16]Unpublished correspondence dated July 21, 1988, from Dr. Robert E. Wren (Director, Office of Coverage Policy, Health Care Financing Administration) to Stephen C. White, Ph.D. (Director, Reimbursement Policy Division, ASHA).

assignment on a claim that was denied as not reasonable and necessary, and the beneficiary did not know and could not know that the service would *not* be covered. Appeals should *not* be made on the basis of "fairness," but on whether an error was made in claim processing or an extenuating circumstance was overlooked.

Medicare procedures for appeal are as follows:

1. *Request a review in writing.* It must be filed with the carrier within 6 months of the date of initial determination.
2. *Request a fair hearing.* Do this only if step 1 fails and the amount in question is at least $100. File the request in writing within 6 months of the date of review determination. Request a hearing in person, by telephone, or on-the-record.
3. *Request a hearing before an Administrative Law Judge of the Social Security Administration.* Do this only if step 2 fails and the amount is at least $500. File a written request within 60 days of the date of the fair hearing decision of record.
4. *Appeal to the Appeals Council.* Do this if step 3 fails. If the Appeals Council also fails and the amount is at least $1,000, the final recourse is to seek judicial review.

In registering an appeal, the audiologist should furnish relevant items, such as documentation of severity or acute onset, referrals, test results, consultation reports, medical history, billing forms, and copies of communications between the audiologist and/or physician, beneficiary, or hospital.

Managed Care

Managed care organizations are rapidly outmoding indemnity health insurance plans because they offer the promise of cost control for health services. Unlike indemnity insurance, managed care does not reimburse patients or providers on a straight fee-for-service basis. Instead, managed care organizations control costs by controlling how, where, when, and by whom services are provided. Providers negotiate agreements with the managed care organization to accept a fixed reimbursement amount per patient (capitation), a reduced percentage of their fees, or some other variation that reduces the managed care organization's cost of paying for care. Managed care organizations take many forms, among them HMOs, PPOs, PHOs, and IPAs. These acronyms were defined in the glossary earlier in this chapter. It is not uncommon for a single managed care organization to contract to manage care and costs for several medical groups,

Providers negotiate agreements with managed care organizations

resulting in a "hybrid" HMO/PPO, for example. In such cases, providers may be contracted to only one "branch" of the managed care organization. In the newest development, some HSMOs are attempting to anticipate and capture entire health care markets by becoming state-licensed insurance agencies as well. In this way, the organization jumps beyond the HSMO concept, by-passing traditional health insurers by offering POS, PPO, and 80-20 policies on an in-house basis.

How Audiologists Fit or Don't Fit into Managed Care

More and more, audiology services will become a part of managed care as it continues to grow and become the standard for health care in the United States. Breske (1994) states:

> Because employers are searching for ways to reduce their health care costs, the focus for the past decade has been on the hospital and physician sectors, . . . where about 65 percent to 70 percent of the dollars are going. With those sectors heading toward capitation, HMO and staff modeling, *the focus is shifting toward non-hospital-based services in diagnostics, surgical procedures, psychological services and physical medicine and rehabilitation.* (p. 9, italics added)

The focus of managed care on diagnostic and rehabilitation services presents an opportunity to our profession, if we can negotiate agreements with health care organizations and achieve legislation that recognize audiologists as independent providers (American Academy of Audiology [AAA], 1993a). Depending on the managed care organization's structure, audiologists may be enrolled as providers or be salaried employees of the organization. In less desirable organizational models, audiologists may be contracted as "outside specialists." In the least desirable models, they may not provide audiology services unless they are employed by physician specialists who are providers for the organization. The latter is unique and reprehensible because the managed care organization offers patients a professional service but refuses to acknowledge the professional existence of the provider. For example, a PHO's bylaws may stipulate that all members must be physicians. The PHO sets up a managed care service called "Elderly Care." Next, the PHO negotiates a contract with Medicare to provide services on a capitated basis (95% of Medicare's cost) to Medicare beneficiaries who transfer their benefits to Elderly Care. The result is a situation in which Medicare beneficiaries who enroll in Elderly Care may receive audiology services from an audiologist only if the audiologist is employed by an otolaryngologist or otologist member of the PHO. Medicare is satisfied because the service is provided and the cost of service is reduced. No laws are broken,[17] but the threat to the autonomous practice of audiology is clear and very real.

Some forms of managed care have the potential to lock out autonomous audiologists

How Audiologists Need to Approach Managed Care

Autonomous audiology practices need to get provider contracts with managed care organizations. To accomplish this, audiologists must market their services to managed care organizations just as they would any other target market.[18]

As with all successful marketing efforts, the key to success is to satisfy the market's need by providing the highest quality product in the most efficient manner at the best price.[19] Recalling the "four Ps" discussed in Chapter 13, the marketing approach must be tailored to the needs of the particular organization. Is the organization in need of hearing care providers (Product), or do they need a provider in a new area of the community (Place)? Are they more interested in the bottom line (Price) or quality (Promotion)?

Audiologists need to research each managed care organization and then send a letter of introduction to its director, requesting enrollment as a provider. Depending on the audiology practice and the needs of the organization, use the letter to stress:

■ the range and quality of hearing care products that the audiology practice is offering,
■ the competitive pricing and any other cost savings (e.g., eliminating a percentage of otolaryngologic examinations),

---

[17]Anti-trust implications of such arrangements have not been examined closely.

[18]As of this writing (1994), ASHA is preparing two products for sale to its membership: (a) *Promoting Your Services to Health Plans* and (b) *Managing Managed Care: A Practical Guide for Audiologists and Speech-Language Pathologists.*

[19]To be successful in managed care environments, audiologists must increase efficiency to reduce costs and improve quality. They should not expect fees to increase over time or even to stay at current levels, in managed care environments. Johnson and Anderson (1994) show that audiology fees remained almost flat over a 20-year period in a robust managed care market. They speculate that competition and rapid HMO expansion have kept fees stable while health care administration costs increased by 12–14%.

- convenience to the patient (e.g., easily accessible location, appointment availability, promptness), and
- convenience to the organization (e.g., 24-hour turn-around on reports, knowledgeable staff).

The letter should include curriculum vitae for all professional staff and end with a promise to follow-up by telephone within a week.

Whenever possible, negotiate as global an agreement as possible. Include services that the practice provides, even if they are not covered services at present. For example, hearing aids may not be a member benefit when the agreement is written, but may become a benefit at a later date. If and when that happens, the audiology practice will want to be in position to provide hearing aids to members. Ask that the agreement use "covered persons" language, allowing any or all of the medical groups within the organization to name the audiology practice as a provider.

Once an audiology practice becomes a provider, it needs to tend the relationship carefully by doing the following:

- develop close working relationships with the organization's Provider Relations Department;
- stay abreast of changes in the organization's structure and policies;
- make sure billing is performed promptly, accurately, according to the organization's guidelines; safeguard the agreement by staying alert to opportunities to update or expand it.

Managed Competition

This topic is addressed in detail in Chapter 16 and is only briefly touched on here. According to this chapter's glossary, managed competition is government's approach to health care cost containment.

Some aspects of managed competition are already in place. For example, Medicare carriers are moving to "focused medical review" to make certain that payments are made only for services that are medically reasonable and necessary (Whigham, 1993). Other aspects are being developed in anticipation of more services coming under the auspices of managed competition. For example, ASHA's Preferred Practice Guidelines (ASHA, 1990) and Scope of Practice statement (ASHA, 1993a) and AAA's Scope of Practice (AAA, 1993b) were developed in part to define and protect audiology "turf" as audiology is absorbed into managed competition.

The question of how audiology will be assimilated into managed competition remains unanswered in the mid-1990s. The fearful specter of the Medicare statute continues to haunt our profession—will audiology be designated as a health care profession by federally regulated boards or health plans? The best way to address this question is to show the cost-effectiveness of autonomously provided audiology services. Toward that end, the AAA has provided compelling statistics to the federal government demonstrating costs reductions of 45 to 60% when audiologists are the entry point for hearing health care, rather than primary care physicians or otolaryngologists (AAA, 1993a).

SUMMARY

Audiologists deal with internal and external reimbursement issues. Internal issues have to do with fee for service credit and collection decisions, which are largely related to hearing aid sales. Audiology practices address internal reimbursement issues by developing credit and collection policies, committing them to writing, posting them, and discussing them with staff and patients.

External reimbursement issues center around insurance claims. Claims used to be treated as fee for service, leaving the responsibility for reimbursement to the patient. As coverage has moved from the insurance indemnity model to a managed care model, external issues have proliferated. Audiologists must be familiar with many different insurance company requirements for indemnity plans. To obtain patients, they must market their skills and advantages to managed care organizations in order to obtain patients. They must prove that their services are cost-effective and responsibly priced. They must learn to live with lower reimbursements per patient and higher accounts receivable.

Most importantly, audiologists must guarantee future reimbursements by taking every opportunity to establish their professional entity at local, state, and federal levels.

REFERENCES

Aetna. (1992, July). Questions and answers physician payment reform (cont.). *Aetna Medicare Newsletter*, p. 24.

American Academy of Audiology. (1993a). *Statement of the American Academy of Audiology: Hearing care services and health care reform.* Washington, DC: Author.

American Academy of Audiology. (1993b). Scope of Practice. *Audiology Today, 5*(1), 16–17.

American Speech-Language-Hearing Association. (1990). Scope of practice, speech-language pathology and audiology. *Asha, 32*(Suppl. 2), 1–2.

American Speech-Language-Hearing Association. (1992). Strategies for responding to the Medicare resource-based relative value scale (RBRVS). Report of the Task Force on Resource-Based Relative Value Scale. *Asha, 34*(4), 63–68.

American Speech-Language-Hearing Association. (1993a). Preferred practice patterns for the professions of speech-language pathology and audiology. *Asha, 35*(Suppl. 3), 1–102.

American Speech-Language-Hearing Association. (1993b). Medicare billing for nondirect client care. *Asha, 35*(11), 14.

American Speech-Language-Hearing Association. (in press). Report of the task force on audiological relative work values. *American Journal of Audiology.*

Breske, S. (1994, June 13). Accepting the challenge of managed care. *ADVANCE for Speech-Language Pathologists & Audiologists,* p. 9.

Cherow, E., & Thompson, M. (1994). ASHA task force recommends CPT revisions. *Audiology Update,* 13(2), 12–13.

Colan, B.J. (1994, August 8). Steps to taken when it's time to collect. *ADVANCE for Speech-Language Pathologists & Audiologists,* p. 19.

Johnson, D. W., & Anderson, V. M. (1994, March). Stability of core audiology procedure fees for 1972-1991 in the Minneapolis-St. Paul metropolitan area. *American Journal of Audiology,* pp. 37–42.

Kander, M., Martin, P., & Hosford-Dunn, H. (1994). Sources and methods of reimbursement. In H. Hosford-Dunn, J. Baxter, A. Desmond, G. Jacobson, J. Johnson, P. Martin, & E. Cherow (Eds.), *Development and management of audiology practices* (chap. 9, pp. 57–66). Rockville, MD: ASHA.

Marion Merrell Dow, Inc. (1993). *Managed care digest* (update ed.). Kansas City, KS: Author.

Scott, G. G. (1990). *Positive cash flow.* Holbrook, MA: Bob Adams Inc.

Thompson, M. (1993). When insurers deny claims, don't give up! *Asha, 35*(6/7), 10–11.

Whigham, C. H. (1993). From the medical director's desk. *Aetna Medicare News, IX,* 1.

White, S. C., & Kander, M. L. (1992). Medicare resource-based relative value scale (RBRVS). Summary and guide. *Asha, 34*(4), 60–62.

SUGGESTED READING

American Speech-Language-Hearing Association. (1994). *Medicare handbook for speech-language pathology and audiology services.* Rockville, MD: Author.

APPENDIX 15-A

Commonly Used HCPCS Codes and Proposed HCPCS Procedures for Audiology and Their Medicare Status

HCPCS Code	Description	Status
92541	Spontaneous nystagmus test	Active procedure
92542	Positional nystagmus test	Active procedure
92543	Caloric vestibular test	Active procedure
92544	Optokinetic nystagmus test	Active procedure
92545	Oscillating tracking test	Active procedure
92546	Torsion swing recording	Active procedure
92551	Pure tone screening test, air	Noncovered service by Medicare
92552	Pure tone audiometry, air	Active procedure
92553	Audiometry, air and bone	Active procedure
92555	Speech threshold audiometry	Active procedure
92556	Speech audiometry, complete	Active procedure Change "threshold and discrimination" to read "speech recognition"[a]
92557	Comprehensive hearing test	Active procedure Change to "threshold evaluation and speech recognition"[a]
92559	Group audiometric testing	Noncovered services by Medicare
92560	Bekesy audiometry, screen	Noncovered service by Medicare
92561	Bekesy audiometry, diagnosis	Active procedure
92562	Loudness balance test	Active procedure
92563	Tone decay hearing test	Active procedure
92564	SISI hearing test	Active procedure
92565	Stenger test, pure tone	Active procedure
92567	Tympanometry	Active procedure
92568	Acoustic reflex testing	Active procedure
92569	Acoustic reflex decay test	Active procedure
92571	Filtered speech hearing test	Active procedure

continued

HCPCS Code	Description	Status
92572	Staggered spondaic word test	Active procedure
92576	Synthetic sentence test	Active procedure
92577	Stenger test, speech	Active procedure
92582	Conditioning play audiometry	Active procedure
92583	Select picture audiometry	Active procedure
92584	Electro-cochleography	Active procedure
92585	Brainstem evoked audiometry	Active procedure Change to "auditory evoked potentials/response"[a]
92589	Auditory function test(s)	Active procedure
92590	Hearing aid examination, one ear	Noncovered procedure by Medicare
92591	Hearing aid examination, both ears	Noncovered procedure by Medicare
92592	Hearing aid check, one ear	Noncovered procedure by Medicare
92593	Hearing aid check, both ears	Noncovered procedure by Medicare
92594	Electro hearing aid test, one	Noncovered procedure by Medicare
92595	Electro hearing aid test, both	Noncovered procedure by Medicare
92596	Ear protector evaluation	Noncovered procedure by Medicare
00000	Loudness tolerance (MCL, UCL, LGOB [Loudness Growth Octave Band])	Potential New Code[c]
00000	Evoked otoacoustic emissions; limited	Potential New Code[b]
00000	Evoked otoacoustic emissions; comprehensive	Potential New Code[b]
00000	Visual reinforcement audiometry (VRA)	Potential New Code[c]
00000	Computerized dynamic posturography	Potential New Code[c]
00000	Cochlear implant evaluation; initial 1 hour, each visit; 00000 each additional 15 minutes	Potential New Code[c]
00000	Cochlear implant rehabilitation; initial 30 minutes, each visit; 00000 each additional 15 minutes	Potential New Code[c]

HCPCS Code	Description	Status
00000	Probe microphone measurement	Potential New Code[c]
00000	Electroneurography	Potential New Code[c]

[a]Proposed CPT revisions recommendations made by ASHA Task Force on CPT Code Revisions. Currently in the peer review process, the final recommendations will eventually be submitted to the AMA CPT Editorial panel (Cherow & Thompson, 1994).

[b]New CPT codes for these procedures were submitted by ASHA to the AMA CPT panel and are to be printed in the 1995 CPT manual (Cherow & Thompson, 1994).

[c]New CPT procedures proposed by the ASHA Task Force on CPT Code Revisions (Cherow & Thompson, 1994).

Sources: HCPCS Codes from Federal Register, Nov. 25, 1991, pp. 59752–59753. All numeric CPT HCPCS copyright 1991, American Medical Association. Proposed codes adapted from American Speech-Language-Hearing Association (1992) Strategies for responding to the Medicare resource-based relative value scale (RBRVS). Report of the Task Force on Resource-Based Relative Value Scale. Asha, 34(4), 63–68; and Cherow, E., and Thompson, M. (1994). ASHA task force recommends CPT revisions. Audiology Update, 13(4), 7–8.

16

Implications of the Evolving Managed Care Environment for Audiologists

Jack T. Diamond, J.D.
David A. Weil, J.D., M.B.A.[1]

[1]Jack T. Diamond is a Partner of Buckingham, Doolittle and Burroughs. David A. Weil is an Attorney employed by Buckingham, Doolittle and Burroughs. Jack and David practice within the firm's Hospital and Health Law Department and address numerous issues and serve health care providers and practitioners throughout the country. Their mailing address is 50 South Main Street, Akron, Ohio 44308. They can be reached at 1-800-686-2825.

This book is not an edited text. However, the principal authors felt that the issues addressed in Chapters 16 and 17 were central to the theme of the book, but required the expertise of outside professionals. Mr. Diamond and Mr. Weil are nationally recognized consultants to hospitals and managed care groups. They graciously agreed to look at the "big picture" from the vantage point of audiologists and write Chapter 16 for this handbook. For a deliberate reason, the style of this chapter differs from the rest of the book. We asked the authors to compose brief "snapshots" of different national managed care issues, concluding each discussion with comments on how the issue pertains to the future of audiology. These comments appear as italicized paragraphs throughout the text.

The discussions are technical and dynamic, using a number of terms and acronyms to describe concepts that are new and often unfamiliar to audiologists. As the chapter makes clear, it is in our best interests to make these our own as soon as possible. In coming years, audiologists who plan to practice with some degree of autonomy will find many of these concepts commonplace.

Improve quality and reduce costs

The purpose of this chapter is to discuss managed care in general terms of continuous quality improvement (CQI),[2] stressing increasingly demands health care providers and practitioners to improve the quality and reduce the costs of hospital and professional services through integration and managed care.

> *The steps taken by audiologists to improve quality and reduce costs must be directly linked to risk management and proven methods of functional assessment*

---

[2]See Chapter 13 for a discussion of CQI.

CQI AND PREFERRED PRACTICE GUIDELINES

The concepts of CQI are being applied to health care through both governmental and private sector efforts. For example, the Health Care Financing Administration (HCFA) is implementing CQI through its *Health Care Quality Improvement Initiative* (HCQII) to decrease variance among practitioners and in the outcomes of the care rendered to Medi-care beneficiaries. The general idea of this initiative is to move State Utilization and Quality Peer Review Organizations (the corporate entities that contract with HCFA to review the utilization and quality of services provided to Medicare and Medicaid beneficiaries) and providers and practitioners into a more collaborative and less punitive relationship through pattern analysis and the application of objective criteria to improve quality.

Part of this effort is HCFA's *Uniform Clinical Data Set System,* which is a computerized quality and cost audit review program. This system will be applied by the review entities to abstract information from medical records throughout the country. This information will be used to profile the quality of care rendered to Medicare beneficiaries and compare how well practitioners are complying with nationally recognized clinical practice guidelines (the "best practices") and how well hospitals are comparing with the "most successful medical centers." An early application of the system is the Cooperative Cardiovascular Project, in which the quality of care rendered to cardiovascular patients through the application of guidelines developed and published by the American College of Cardiologists and the American Heart Association. The federal government is already developing similar projects to apply objective criteria based upon guidelines for numerous other procedures that are common among Medicare beneficiaries.

> HCQIIs use "best practice" standards to objectively profile individual practitioners

Therefore, it is important that audiologists embrace the use of Preferred Practice Patterns for the Professions of Speech-Language Pathology and Audiology, or similar guidelines, with a view toward the application of objective criteria by the federal government to the care of patients treated by audiologists.

Criteria, or standards of care, for audiologists are set forth in the American Speech-Language-Hearing Association's Scope of Practice and "Best Practice" Guidelines and Preferred Practice Patterns.

In order to survive in the evolving managed care environment and to manage risk within their practices, a goal of audiologists will be to concentrate on operating and marketing their practices based upon sound processes and favorable outcomes through compliance with preferred practice patterns, especially those which will be endorsed by public and private payors.

THE CONCEPT OF MANAGED COMPETITION

Historical Perspective

Managed competition was first spelled out in major legislation and debated nationally in 1993 when President Clinton compiled the Health Security Act. Although the legislation did not pass into law, it and the debate it spawned were framed in six principles that define the concept of managed competition.

Six Principles of Managed Care

- *Security*
- *Simplicity*
- *Savings*
- *Quality*
- *Choice*
- *Responsibility*

The basic premise of the 1993 legislation was universal access to health care for all Americans through an employer mandate and governmental subsidies. The Clinton administration proposed to raise the additional funds required for this plan, in part, by cutting gross Medicare and Medicaid spending. Even without a universal health care program in place, reductions in reimbursement have compelled health care providers and practitioners to compete based on quality improvements and cost reductions for fewer dollars.

Proposed Methods to Meet Managed Care Objectives

Providing health care services on a prepaid basis, or at capitated rates, and managing utilization are the most widely used means of addressing the objectives of quality improvement and cost reduction. One significant method of managing utilization while providing quality care is to use primary care physicians to serve as "gatekeepers." In other words, all patients who are covered by a particular health care insurance plan or present to the hospital with coverage based on capitation (usually, a set monthly premium per patient per month for certain enumerated services) are initially examined, or screened, by a primary care physician, usually a board-certified family practice physician, before being assessed by any specialists. Providers and practitioners as well as payors, for the most part, have acknowledged the advantages of capitated systems and the use of primary care physicians as gatekeepers to manage utilization and are either contracting for or creating their own managed care plans with these objectives in mind.

According to the concept of managed competition, practitioners would be reimbursed through either regional or corporate alliances for non-Medicare patients on a reasonable charge or fee schedule basis. Each corporate alliance, which would be an alliance formed voluntarily by a company which has at least 5,000 employees, would be required to offer its enrollees at least one plan organized around a fee-for-service system in which the enrollees have the option to consult the physician or practitioner of their choice, subject to utilization review and prior approval for certain services. Fee-for-service options would be available to other employees and the remainder of the population. Practitioners would be required to accept the fee schedule or allowed charge amount adopted by each patient's alliance or health plan as payment in full for their services, and would be prohibited from "balance billing" patients for any amounts in excess of those amounts. Regardless of the creating of alliances on a national basis, most providers and practitioners have already prepared themselves for a similar reimbursement scheme.

Audiologists will want to take advantage of this opportunity on an ongoing basis and demonstrate how their services can be provided in a manner which complements the services provided by primary care physicians, including family practice physicians and pediatricians, and specialists, including oto-

Gatekeepers and capitation

laryngologists, and the hospitals at which these physicians serve as medical staff members.[3] Audiologists are in a favorable position with regard to the cost-effectiveness of health care resources and, therefore, the utilization management function within the hospital.

INTEGRATION

Hospitals and practitioners are integrating their services to pool their resources, to reduce costs and manage their utilization of resources while maintaining the quality of their care. This movement entails the bringing together and packaging of hospital and professional services. The incentives driving integration include:

Corporations are offering hospital and private practice services as one "product"

1. Maintaining access to patients through direct contracting.
2. Gaining leverage in the health care market.
3. Getting control over costs and availing providers and practitioners of economies of scale.
4. Engaging in a well-reasoned and carefully planned response to the call from insurers, employers, and other payors for managed care plans, discounted fee schedules, and capitation.

Audiologists, in addition to other practitioners, can best position themselves for integration and the movement toward managed care by complying with the preferred practice guidelines developed by nationally known experts in audiology. By working toward the "best practices" and improving their outcomes in comparison to the most highly regarded practitioners, audiologists will more effectively be able to demonstrate the quality of their services, control costs through managing their utilization of resources, and market themselves by fitting their services into the quickly developing managed care plans.

The movement toward integration is permanently influencing how health care services are provided. The health care

---

[3]Audiologists who have clinical privileges to render care to patients within a hospital are usually considered members of the hospital's allied health professional staff rather than the hospital's medical staff. The medical staff is usually credentialed and granted privileges and otherwise governed by the hospital's medical staff bylaws. Allied health professionals may be governed under particular provisions of the medical staff bylaws but are preferably granted privileges and governed under a separate document which sets forth the relevant policies and procedures expressing the requirements, duties or obligations and privileges of such professionals based on their qualifications and capabilities.

industry has instituted aggressive efforts toward reform regardless of, or in addition to, various legislative proposals at both the state and federal levels. The health care industry has progressed far beyond the basic parameters of many legislative proposals. Collaboration and the concomitant creation of new corporate entities which can provide the services of both the hospital and practitioners as a single "product" is a reality.

Audiologists can take advantage of these changes by demonstrating the value of their services and offering services that will improve the quality of patient care on a cost-effective basis.

Legal Issues Relevant to Integration

There have been a number of changes in the law which have an impact on the efforts of providers and practitioners in their efforts toward integrating.

Antitrust Guidelines

On September 15, 1993, the Department of Justice and the Federal Trade Commission published guidelines establishing "safety zones" within which practitioners may bargain collectively with health plans about payment and coverage issues, decisions about medical care, and other matters without fear of prosecution under federal antitrust laws. Several states have enacted legislation that also protects related activities, such as the exchange of price information, under certain circumstances which enable providers and practitioners to coordinate services. The FTC guidelines also provide for an expedited advisory opinion mechanism under which providers and networks can obtain advice and assurances within ninety (90) days as to whether a proposed joint venture would be challenged.

Antitrust liability can arise where a professional group, such as a medical group practice, or an organization or arrangement among providers or hospitals, sets prices or behaves in an anti-competitive manner. Such behavior can occur where practitioners or providers corner the market or provide services to a large percentage of the patients within a particular geographic area and, thereby, exclude competitors or invoke barriers to new market participants.

Exclusionary ventures may be challenged

Audiologists should keep in mind the restraints imposed on physicians and hospitals by federal and state antitrust laws. These restrictions have an impact on what types of arrangements and agreements audiologists can reach with practitioners and providers.

Malpractice Reform

Malpractice reform is under consideration to help providers and practitioners keep their costs down. Patients with claims against providers and physicians are increasingly required to first present the claim through an *alternative dispute resolution* mechanism before proceeding to court. Some agreements require that malpractice suits filed in court be accompanied by an affidavit signed by a specialist practicing in a field relevant to the claimed injury, with an attestation that the procedure or treatment that produced the claim deviated from the established standard of care.

Some states have already passed legislation that allows physicians to demonstrate compliance with certain clinical practice guidelines or practice parameters as an affirmative defense to medical malpractice claims. The federal government is moving toward the enactment of similar legislation based on clinical practice guidelines published by the federal Agency for Health Care Policy and Research as the entire country moves toward nationally recognized and accepted standards of care. *Audiologists can expect preferred practice patterns to be endorsed and used in a similar manner to limit their liability as well.*

Following Preferred Practice Guidelines is good protection

Fraud and Abuse

The federal government has expanded the fraud and abuse enforcement program. For example, the self-referral prohibitions regarding clinical laboratory services have been expanded in "Stark II," §13562 of the Omnibus Reconciliation Act of 1993 (OBRA '93), to the payment for certain "designated health services" which are provided by an entity with which the physician ordering the service has a financial relationship and where such physician does not render that item or service. Also, Stark II has expanded the rules prohibiting physician ownership and referral to cover Medicaid as well as Medicare payments for these services.[4]

Most of the exceptions to the prohibition have been retained, but the group practice exception has been narrowed to prevent the operation of sham groups. The Stark II provisions for physician ownership and referral are effective after December 31, 1994. At the time of writing (1994), HCFA is scheduled to develop proposed regulations for the self-referral amendments of OBRA '93 in spring of 1995. According to

[4]At the time of writing (1994), a "Stark III" set of amendments could be included in future Medicare and Medicaid legislation, which would expand self-referral prohibitions to all payers, not just Medicare and Medicaid.

Designated Health Services

- *Clinical laboratory services*
- *Physical and occupational therapy*
- *Radiology or other diagnostic services*
- *Radiation therapy services*
- *Durable medical equipment*
- *Parenteral and enteral nutrients, equipment, and supplies*
- *Prosthetics, orthotics, and prosthetic devices*
- *Home health services*
- *Outpatient prescription drugs*
- *Inpatient/outpatient hospital services*

the American Speech-Language-Hearing Association (ASHA), HCFA expects that audiologic tests and hearing aids will fall under two categories of the designated health services: (1) radiology or *other diagnostic services* and (2) prosthetics, orthotics, and *prosthetic devices.* However, HCFA "will not confirm or deny the ban on audiology referrals where there is a physician ownership interest until the proposed regulations are printed" (ASHA, 1994, p. 24).

Under the "In-Office Ancillary Services" exemption, audiology services are exempted from the self-referral amendments if they are provided by an audiologist who is an employee of the referring physician(s) and if the services are:

1. supervised by the referring physician or by another physician in the group practice;
2. rendered in a building in which the referring or group physician furnishes services unrelated to the "designated health services;" and
3. billed by the physician supervising the services, by a group practice of which the physician is a member, or by an entity that is wholly owned by such physician or such group practice. (ASHA, 1994, p. 24)

In summary, a physician may refer a patient to an audiologist with whom the physician has a financial relationship provided that (1) such services do not fall within any of the designated health services (which seems unlikely, given ASHA's interpretation of HCFA's intent) or (2) such audiologist is a supervised employee operating on-site within the physician's group practice.

At the same time, audiologists must be careful to avoid anti-kickback laws[5] when they accept patients and bill for tests that are referred by physicians with whom the audiologists have financial arrangements.

FINANCIAL CONCERNS AND BUDGETARY CONSTRAINTS

Price pressures will increase

The creation of a single large health alliance, as contemplated by the reform initiatives encompassing the concept of managed competition, in each geographic area would create an entity with the market power of a very large employer. The market power of these alliances would also be reinforced by the regulatory provisions of the health care budget. The combina-

---

[5]Although the self-referral amendments apply only to physicians, physicians are not the only ones who come under scrutiny. Anti-kickback regulations apply to anyone who "knowingly and willfully offers, pays, solicits, or receives remuneration in order to induce business reimbursed under the Medicare or Medicaid programs." (ASHA, 1994, p 24)

tion of a large enrollment with regulatory controls on rate increases would restrain increases in the prices of hospital and professional services. The price pressure is likely to increase as time goes on because the anticipated price increases under the budget system are substantially less than historical increases in the costs of hospital services.

Hospitals seeking relationships with corporate payers or employers must demonstrate that they can provide a product, or package of hospital and professional services, that is more attractive than those offered by competitors. Even if a hospital has had a direct contracting relationship with large corporate employers in the past, the existence of regional purchasing payers creates downward pressure on health care prices because those payers are an alternative for employers who have previously sponsored their own health plans.

Any national health care budget, although identified as a "backstop" to market forces, is calculated to establish a maximum payment rate within a short time. Any budget system heavily penalizes any provider whose bids contribute to an excess of cost over the payer's weighted average premium target. Because the cost control mechanism is backed up not only by market forces, but by a regulatory structure, the de facto price control in such a system could emerge not from negotiations, but from the regulatory system within a brief period.

Hospitals' Strategies

Hospitals are using several different strategies to succeed in the face of negotiations with payors and the health plans with which they are contracting. Hospitals often use a combination of these strategies in order to compete.

Low-cost Provider

One strategy is to negotiate as a low-cost provider, because the primary goal of payers, alliances and health plans is to minimize the price paid for hospital services. Although very low cost providers should be able to obtain patients through this mechanism, the competition to deliver services at the low cost end of the hospital service scale is likely to be intense. If the management of utilization by health plans is successful, hospitals will be willing to compete for patients on a very low margin. Hospitals without the financial strength to bid aggressively may find the low cost-provider strategy difficult to sustain in the face of intense provider competition.

Affiliate with financially strong institutions

Niche Marketing

Audiology is a niche market

A second strategy is to focus the hospital's attention on patient populations or types of services which have not been the focus of competition among health care providers in the past. The scope of coverage in the contemplated guaranteed national benefit packages contains a number of significant expansions of benefits now paid by insurers. Home health care, hospice care, and mental health services are areas in which hospitals have the ability to bring substantial efficiencies and provide quality service. Focusing on services that are to receive substantial new amounts of payment and organizing these services in a comprehensive manner may help institutions benefit from health reform.

Another way of optimizing utilization is to seek patients who have not been the source of provider competition in the past. The expansion of benefits to the uninsured population and the changes in benefit provisions for Medicaid patients will create new demand from such patients for health care alliances. However, subsidies for such patients are unlikely to reimburse the cost of higher level health benefits. Hospital-affiliated services which seek to capture the expanding marketplace, therefore, would need to be organized in a highly efficient and cost-effective manner.

Audiologists can contract their services to the hospital in a manner that is attractive from the niche marketing perspective.

Integration of Hospital and Practitioner Services

This strategy uses "one stop shopping" to control costs

A third strategy involves the formation of an integrated delivery system (IDS), or network, either on a single institution or a multi-institutional basis. Each payer contracts with providers, or networks of providers, that offer a substantial portion of health care coverage throughout the payer's service area. Those institutions that can provide the full range of services and assume the risk for controlling the cost of those services through integration appeal to health plans for selection by each payer.

The strategies for establishing these organizations differ depending on urban or rural location and the breadth of services that the providers are willing to offer. Particularly in rural areas, hospitals that can offer a full range of services would be favored by the alliances.

Audiologists can use the incentive for hospitals to provide this full range of services and demonstrate that they can provide hospitals with services needed to render comprehensive care.

Hospitals' Efforts and How Audiologists Can Contribute

Hospitals are negotiating their rates and services through evolving means. Hospitals that successfully package both hospital and professional services, negotiate rates, and provide convincing evidence of their ability to deliver comprehensive and cost-effective care, especially through capitation, are most likely to succeed in the evolving managed care environment.

In order to compete more effectively, hospitals are moving away from the traditional hospital-medical staff relationship toward integrated structures such as:

- hospital-based, or management, service bureaus
- hospital-based IPAs
- physician hospital organizations (PHOs)
- hospital-based, or comprehensive, management services organizations (MSOs)
- foundations
- hospital-based clinics
- physician equity models
- hospital employment models

Audiologists will want to consider developing and implementing a basic strategic business plan to manage their practices and market their services to these entities with a view toward managed care and integration. This involves the following steps:

- *Calculate the costs of services.*
- *Determine reasonable fees and minimum rates based on the most efficient utilization of health care resources.*
- *Evaluate the feasibility, advantages and disadvantages of forming an integrated group practice among audiologists and in conjunction with physicians, especially family practitioners and pediatricians.*
- *Formulate a strategic business plan, taking into consideration the value, quality, and costs of the audiology services that can be provided.*
- *Demonstrate to appropriate hospitals, clinics, and other providers how audiology services can be used to complete the package of hospital and professional services provided.*

Capitation and integration are cornerstones of success

PHYSICIANS AND HOW AUDIOLOGISTS CAN WORK WITH THEM

> *Independent audiologists can pursue the same paths as hospitals and physicians*

The manner in which patients ultimately come to physicians will dramatically change in the evolving managed care market. Traditionally, each patient selected his or her physician of choice, but in the future the managed care plans under which patients obtain coverage will dictate the choices regarding physicians and other practitioners. As a result, physicians are evaluating and implementing methods to retain control over their own practices and maintain, if not gain, the bargaining power needed to compete in the evolving managed care environment.

Like hospitals, physicians are using a wide range of practice structures to integrate and market professional services packages. Professional practice structures range from the traditional preferred provider organizations (PPOs) to the newer independent practice associations (IPAs), group practices without walls (GPWWs), integrated medical group practices, IPA affiliation models, freestanding group practice-related MSOs, and freestanding clinics.

Physicians are undertaking integration in large part to implement the "one stop shopping" concept for professional services. The more services that physicians can bundle, the greater their leverage with hospitals in more comprehensive integrated structures. The integrated structures often offer services that include billing, collection, financial planning, handling of real estate transactions, recruitment, practice management, marketing, cross coverage, and legal and group purchasing discounts.

Managed care plans are expected to negotiate with integrated systems of providers and practitioners who, through their organizational efforts, have realized significant economies of scale, meaning that the overall price for comprehensive professional services offered should be lower. Managed care plans find these integrated networks attractive for building or expanding their provider networks in particular communities.

Therefore, independent audiologists have an opportunity to become equal members of integrated networks. They can offer their services to augment the professional service packages that physician groups are putting together in order to survive in the managed care environment.

SUMMARY

Managed care and the integration of hospital and professional services is affecting the utilization and the quality of professional services. Although control over the costs of care tends to be the major issue driving integration, the quality of care will remain a significant factor in managed care. Quality will be increasingly measured through the application of objective criteria. *For audiologists, these criteria will be based, in large part, on preferred practice patterns.* Compliance with these practice patterns and the generation of favorable patient care outcomes will be profiled to ascertain who will be paid for what services and used as a factor in the negotiating process. *Audiologists have a strong incentive to follow through with the following: (a) focus on processes of care and patient outcomes through preferred practice guidelines, (b) manage risks through strict adherence with the appropriate standard of care and proper documentation of all audiology services rendered, and (c) compete in the evolving managed care environment and the movement toward integration of hospital and professional services by demonstrating that his or her practice is the best practice.*

REFERENCE

American Speech-Language-Hearing Association. (1994). Physician self-referral. *Asha 36*(11), 24.

SUGGESTED READINGS

American Speech-Language-Hearing Association. (1994). *Introduction to managed care for audiologists and speech-language pathologists.* Rockville, MD: Author.

American Speech-Language-Hearing Association. (1994). Managing managed care: *A practice guide for audiologists and speech-language pathologists.* Rockville, MD: Author.

Harrison, M. (Ed.). (1994). Total quality management: Application to audiology. *Seminars in Hearing, 15*(4), 259–330.

17

Risk Abatement in an Audiology Practice

Alexander Woods, M.D., J.D.[1]

[1]Dr. Woods can be reached at his home address: 5805 Cerrada Chica, Tucson, AZ 85718. (602) 299-3646.

This book is not an edited text. However, the principal authors felt that the issues addressed in Chapters 16 and 17 were central to the theme of the book, but required the expertise of outside professionals. Dr. Woods was invited to write Chapter 17 because of his long and varied background in medico-legal issues. He is an Emeritus Professor at the University of Arizona Medical School and a practicing attorney, specializing in Health Law. He continues to practice medicine on contract to Hughes Missile Systems. Of particular importance, he is a strong proponent of amplification, based on his own experiences wearing binaural hearing aids in classrooms, clinics, and courtrooms.

This chapter differs in style from the rest of the book for two reasons: (1) The Marketing Chapter admonishes audiologists to view their practices through the eyes of their customers. Dr. Woods gives us the rare opportunity to simultaneously view our field through the eyes of a customer <u>and</u> an outside expert. (2) It was unlikely that we could improve on Dr. Woods' inimitable style without detracting from the commentary and losing the intimacy of his message.

> ### *"Most of the principles hammered out in medicine do not yet exist in audiology: it is too new."*

I have approached this chapter on risk abatement in a book devoted to practice management in audiology as an outsider (i.e., as a consumer not specially versed in audiology). Knowing something of both medicine and law and having spent several years practicing in the area between them, I found that most of the principles which have been hammered out by decades of litigation in medicine do not yet exist in audiology[2]: it is too new. What we know today by the term "audiology" is in fact the merger of two previously independent occupations, the purely scientific and technical study of hearing and its defects and the frankly commercial dispensation of hearing aids by dealers. This merger is still far from complete, and much ethical and legal conflict is arising in the process. The use of product sales to support a professional practice, as in dispensing audiology, is fraught with the taint of commercialism, and the dealers whose turf is being invaded will fight back. Likewise, otolaryngologists will lose turf as autonomous audiologists continue to emerge as entry points for hearing health care management, including hearing aid sales. The ground is in constant motion as these forces shift and develop, particularly as the trend to concentrate hearing aid dispensation in audiologist's offices gathers momentum (American Academy of Audiology, 1993; O'Toole, 1993) and public discontent accumulates from years of fraudulent and incompetent sales by some hearing aid dealers.[3] Much of what I have to say will focus on this conflict as it might contribute to legal proceedings, and will be borrowed largely from parallel experiences of sister professions.

I have been provided an ASHA communication dated September 22, 1993, discussing recent testimony before the U.S. Senate Special Committee on Aging (O'Toole, 1993), which illustrates this. Beginning with the panoply of customer complaints regarding hearing aids, now familiar to most of us, concerning misleading advertising, coercion for sales, variation among federal and state regulations, and dissatisfaction with results, the ASHA mounted a plea for uniform state licensing and federal recognition of audiologists permitting dispensation of hearing aids and consumer education on the benefits to be expected from them. In a similar vein, the American Academy of Audiology (AAA, 1993) recommended to the President's Task Force on National Health Reform that legislation be enacted to:

- Provide appropriate recognition of audiology as an entry point into hearing care.
- Ensure appropriate service provider status for audiologists.

---

[2]For a list of the few professional claims that have been filed against Speech-Language Pathologists and Audiologists, see American Speech-Language-Hearing Association (ASHA), 1994.

[3]Remarks by Rep. William Cohen (R-ME) contained in O'Toole (1993).

■ Prohibit any unjustified action to limit the practice of audiology on the part of physician providers.

Unsurprisingly, hearing aid dealers oppose regulations limiting their power to dispense, and otolaryngologists oppose regulations that diminish their gatekeeper role. Audiologists thus find a contested trend toward redirecting dispensation of hearing aids to certified audiologists, which, if completed, will bring with it as the price of victory a redirection toward them of the existing consumer mistrust and increased efforts on the part of some otolaryngologists to relegate audiology to a technical support role.

Audiologists do not start with a clean slate

Audiologists do not, therefore, start with a clean slate. They must shed their long-standing technician status in the medical environment. At the same time, they inherit consumer hostility especially among the geriatric set which includes the majority of audiology patients and is ably represented by the American Association of Retired Persons (AARP),[4] which demands even more meticulous attention to professional and ethical principles. After all, juries are composed of these people.

Definition of a clinical professional

The essential thing to remember is that audiologists are independent professionals who also dispense hearing aids. They are not hearing aid dealers who also provide testing services. The difference is crucial to the discussion of professional and legal responsibilities that follows, as I hope will become clear as the chapter progresses. Let's start with the definition of a clinical professional. This is a person possessing special skills to be used on people, gained through training and attested to by appropriate diplomas. A clinical professional has generally also been certified by a group of peers as competent to practice a defined clinical specialty. Virtually all will have an advanced degree, and most will operate in an area where their state has defined the scope of their practice, licensure, and governing bodies. Audiology is clearly such a profession, but it exhibits peculiarities due to its still incomplete merger with hearing aid dispensing and its vestigial ties to otolaryngology. In a few states, for example, there are regulations affecting hearing aid dispensation but none concerning the practice of audiology. I shall nevertheless consider audiology as a clinical profession whose rules and definitions are still in a formative stage (ASHA, 1994a; 1994c; 1994d).

Up to this point, most of what I have said has probably been obvious; what may not be obvious is the way society

---

[4]See the AARP testimony reported in O'Toole (1993).

Clinicians' Privileges and Responsibilities in Society

- *Right to practice a profession*
- *Meet or exceed national standard of care*
- *Duty of trust to patients*

behaves with regard to professionals, what privileges it grants them, and what duties and responsibilities it imposes on them in return. First, it permits them the privilege of practicing their professions. Second, it requires them to perform this practice at a level of competence at least equal to that of others in the same profession. Third, it imposes on them a duty of trust, a responsibility that they will not abuse the confidence of their patients, that they will be motivated only on the behalf and for the benefit of these patients, and that they set their patients' interests above their own. This type of trust is known as a fiduciary responsibility. Legally, it applies whenever one side of any transaction possesses immensely more knowledge or power than the other, an inequality that puts the ignorant side at a disadvantage and can breed abuse. The concept of fiduciary responsibility protects against this, and can be a potent legal argument if breached. Already, many in the audiology profession are anticipating increased malpractice risk (Kirkwood, 1994). ASHA (1994b) has developed a patient's "Bill of Rights" delineating 12 areas of fiduciary responsibility that are incumbent on audiologists and speech-language pathologists who provide services to patients (see Appendix 17-A).

Applying these principles to audiology says that you will be held to the performance standards of a trained professional audiologist in everything you do, including the dispensation of hearing aids. In return for this high level of performance, people like FDA Commissioner Dr. David Kessler have suggested strengthening hearing aid rules by discarding the current [1994] mandatory examination by a physician before a hearing aid is dispensed. In its place, the FDA has proposed a nonwaivable hearing examination by a health professional licensed by the state to do hearing aid examinations. Consumer organizations such as AARP and Self Help for Hard of Hearing People (SHHH) acknowledge the preeminent role of audiologists in hearing aid dispensing, noting that prospective hearing aid purchasers are best served by obtaining a hearing evaluation by an audiologist, and that current FDA law preempts the rehabilitation role of audiologists in fitting hearing aids.

With this background I have attempted to develop a set of guidelines for practicing audiologists which would reduce their overall risk of litigation and at the same time enrich the quality of practice.[5] These are drawn partly from experience with other clinical professions and partly from general ethical principles. There are twelve guidelines; each is stated in brief, followed by the reasons for suggesting it and the specific risks it attempts to abate. The guidelines are divided into five sections as follows.

I. Ethical Principles
   Guideline 1: "Above All, Do No Harm"
   Guideline 2: Professional and Fiduciary Responsibility
   Guideline 3: Avoidance of Criticism
II. Professional Personnel
   Guideline 4: Competence and Compliance
   Guideline 5: Training and Vicarious Liability
III. Equipment
   Guideline 6: Operation and Maintenance
IV. Relations with Patients
   Guideline 7: The Written Record
   Guideline 8: Financial Arrangements
   Guideline 9: Informed Consent
   Guideline 10: Predictions and Warranties
V. Medico-Legal Audiology
   Guideline 11: Referral or Not?
   Guideline 12: Basic Legal Knowledge

---

[5]Chapter 18 lists of the types of insurance protection that were available to audiologists through the American Speech-Language-Hearing Association in 1994.

ETHICAL PRINCIPLES

Guideline 1. "Above All Do No Harm"

This is the oldest medical principle of all. Literally, it means physical harm — if you can't heal, don't hurt — but the same principle extends itself easily to cover financial harm as well. The cardinal rule is that all your professional activities must be directed solely toward your patient's benefit; and that none of them be for secondary gain, such as the enrichment of yourself or others. This seems an elementary principle, yet its abuse led Congress to enact the Health Care Quality Improvement Act of 1986 (HCQIA) to limit the undue profit made by some physicians through kickbacks or partial ownership of the health facilities to which they referred patients. Examples were Computed Axial Tomography (CAT) and Magnetic Resonance Imaging (MRI) scanners partially owned by physicians who used them more frequently than similar nonowned facilities. In some cases, the extra use was needless and not indicated. Two things stood out: that the physicians were biased toward their own self-interest and that they would occasionally manufacture such referrals for their own profit with no benefit to the patient.

Patient benefit is paramount

Audiologists who dispense hearing aids are at risk for a similar ethical lapse. They must make their choice of the appropriate hearing aid for a given patient solely because it is the best match for the hearing defect encountered, not because of any external influence such as a commercial tie-in with the manufacturer. To do otherwise would be unethical *unless* the hearing aid dispenser is a dealer in only one brand and this is made immediately apparent by advertising so that the public is duly warned that the choice will be biased. Otherwise the public is entitled to assume that an audiologist is free from commercial taint and will choose the best instrument for the purpose, whoever the manufacturer may be.

The HCQIA defined certain "safe harbors" among health facilities into which physicians could safely invest their money. These are mostly multi-million dollar concerns with hundreds of investors, enough so that the actions of one person or a group are diluted out. Suffice it to say that various investigative government offices now have a body of law to back up their curiosity in any scheme that enriches a practitioner without conferring an equivalent benefit to the patient.

Guideline 2. Professional and Fiduciary Responsibility

Society sees fit to impose on individuals who have become experts in their fields an extra measure of responsibility based on public trust. This trust takes two forms:

- First, that these individuals will maintain their skills at a high level.
- Second, that they will use these skills for the benefit of others above personal concern.

Skill is the defining factor

In a way, this is a corollary of the guideline above, but there are important differences. For one thing, the matter of "skill" becomes a crucial definition. You are charged not only with maintaining your own skill at least on a par with other audiologists, but also with knowing when your skills are not adequate for the case before you (i.e., when the patient must be referred to some other practitioner). Knowingly to perform procedures in which you are not competent, or operating equipment in which you are not trained, are lapses of professional responsibility and may be actionable. Often the limits of what you may and may not do are set out in your license, if any, and frequently they are spelled out in the form of clinical privileges set by the hospital or clinic. As a solo practitioner, you must be the final judge of your own clinical competence, and you may have to defend this if it is challenged.

The second aspect of this guideline is that society trusts you to deliver your services only when, in your opinion, they are necessary for the patient you are seeing. Many situations exist in the health fields where the person who decides whether a service is needed is also the one who performs it, a potential conflict of interest which may be inevitable in some situations. Cardiac surgeons are a good example. Here, society requires that you place the patient's interest first. Your judgment of this must be paramount and should be rooted in your training.

It is public policy that such trust be placed in professionals, and a breach of such trust may be subject to suit as being against public policy. It is well to keep these principles in mind. They are embodied in the Codes of Ethics of the ASHA (1994a) and the American Academy of Audiology (AAA) (1991), which proscribe exploitation of patients for services that are not professionally indicated.

Guideline 3. Avoidance of Criticism

Another ethical consideration is the avoidance of gratuitous derogatory statements about other practitioners or their equipment. A comparison is valid, as long as your facts are true, but more than this may be unethical and a cause of action in addition. Such criticism is expressly banned in many state regulations.

Derogatory remarks about other professionals are unethical and grounds for legal action

PROFESSIONAL PERSONNEL

Guideline 4. Competence and Compliance

It is essential that you become familiar with state or local regulations pertaining to audiology and hearing aid dispensing. In most states these are still separate and will remain so if the existing dealer-dispensers have their way. You will need to keep your licensure(s) current and meet any continuing education requirements because, wherever a license is required, practicing without it is prohibited.

Beyond this lies a level of professional performance that is not set by law but by the standards of the average practitioner of your profession. In past days when rural practitioners were felt less able than urban ones, the standard used was that of the community (i.e., rural or urban). Today the standards used are national ones with no exceptions for local variations. You will be expected to meet or exceed these. As the level of practice changes with the introduction of new methods, you will be expected to change with it. If you fail to do so and an injury results, you can be sued for negligence (i.e., malpractice). This is what is meant by having *"a duty of reasonable care."* The level of care that is reasonable is defined by the standard of performance set by other practitioners in the field.

National standard of care prevails

The duty of reasonable care begins directly after the formation of a professional relationship with the patient. This clearly occurs after an office visit in which some services have been rendered; it may also occur with a patient you have never seen who is given advice over the telephone. Exchange of money is not necessary, all that is needed is for some professional advice to be given, paid for or not. Once made, this is a continuing relationship; it cannot be broken by you without first giving adequate notice and making sure that any urgent pending care or follow-up is arranged with another audiologist. The patient, of course, can break it any time; that is his or her privilege, it is not yours.

What constitutes reasonable care?

Guideline 5: Vicarious Liability

Should any of your employees cause an injury, you will probably also be liable for it under the legal principle of *respondeat superior*[6] which extends the liability to the employer: this is vicarious liability. Protection against it should be written into your insurance, and often this insurance will specify what the employee can and cannot do. To abate the risk of vicarious liability means taking extra pains during employment and training. These are important concepts and are discussed separately.

Employment

With regard to employment, bear in mind that if one of your employees causes an injury through some defect of personality or training that you either knew about or *should have known about,* you are liable. This is not limited to audiologic procedures but includes any interchange or contact. *You are expected to do what is reasonable to discover potentially dangerous defects in your employees.* Previous aberrant mental behavior can often be tracked down through prior employers. Testing for communicable diseases such as AIDS and Hepatitis B occupies much discussion today but cannot yet be used as a condition of employment. Some former employers may be reluctant to give derogatory references in this litigious age, especially in writing, for fear they may be liable for defamation for a poor reference. Equally, if they *fail* to provide information regarding a dangerous characteristic which later causes injury, they are again liable for failure to warn.

Avoid the appearance of discrimination

If you seek an employee through advertisement, and then choose one of several equally qualified candidate, there can result accusations of sexism, racism, or some other form of discrimination. You can avert some of this by making clear to all the basis of your choice; also make a written reminder of this. Discharging an employee also calls for care, making sure the grounds are understood and written down. With Worker's Compensation and Unemployment Insurance,

---

[6]Literally, "let the master answer." A legal term which sums up the following: A master is responsible for the want of care by his servant toward those to whom the master owes a duty to use care, provided this occurs during the course of the servant's employment.

whether an individual is paid or not depends on whether the separation was the employee's fault or not.

Training

Some of your employees may require licensing, and you will need to ensure that their licenses are kept current. Whether employees are capable of performing a service to a patient, however, is seldom adequately vouched for by a license. You should observe their skills and, where needed, improve them with training. The skill of your employees is your responsibility. Technicians and assistants must be experienced in infection control procedures. They must also be familiar with the audiological or hearing aid equipment in your office, or at least the equipment they either use or maintain. The best way to ensure this is have a formal training and maintenance program described on paper, with scheduled refresher sessions, and an initialed list of those present. This can be combined with maintenance on the equipment itself, as noted below.

Have a training manual and training sessions

EQUIPMENT

Guideline 6. Maintenance and Currency

Your employees (and you) should be familiar with any maintenance, cleaning, or updating required for any equipment used on patients. All such routine service should be listed on a schedule and signed off. Keep adequate records concerning quality controls, maintenance, updating, and so on. A routine should be established. You must be able to show, in case an injury or an erroneous reading is received, that you have done everything required to prevent it. This is necessary, for example, to transfer liability for an injury to the manufacturer of an instrument; any failure of maintenance or other misuse may exonerate the manufacturer.

You also are responsible for knowing any dangers in the operation of your equipment, coming from at least three places: the manufacturer, your own experience, or other audiologists' experience with it communicated to you in a journal, a meeting, or personally. Where a danger in a procedure exists and cannot be removed, suitable warning of patients must be given. If it is still necessary to use the equipment or do the procedure, informed consent of the patient must be obtained (see below).

PATIENT RELATIONS

Guideline 7. The Written Record

The cardinal rule is to make notes of what you have done or said to the patient, and your reasons for it, as part of the written record. Although the reasons for this may seem obvious, it is alarming how many practitioners' records are abysmally incomplete. Unfortunately this omission, perhaps forced by constraints of time, becomes most glaringly obvious in the courtroom where it may be all you have to prove you did or did not do something you are alleged to have done or not done. Whether you take a complete medical history depends upon your training, the nature of the complaint, and whether the patient comes to you with a physician's referral, as discussed below. There are dozens of hearing problems that arise from systemic conditions, ranging from antibiotics to such drugs as diuretics or aspirin. The observation of pigmented skin tumors may suggest an acoustic neuroma; there may have been a recent flight with barotrauma, and so on. Your history must be such that any reversible cause for hearing loss is identified and any progressive disease whose sign may be hearing loss (e.g., hereditary nephritis), is discovered and referred appropriately or the physician is notified of any change in hearing that may be associated with ototoxic drug intake.

There are a few rules for the written record:

- Never erase or obliterate any writing. If you wish to change a prior entry, draw a single line through it so that it is still legible and connect this to a revised comment, giving the reason for the revision.
- Make the record inclusive; one of my professors used to say, "If it isn't written down, it wasn't done."
- Make a note of any promises or disclaimers you made to the patient, as emphasized below.
- Finally, make the record legible.

Computer records require special procedures

A last point about patients' records concerns the increasing use of computers to contain clinical information. Computerized records can be altered at will while they remain on the disk or hard drive, therefore their weight as evidence is correspondingly reduced. I have found the best way to handle such data is to transcribe daily from the disk to the individual charts the notes you wrote that day. There are sheets of printer paper which contain one or more sticky-backed panels. You can print the note on the panel, then peel it off and stick it in the chart. Also, remember you must maintain privacy of patients' records. When these are in a computer it is more difficult to protect them than simply locking a file; you must use suitable code words and limited access measures.

Guideline 8. Financial Arrangements

Put all financial arrangements in writing, initialed by both the practitioner and patient, if possible, with a copy to the patient. Some patients shop for prices and may ask you to undercut another practitioner, especially with hearing aids. Others may be concerned whether their health insurance covers them. Both of these can be sources of trouble with patients, putting you in court either to recover what is due or to defend yourself from what a patient remembers your saying. A clear summation of costs turns away much wrath. The whole subject of financial arrangement also touches on promises or guarantees you may have made or are alleged to have made, and which you may later be accused of not fulfilling, this nonfulfillment being the reason given for not paying. Criticisms of other instruments or dispensers may also come back to haunt you in the hassle of collecting refractory payments, as noted above.

One of the chief causes of discontent for both patients and practitioners comes from time-payment contracts. These are best avoided; use credit cards even though they raise costs by a few percent. Avoiding collection problems is worth the price. Most states have small claims courts where amounts up to $5,000 or so can be adjudicated without a lawyer. Even then, try to avoid it; your business is audiology, not collection of debts.

Guideline 9. Informed Consent

Get informed consent for any procedures that require it. You may well ask, what are they? The answer is that any procedure which carries any risk probably needs an informed consent. How much risk, you ask? The answer is any amount of risk that might make the patients change their minds; this also means anything that might make the *jury* change its mind. In an audiology practice, something like a deep impression for a completely-in-the-canal hearing aid might qualify as needing informed consent, as would caloric stimulation, intraoperative monitoring, or canal and tym-

How much risk?

panic electrode placement. Anything out of the usual routine of your office such as research activities, use of an experimental drug or device, teaching activities, or students who may come in contact with the patient may require extra caution and a consent form.

Guideline 10. Prediction and Warranties

Disclaimers, warranties, maintenance contracts

The written record may be most important when you make a diagnosis, a recommendation for treatment, or a prediction about the results of this treatment. Many lawsuits are based on the patients' dissatisfaction with the results they actually get compared with what they remember you "promised." Expectations almost always exceed reality. Guard against this with a written note. A general disclaimer, printed in advance, can also be used describing the varied results obtained with hearing aids, plus the fact that the signal-to-noise discrimination so often lost in presbycusis will not be entirely restored. Copies of the manufacturer's warranty with the type of preventive maintenance needed and who will supply it can be enclosed with the disclaimer.

MEDICO-LEGAL AUDIOLOGY

Guideline 11. Referral or Not?

Presently, it is the practice for many audiologists to receive their patients either by referral from physicians, especially otolaryngologists, or to refer the patient to them for clearance. The question is whether this is the ideal situation, or whether the physician cannot be dispensed with in many cases. I listed above a sampling of systemic conditions that can cause hearing problems, some of which may be the first manifestation of the underlying disease. Clearly, having a physician clear the patient medically before or during his visits with you can bring peace of mind and abate your risks. Should any medical condition later become apparent, its detection lay primarily in the physician's purview, not yours, and the physician's presence will aid your legal defense immeasurably.

Guideline 12. Basic Legal Knowledge

The best way to abate medico-legal risk is to acquire enough legal knowledge to provide advance warning of potential problems. Foreseeing trouble is more difficult in law than in science, because science reposes on an immutable body of facts in the form of the laws of nature. By contrast, mutability is the hallmark of the laws of man, changing from week to week and case to case. Given a particular set of facts, most engineers can predict an outcome, even guarantee it. No lawyer would dream of doing such a thing. All a lawyer can offer is opinions, intelligent guesses based on recent court decisions where the facts were similar, and even this ground is unstable. Worse, emotionally inflamed juries have been known to ignore concrete facts and make decisions that defy reason. This legal quagmire provides unsteady footing, even for those experienced in the law. To make it, perhaps, more understandable, I have isolated below four principal areas of a typical civil legal proceeding for brief study:

1. the plaintiff and the plaintiff's attorney,
2. the cause of the action,
3. the jury, and
4. the defendant's attorney and insurer.

The Plaintiff and the Plaintiff's Attorney

To begin, the injured party (the plaintiff) must find a lawyer.[7] This is not as simple as television ads suggest. There are far more people wanting to sue than lawyers willing to represent them, especially in malpractice cases. Over 85% of potential malpractice plaintiffs are turned away by lawyers. Two reasons exist for this paradox: the high cost of litigation and the lack of merit of most cases, where "merit" is a term composed of two things: the lawyer's estimate of the chances of winning the case and the amount of money that might be recovered. Lawyers may gamble on a long shot, a case where the outcome is very much in doubt, if there is enough money at stake, but they prefer "shoo-in" uncontested cases where the rewards may be small but the outcome is sure. As the number of lawyers rises, more cases may be accepted, but Rule 11 of the Federal Rules of civil Procedure[8] acts to keep the lid on. It requires the plaintiff's lawyer to sign the initial complaint to signify the lawyer has studied the facts of the case, made reasonable inquiry as to their accuracy, and certifies that the

A question of merit

---

[7]Claims below about $5,000 can be pursued in Justice Court without a lawyer in most jurisdictions.

[8]*Federal Rules of Civil-Appellate Procedure*, St. Paul, MN: West Publishing Co. Issued yearly.

suit is neither frivolous nor intended solely to intimidate or harass. If the case turns out to be frivolous, heavy penalties may hit both the plaintiff and the plaintiff's lawyer. To satisfy this rule in malpractice cases, the plaintiff's lawyer must consult an expert such as an audiologist, to advise him as to the scientific validity of the facts. Without using such an expert, most lawyers would be in violation of Rule 11 because they are not considered adequate judges of technical matters. The fees for such consultations may run into the hundreds before the attorney has enough information just to decide whether or not to represent the plaintiff. These legal costs are borne by the plaintiff. These costs are outside the contingency agreement and are paid by the plaintiff; however they are usually advanced by the attorney for later recovery out of the judgment. Should the case be lost, however, there is no judgment from which to recover costs. If the plaintiff is unable to pay them, the attorney winds up paying them out of pocket, a chilling prospect for a trial lawyer which acts as a deterrent to accepting any but open-and-shut cases from truly impecunious plaintiffs.

The other component of merit is how much money can the suit reasonably ask for or expect to win. This goes to the extent of the injury, the degree of culpability of the defendant, and how much money the defendant has or is insured for. No lawyer sues an uninsured taxi driver. Instead, he or she tries to reach a deep pocket by contriving a way to sue the manufacturer of the taxi, or its tires, or its brakes. Why are the malpractice insurance rates for obstetricians so high while those for geriatricians are among the lowest? Let's see. Say two individuals die due to alleged medical negligence and wrongful death suits are filed in each case. One individual was 80 years old, the other 80 days old. The amount to be claimed in each case is estimated by the loss of income that would have been earned. Thus, the 80-year-old, who had retired on a $25,000 annuity and had a remaining life expectancy of 5 years, had a projected income loss of $125,000. The newborn is imagined to be a future college graduate with a salary of $100,000+ for a period of 40 years, or $4 million. The American contingency system usually grants the attorney one third of this. The attorney for the baby therefore earns $1.33 million, whereas the attorney for the 80-year-old may not even cover his costs with $40,000.

No wonder the obstetrician is at greater risk for suit; it is the bottom line that counts. It is clear that the contingency fee arrangement is not the poor man's key to the courthouse, as maintained by trial lawyers, at least if he is a poor old man. An audiology practice will often include many older patients, to whom this rule might apply. This is a simplified calculation that ignores such major components as pain and suffering, loss of consortium, and punitive damages. These vary greatly among cases.

The Cause of the Action

Malpractice actions, like others based on negligence, have four elements:

1. A duty exists to cover the situation at hand;
2. This duty is breached by the defendant;
3. The plaintiff is injured;
4. The breach of duty was the proximate cause of the injury.

Most duties are fairly obvious, but their breach may be more subtle. A trustee, for example, has a fiduciary duty to invest monies left in trust wisely. Thus, if a trust earns only 3% when the prime rate is 8%, the trustee has breached his or her fiduciary duty and can be sued for it. The duty in the medical sciences, as discussed above, is for practitioners to perform their jobs with at least the same degree of skill as the average similar practitioner, nationwide. Endless courtroom disputes have revolved around defining this duty and whether it was breached. Such discussions may elicit testimony from multiple experts, but the ultimate decision as to exactly what the professional standard was and whether it was breached is left in the hands of a body chosen neither for its knowledge nor for its decision-making ability, the jury.

Another term difficult to grasp is "proximate cause." This means that there is an unbroken chain leading from the breach of duty to the injury; that no unforeseen intervening event has occurred to break this chain. For example, suppose you rear-end someone, causing a whiplash. The victim is taken to a hospital by ambulance for x-rays. There, the stretcher collapses and the victim's head strikes the floor. Does this break the chain and release you from liability? No, it does not. Events like the faulty stretcher (even medical malpractice in the receiving hospital) are predictable risks the victim would not have encountered without your faulty driving. Suppose again that the ambulance, on the way to the hospital, is seized by a sudden earthquake and falls into a crevasse, further injuring the victim's neck. This probably will break the chain of proximate cause, it is both unpredictable and intervening.

Proximate cause

The Jury

Audiologists, like other practitioners, must be aware that their skills and performances will ultimately be judged not by their peers, but by a group of people possessing no information or training on the subject. Furthermore, these people, the jury, may decide directly contrary to indisputable scientific evidence. Experts are employed only to advise the jury; their opinions are in no way binding upon it. The jury's freedom to ignore demonstrated facts allows it to be emotionally swayed by rhetoric or by the sight of a pitiful plaintiff displayed huddled in a wheelchair. The presence of juries in civil suits has been done away with in other countries for precisely this reason. The inconsistency of juries often stands in the way of justice.

The Defendant's Attorney and Insurer

A defendant, especially a doctor, has a large interest in clearing his or her name of any taint of malpractice. Such taint, registered in the National Physicians' Data Bank,[9] can raise the physician's insurance rates and result in lost hospital privileges or ejection from HSMOs, all cataclysmic events. The physician's insurer, however, is interested only in saving money. If it proves cheaper to settle than to litigate, that is what the insurance company will do, but settlement will not clear the physician's name. The defendant's lawyer, usually employed by the insurance company, has a natural bias in their favor. Lawyers for the plaintiffs are well aware of these things and are not above filing a suit just below the level at which they think the company will settle, hoping for an uncontested small windfall and leaving the professional dangling.

THREE CASE STUDIES

The following cases illustrate different facets of the guidelines. In each, someone is harmed, and the job set before the reader is to determine if the harm was due to negligence and, if so, on whose part. The reader may have to determine both the duty and the breach. *Remember always that no professional is perfect, that honest mistakes will happen, some of them unavoidably. Such mistakes are not or should not be a basis for a suit.* Some examples are real, some contrived.

---

[9]Set up by the Health Care Quality Improvement Act of 1986, this records all suits or other actions such as denial of privileges against physicians nationwide. The potential of expanding this to other health care providers exists.

Case 1

A male, 54, comes to you for loss of hearing over the past 6 months. He has a history of congestive heart failures, and, during the same period, he also experienced his first attack of gout. His otolaryngologist suggested a hearing aid and referred him to you. On examination you find a moderate bilateral sensorineural loss with no objective changes in the ears. You recommend hearing aids in both ears and discuss types and costs. He accepts and you fit him with aids costing a total of $1,500, which he pays up-front. On a return visit in 3 months he expresses satisfaction with the hearing aids but notes that he does not seem to need them as much. You repeat his audiogram and confirm that his hearing loss has improved markedly. On further questioning you find that his internist has discontinued the loop diuretic he was taking for congestive heart failure, blaming it for the gout. You then realize that his hearing loss was probably on the same basis (i.e., a reversible ototoxic effect of the diuretic).

Question 1. Are you ethically bound to return his $1,500, recognizing that if you had taken a more complete history, you would have told him that diuretics may cause hearing loss (and gout) which is often reversible, and that he should ask his doctor to stop his diuretic first, then return to you in a month or two?

Suggested Answer: This is a purely ethical question; nothing is forcing you to return his money, and the probability is nothing ever will since the patient is unaware of the situation. We would like to think that, under similar circumstances, all of us would return the money or at least counsel the patient that he might have bought something he did not need. If the patient brings up the matter, of course, it passes beyond the purely ethical.

The root issue here is that hearing aids were sold that proved to be unnecessary, and this fact should have been appreciated from the beginning, but was not. The standard of practice for audiologists certainly includes taking a history for ototoxic drugs, so your performance fell below this standard (i.e., there was a duty and it was breached, causing $1,500 injury). If these facts are introduced in court, the issue will almost certainly go against you, so much so that the insurance company will settle as quickly as it can.

The thing that makes this question ethical is simply that the patient has not complained. If he never does, the matter may never come up. You could elect, of course, to delay until it *does* come up somehow, and then make good. This is entirely reasonable and also unethical.

Question 2: Does the fact that his otolaryngologist cleared him for a hearing aid exonerate you so that you can keep the $1,500, knowing the otolaryngologist made the same error you did?

Suggested Answer: The otolaryngologist is in the same boat you are in and should, ethically, return any fees charged for services. The otolaryngologist is primarily to blame for prescribing an unnecessary hearing aid. Should you choose (or need) to do so, you could probably recover part of your loss from the physician. What effect this might have on your practice is problematic.

Question 3: Should you just keep quiet about the whole thing, explaining to the patient that hearing losses can fluctuate, so he should keep the hearing aids against that probability?

Suggested Answer: We covered this pretty well under Question 1. The answer is: say this only if *you* believe it.

Question 4: This time, the patient tells you his physician told him his hearing loss might have been caused by the diuretic, like the gout, and wants to know if he can return the hearing aids and get his money back. Will you give it to him or refuse, defending your performance as meeting the professional standards of your peers and claim, furthermore, that there is no proof that the diuretic was at fault?

Suggested Answer: It depends on what you believe is the truth. If you choose to deny the connection, you will be faced with the probability of having to prove it, both to your insurer and to a court. The other side will surely have an audiologist whose expert opinion will oppose yours. You may have one of your own to support you. All this could then go to a jury, with uncertain results. Another possible scenario, since the amounts here are small, is that a complaint against you for the $1,500 could be lodged in a Justice Court, where it is heard without lawyers on either side. Or it could be sent for binding arbitration in front of a single arbiter, depending on local rules. Under any of these scenarios, follow the course indicated by your own firm beliefs and common sense.

Case 2

A patient is referred to your office by an otolaryngologist for a hearing aid evaluation. The transfer note and your examination disclose that she has a ventilating tube in one ear, placed for persistent serous otitis following barotrauma. In your absence, your employee, a licensed dispenser, decides to make a deep ear impression without first examining the external canal or noting the tube, which becomes displaced by the impression, resulting in secondary infection, a prolonged course of antibiotics, and a greater conductive hearing loss in that ear.

Question 1. You have repeatedly told your employee to inspect the external canal before making a mold and reinspect after removing the impression; in fact, this is written down as one of your office procedures which the employee initialed. Does this remove your responsibility (i.e., is the employee the only one at fault and liable for the injury produced)?

Suggested Answer: Telling an employee to do something—even doing it repeatedly, even writing it down and getting initialed—none of these things insulates you from ultimate responsibility for what is done in your office and under your name and authority. Were this not true, your employee would have to carry his own malpractice insurance, something that some nurses are now finding necessary even though they, for centuries, have been covered by the physicians' coattails.

Question 2: Does the principle of <u>respondeat superior</u> apply here?

Suggested Answer: Yes, of course. This is just legal shorthand. It includes what is also called the "Captain of the Ship" doctrine, although this applies more to a surgeon's operating room crew. The legal term respondeat superior which means "let the master answer" sums up the following[10]: an employer is responsible for negligence by his or her employees toward persons to whom the employer owes a duty of reasonable care. A further consideration is that the employee not be an independent contractor, and this may be a fine distinction. An independent contractor is paid for doing a specific job, using his or her own tools, methods, and workers over which the employer has no control; while an employee may also be paid for a specific job, the employer retains control over the tools, methods, and assistants.

Question 3: This is the second time this employee has violated your instructions. You gave him a warning the first time not to do it again, so now you fire him. A week later you get a questionnaire from the Unemployment Insurance Office, asking

---

[10]See footnote 6.

whether the employment was terminated for cause (i.e., misbehavior); how do you answer?

Suggested Answer: You should have dictated a complete description of your difficulties with this employee as soon as you fired him, indeed beginning with his first warning. You can supply a copy of this to the Unemployment Insurance office. Parenthetically, if your previous problems with this employee had become known during the present case, the fact that you had neither fired him nor put in place a safety net to prevent further insubordination would be a mark against you suggesting gross negligence, a factor often used to support punitive damages. In other words, if something goes wrong, fix it and also take steps to see it does not happen again.

Question 4: You answered the inquiry above that the termination was for cause, and Unemployment Insurance was denied. Now you are served with a summons and complaint by the employee's attorney stating that your tyrannical attitude in the office so increased the employee's stress level that he became unable to think clearly and this caused him to overlook inspection of the external canal. Now he is unable to get another job and cannot even get Unemployment Compensation due to the stress that you caused. He now wants Worker's Compensation for the job-related stress and damages from you for defamation. What do you do now?

Suggested Answer: This illustrates what happens when there are too many lawyers. This is a nuisance suit, trying to get a settlement from your insurance company which might pay $5–10,000 in settlement to avoid the greater expense of having to litigate, no matter how absurd the charge. If you do litigate and win, you could countersue for false and malicious prosecution (i.e., a breach of Rule 11 referred to above), but most nuisance suits do not reach this level.

Case 3

A 62-year-old laborer is referred to you by his family physician for moderate bilateral hearing loss. The patient had some tinnitus, some recent dizziness, and a history of noise exposure. Audiometry showed an asymmetrical, high-frequency sensorineural hearing loss, poorer in the right ear. Word recognition scores were symmetrical, with no roll-over bilaterally, and there were no retrocochlear signs on acoustic immittance testing. The referring physician was informed of the results and subsequently signed a medical clearance for amplification. A right ear hearing aid was dispensed.

Two years passed, during which the patient returned for battery purchases. On one occasion, he complained of reduced benefit from the hearing aid, but did not come in for audiometric follow-up. Finally, you learn that shortly after his hearing aid fitting, he experienced a severe vertiginous episode and saw an otolaryngologist. The otolaryngologist diagnosed an acoustic neuroma on the right, ordered an MRI scan, and obtained a neurosurgical consultation, the upshot of which was the decision not to operate because the neuroma was small and stable and surgery would sacrifice the remaining hearing in that ear. The patient had not offered this bit of history to you spontaneously, and your notes do not indicate that you ever asked him about it or took an interval history. You repeat his hearing test and document an asymmetrical hearing loss with decreased sensitivity and word recognition in the right ear, compared to the initial audiometric evaluation.

Question 1. The patient had a retrocochlear lesion that you missed on initial evaluation. If your equipment now tests according to specifications and is apparently okay, is this failure to diagnose the neuroma actionable (i.e., is it below the standard of performance expected)?

Suggested Answer: Even with properly functioning equipment, the chance of having a misleading result may be large enough to remove negligence; the state of the art for basic audiometric testing is simply not good enough. Your results were within "the state of the art," as you practiced it, and that is all you could be held responsible for. If, however, accuracy had been vital and you knew that better tests exists elsewhere (e.g., electrophysiologic tests), you had a duty to inform the patient and the patient's physician of this. Otherwise, knowing the information to be critical, you failed either to advise the referring physician of the limitations of your equipment or to refer the patient elsewhere for more definitive testing, and this lapse would have been below a reasonable standard of performance. It might, also have cost the patient a loss of a chance, explained more fully below.

Question 2. Suppose that your test equipment does not test up to specifications and you cannot find any record of its having been serviced in the year of the original test. Any change in the answer for the question above?

Suggested Answer: This is plain sloppy housekeeping. You are derelict in the maintenance of your equipment, and this performance could be shown to be below acceptable standards.

Question 3. Does the fact that you took no interval history during a 2-year follow-up period fall below expected standards, noting that his hearing in the right ear continued to worsen?

Suggested Answer: I doubt that failure to take an accurate interval history would be actionable, given the facts here. If, however, the patient's course over the two years had been such that you were concerned over the changes, then a failure to take an interval history might be actionable, especially if damage resulted which could have been avoided by asking questions earlier. One type of damage increasingly sued for is "loss of a chance" injury. This occurs when missing a diagnosis or other observation has cost the patient a window of opportunity during which a result might have been obtained (i.e., the loss of a chance for desired goal). In this case, if the neuroma had achieved such size that extensive surgery was needed, where a lesser procedure would have sufficed initially, this might be considered as the loss of a chance; however, here the decision not to operate had already been made.

Question 4. You are an attorney to whom this patient has come, desiring to sue the audiologist. You (the lawyer) have hired experts who tell you the answers to questions 2 and 3 above are "yes." You now calculate the rest of the merit figure. How would you calculate the injury in dollars, would you ask for an additional amount for pain and suffering, and would you ask the jury to award the plaintiff punitive damages as well, "to teach the audiologist a lesson?"

Suggested Answer: Because negligence has been admitted, the only questions concern the injury (what is it and what is it worth?), the response of the plaintiff (should pain and suffering be claimed?), and the degree of culpability of the defendant audiologist (Should punitive damages be asked?). The patient is a 62-year-old laborer, probably not in a very high income group even if he was rendered unable to work by your negligence, which seems unlikely. He suffered no pain but may have had some inconvenience from hearing loss. Your mistake did not cause him to lose a chance because surgery had already been decided against and, even if done, would have resulted in deafness in that ear. So the injury was small. Pain and suffering is also small. Some punitive damages might be considered to induce you to keep a better equipment maintenance schedule, but this would also be small. Net result of all this: the case probably does not have sufficient merit (not a big enough bottom line) and will be turned down.

EPILOGUE

I am unable to complete this chapter without addressing something that you have undoubtedly perceived already; our civil justice system has reached a sorry state which is getting rapidly worse and demanding change. The force that drives it is no longer truth nor justice, but money. Winning a civil suit may cost almost as much as losing it, and even the winners only see about 38 cents out of each dollar awarded, the rest is consumed by the system. A wastage of 62% is an unconscionable price for justice. Further, this amount of money diverted from its rightful owners into the pockets of lawyers inflames them to perpetuate the system. Do not kill the goose that lays the golden eggs!

Three changes in our legal system, two simple, one complex, would correct many of the existing faults. Not only are most of these changes simple, they represent the current practice in all civilized countries in the world except the United States. Only here are they in force, vigilantly protected by the Trial Lawyers Association. These three changes are:

1. Make the Loser Pay the Winner's Costs

This seems such an elementary concept; it is the custom everywhere else. Such a rule would dry up frivolous and malicious suits faster than Rule 11. If you knew you would have to pay the defendant's legal fees and associated costs if you lost a suit, you would think carefully before filing one. As it is, if you lose, all you pay are your own costs (experts, filing fees, etc). You do not even have to pay your own lawyer because of the contingency system. So the current system encourages suits by making losing them as inexpensive as possible, throwing more coal into the legal furnace.

But now consider the effect on the innocent defendant. Even if she wins, she pays. In a case where a physician blew the whistle on another he felt was implanting cardiac pacemakers unnecessarily (at $15,000 each), they sued him for defamation and lost, but his legal fees still ran over $50,000. Tales like this discourage professionals from policing their own professions, something they are often criticized for. This failure to weed out incompetents permits enough true malpractice by them to escalate professional costs, drive up malpractice insurance fees, and fuel the trial lawyers' claim that professionals protect each other with such a conspiracy of silence that only the lawyers can purify the professions.

2. Eliminate the Contingency System

This system makes the lawyer's *fee* contingent on winning the case; it does *not* include the costs of the trial. It is normally about a third of whatever is won. The plaintiff's bar claims that this is the poor man's key to the courthouse; that without it poor folk could not obtain justice. We have seen above where this claim is untrue, exemplified by the difference in obstetric and geriatric insurance premiums. Somehow, other countries seem not to need the contingency system, obtaining justice effectively and at lower cost without it. In the last analysis, it benefits most lawyers; the rest of the population would be better off without it.

3. Remove the Jury from Civil Trials

The 6th Amendment guarantees a jury trial for criminal cases, and the 7th Amendment extends this right for civil trials where the amount "exceeds $20" (1791 dollars). This is echoed in most state constitutions. The right to a jury can be waived by agreement of both parties, but this rarely occurs where the victim has been disfigured or maimed, because the jury may be an essential target for attempts by the plaintiff's attorneys to influence the decision on emotional grounds. Exhibiting disabled plaintiffs in the courtroom, huddled in wheelchairs at their pathetic worst, can sometimes sway juries to impossible decisions, particularly if the victim is a child. This effect would be lost if the jury were replaced by judges, as in a bench trial, because they are largely immune to such chicanery. The plaintiff's bar, therefore, usually wants a jury trial.

Further, today's complex technological society presents issues in court that the average jury simply cannot comprehend well enough to discharge its duty in a rational manner, whereas an experienced and educated panel of judges is able to approximate justice far more closely (and cheaply). Other countries also feel this way and have made most civil actions into bench trials (i.e., judge only). To do it here, however, would require a constitutional amendment, both for the federal and at most state levels.

These thoughts are included here because those of you who read this handbook will necessarily become involved in them over time. Your practice will include individuals with claims based on various entitlement programs, from SSI[11]

[11]Supplemental Security Income. Administered under the Social Security system, it places an income floor under medically incapacitated persons.

through Worker's Compensation,[12] and these will include some manipulators and malingerers. Sorting these out can be a legally hazardous occupation subject to challenges where your records will be especially important. The fact that 25% of medical costs arise from "defensive" practices, and another 25% from administrative costs, seemingly should force corrective action, but powerful forces protect the existing system. We are a society founded on law, but the next 20 years will see a major restructuring of its mechanisms in places where abuses have become intolerable.

REFERENCES

American Academy of Audiology. (1991). *Code of ethics.* Houston, TX: Author.

American Academy of Audiology. (1993, April 29). *Hearing care services and health care reform* (pp. 1–14). Prepared for the President's Task Force on National Health Reform. Houston, TX: Author.

American Speech-Language-Hearing Association. (1994a). Code of ethics. *Asha, 36*(3, Suppl. 13), 1–2.

American Speech-Language-Hearing Association. (1994b). The protection of rights of people receiving audiology or speech-language pathology services. Task Force on Protection of Clients' Rights. *Asha, 36*(1), 60–63.

American Speech-Language-Hearing Association. (1994c). Professional liability and risk management for the audiology and speech-language pathology professions. *Asha, 36*(3, Suppl. 12), 25–38.

American Speech-Language-Hearing Association. (1994d). Representation of services for insurance reimbursement or funding. *Asha, 36*(3, Suppl. 13), 9–10.

Kirkwood, D. H. (1994). Changes in hearing health care raise specter of increased malpractice risk. *The Hearing Journal, 47*(9), 13–22.

O'Toole, T. J. (1993, September 22). *Memorandum to ASHA audiologists from ASHA President Thomas J. O'Toole.* Rockville, MD: ASHA.

SUGGESTED READING

Scott, R. W. (1994). *Legal aspects of documenting patient care.* Frederick, MD: Aspen.

---

[12]A nation-wide system, shaped differently by each state, designed to provide no-fault insurance for workplace injuries. Abuses of this system in California have been shocking.

APPENDIX 17-A

Model Bill of Rights for People Receiving Audiology or Speech-Language Pathology Services[1]

Customers receiving audiology or speech-language pathology services have:

1. THE RIGHT to be treated with dignity and respect;
2. THE RIGHT that services be provided without regard to race or ethnicity, gender, age, religion, national origin, sexual orientation, or disability;
3. THE RIGHT to know the name and professional qualifications of the person or persons providing services;
4. THE RIGHT to personal privacy and confidentiality of information to the extent permitted by law;
5. THE RIGHT to know, in advance, the fees for services, regardless of the method of payment;
6. THE RIGHT to receive a clear explanation of evaluation results, to be informed of potential or lack of potential for improvement, and to express their choices of goals and methods of service delivery;
7. THE RIGHT to accept or reject services to the extent permitted by law;
8. THE RIGHT that services be provided in a timely and competent manner, which includes referral to other appropriate professions when necessary;
9. THE RIGHT to present concerns about services and to be informed of procedures for seeking their resolution;
10. THE RIGHT to accept or reject participation in teaching, research or promotional activities;
11. THE RIGHT, to the extent permitted by law, to review information contained in their records, to receive explanation of record entries upon request, and to request correction of inaccurate records;
12. THE RIGHT to adequate notice of and reasons for discontinuation of services; an explanation of these reasons, in person, upon request; and referral to other providers if so requested.

These rights belong to the person or persons needing services. For sound legal or medical reasons, a family member, guardian, or legal representative may exercise these rights on the person's behalf.

---

[1]Reprinted with permission from American-Speech-Language-Hearing Association. (1994). The protection of rights of people receiving audiology or speech-language pathology services. Task force on protection of clients' rights. *Asha, 36*(1), 61.

Financial Planning

> *"Financial planning addresses areas foreign to most audiologists, such as insurance, taxes, retirement plans, and estate planning."*

Personal and professional autonomy rely on good financial planning. No matter how much expertise the audiologist brings to a practice nor how much revenue the practice generates, neither the audiologist nor the practice can expect long-term success if basic tenants of financial planning go unheeded. Individuals must develop and attend to *personal financial plans*; practice owners must also create and tend to *employee retirement plans*.

Like other chapters in this book, this chapter addresses topics that are complex and are the subjects of whole books in other treatments. It gives a general overview, but *this chapter is not intended to advise audiologists or practice owners on how to make investments or manage qualified plans.* Advice in these areas should come from financial planners, accountants, insurance agents, and attorneys who are fully versed in the individual's or business's situation.

The chapter begins with a glossary, because many terms used in financial planning may not be familiar or fully understood by audiologists. Next, it describes basic steps for financial planning in six areas. It goes on to describe different types of investments, their risk levels, and ways of combining them to achieve balanced portfolios. It describes qualified retirement plans for small businesses, emphasizing the legal and taxation requirements. The chapter concludes with a discussion of plan development with the help of a financial consultant.

GLOSSARY OF FINANCIAL TERMS

ACRS. Accelerated Cost Recovery System. A method in which the cost of tangible property is recovered over a prescribed period of time. Enacted by the Economic Recovery Tax Act of 1981.

Annuity. A fixed sum payable to a person at specified intervals for a specific period of time or for life. Payments represent a partial return of capital and a return (interest) on the capital investment. An exclusion ratio must be used to compute the nontaxable income until the annuitant has recovered his or her investment.

Bonds. A legal document representing creditorship in a corporation, state, or municipality issued to raise capital. The issuer pays interest at specified dates and eventually redeems the bond at maturity.

Community property state. A state in which all property is deemed either to be owned by the spouse or belong to the marital community. Property may be held separately by a spouse if acquired before marriage. For federal income tax purposes, each spouse is taxed on one-half of the income from property belonging to the marital community (Hoffman, Smith, & Willis, 1994). As this book is published, there are nine community property states: Arizona, California, Idaho, Louisiana, Nevada, New Mexico, Texas, Washington, Wisconsin. All other states have common law property systems (i.e., based on case law).

Depreciation. The deduction of the cost or other basis of a tangible asset over the asset's estimated useful life. Replaced by ACRS in 1981.

Diversification. The spreading of investment risk by investing in enough and varied instruments that the potential for a negative effect on one's portfolio caused by individual company or industry downturns is offset by investments in other areas that may respond favorably to the same events.

Earned income. Income from personal services as distinguished from income generated by property.

Equity assets. Holdings that represent ownership in a tangible asset such as owning a home or owning stock which represents ownership in a company or corporation. A good hedge against inflation, their rate of return is set by the market place, and they present the investors with the opportunity for growth.

ERTA. Economic Recovery Tax Act of 1981, which introduced ACRS as a method of cost recovery based on classification of assets versus useful life cost recovery under the depreciation format.

Fixed assets. Investments where there is a fixed rate of return over a specified period of time (e.g., savings bonds). Their sole source of growth is the interest earned.

401K Plan. A retirement plan named after the section of the tax code that defines it, which allows employees to shelter a portion of their compensation until retirement. Employees tend to favor 401Ks over IRAs because they can shelter more than $9,000 versus $2,000 for an IRA. There are allowances for early withdrawals, lump sum distributions with favorable income averaging and loans can be taken against a 401K.

Growth. An investment with an objective to increase in value versus an investment with an objective to provide income. Younger investors generally focus on growth investments to build their portfolios in order to provide more income in their later years.

Investment grade. A designation placed on municipal bonds, corporate bonds, or corporate paper by one of two rating services. It signifies that these instruments represent a prudent level of risk to the investor.

IRA. Individual Retirement Account. Individual taxpayers with earned income may put up to $2,000 per year into an IRA. Employees not covered by qualified plans and individuals who meet adjusted gross income cutoffs may deduct their IRA contributions. Income in the account accumulates tax free until distribution.

Keogh Plan. A retirement plan for self-employed individuals, who may deduct up to 25% of net earnings from self-employment or $30,000, whichever is less. If the plan is a profit-sharing plan, may deduct 15%.

Load. The portion of an offering price in an open-end investment company that covers sales commissions and all other distribution costs (sales charge).

MACRS. Modified Accelerated Cost Recovery System. Introduced with the Tax Reform Act (TRA) of 1986, it further expanded the length of time required to recover costs of tangible assets.

Maturity. The date on which a loan, bond, or debt instrument comes due. The principal and accrued interest must be paid at that time.

Money market. Short-term debt instruments maturing in 1 year or less (i.e., commercial paper, bankers' acceptances, Treasury bills, certificates of deposit).

Mutual funds. Shares offered by an open-end management company (mutual fund company). There is no limit to the number of shares that can be issued. The investor buys shares from the fund and sells (redeems) shares back to the fund. Mutual funds are a continuous new issue. The fund managers set the direction of the fund based on numerous objectives. Funds can be aggressive or conservative, they can target growth over income or specialize in bonds versus stocks.

Net wealth. For IRS purposes, the sum of assets owned, including face value of life insurance and qualified plan benefits, less outstanding debts. This value is important for estate planning purposes.

Portfolio. The security holdings of an individual or an institution.

Qualified retirement plan. An employer-sponsored plan that meets the requirements of Section 401 of the tax code. If the requirements are met, none of the employer's contributions to the plan will be taxed to the employee until they are distributed, and the employer is allowed to deduct the contributions in the year the contributions are made.

Revocable trust. An estate-planning vehicle used to eliminate probate, avoid conservatorship, minimize inheritance taxes, and control the distribution timing of assets to the heirs. It may be modified or terminated during one's lifetime or a spouse's lifetime.

Risk. The exposure an investor has for loss with a particular investment. Generally treasury obligations are considered the most risk free, but even those investments have varying levels of risk based on the length of the investment. Using a portfolio approach can reduce individual asset risk.

Securities. Any note, stock, bond evidence of debt, interest or participation in a profit-sharing agreement, investment contract, voting trust certificate, fractional undivided interest in oil, gas, or other mineral rights, or any warrant to subscribe to, or purchase, any of the foregoing or other similar instruments.

SEP. **S**implified **E**mployee **P**ension. A qualified plan in which an employer may contribute to an IRA for an employee for the lesser of $30,000 or 15% of payroll compensation. Similar in many regards to other qualified plans but with stricter participation rules and no lump sum distributions or favorable income averaging.

Stocks. Certificates evidencing equity ownership in a corporation. Stocks may yield dividends and can go up and down in value.

Tax-deferred. Monies that will not be taxed until distribution. Could be the compensation that is part of a qualified pension plan or the earnings on a retirement vehicle such as an IRA.

Wealth. All property possessing monetary value.

SIX INTERACTIVE PLANNING AREAS

Developing a financial plan is like developing a business plan. It asks the following questions:

- *Where are you financially?*
- *How much money is needed to meet financial goals?*
- *How much time is available?*
- *What can be done to reach your financial goals?*

It should:

- be initiated as early as possible,
- be designed to address short-, and long-term goals,
- anticipate changing needs, and
- be prepared to handle undesirable events.

To accomplish these feats, the planning process must work in six broad, interactive areas. A schematic of these areas and their interactions is diagrammed in Figure 18–1. Like a juggling act, a good personal financial plan simultaneously monitors and balances needs in all six areas throughout a person's lifetime. The emphasis on these areas is seldom equal at any given time, but each gains in ascendancy at some point during a lifetime.

Review the six areas of financial planning and think about how much thought and effort you have given them. Can you give concrete answers to the following questions in each of the six planning areas?

Present Financial Situation

Always a concern, this category prompts questions such as:

- *What is your current net worth?*
- *What are your income and expenses?*
- *What is the value of your business to you?*
- *What is the value of your business in the market place?*

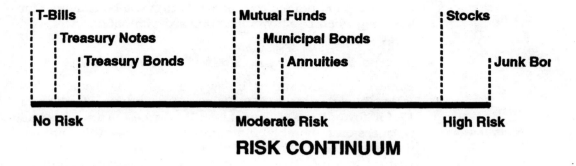

<table>
<tr><td>T-Bills</td><td>Mutual Funds</td><td>Stocks</td></tr>
</table>

T-Bills	Mutual Funds	Stocks
Treasury Notes	Municipal Bonds	
Treasury Bonds	Annuities	Junk Bo

No Risk   Moderate Risk   High Risk

RISK CONTINUUM

Figure 18-1. Six interactive areas of financial planning.

As in a business, these types of questions are answered by constructing a *personal financial statement*, an *income statement*, and doing a *cash flow analysis*.

Personal Financial Statements

A personal financial statement is constructed in much the same way that a business constructs its balance sheet, by itemizing assets and liabilities. However additional information is included on each item.

Begin with an inventory of assets. Alongside each asset, list its current value, purpose, and what it is earmarked for (e.g., *"U.S. Savings Bonds to fund the children's education"*). This process uncovers assets that are not directed toward any financial objective or that are no longer appropriate for today's goals and objectives. Consider any sentimental value attached to assets. For example, you may not be willing to sell the 500 shares of stock or a house inherited from your grandfather, even if they are not performing for you.

Next, inventory your liabilities (e.g., mortgages, bank loans, auto loans, and credit card or charge accounts). For each item, list the current amount owed, the monthly payments, and the interest rates. Rank order liabilities according to which should be paid off first. This ranking provides input to the goal setting portion of financial planning. It also

*Inventory assets
and liabilities*

identifies potential sources of funds that will be available for investing when liability obligations are eliminated.

Income Statement and Cash Flow Analysis

Compare income and expenses

Construct income and cash flow analysis using the same formats a business would (see Figures 12–5 and 12–6 in Chapter 12 for format examples). List all sources of income and expenses on a monthly and annual basis. Once this information is totaled for the month, compare annual expenses to annual income. It is often too easy to dismiss monthly expenses as inconsequential, but in the context of annualized expenses, these numbers take on impact and significance.

Develop a picture of cash flow by comparing expenses and income. Identify any discretionary income that could be tapped to address financial goals.

Insurance Needs

These needs vary according to your age, health, family structure, net worth, and size of the business, if self-owned. Questions in this category include:

- *Is your family covered in case of your death or disability?*
- *Do you have adequate liability protection for yourself and employees?*
- *Are your assets protected?*
- *Is your retirement income protected against long-term illness?*

Insurance protects individuals and businesses from the risks of death, disability, property damage, accidents, employee disputes, and negligence suits. With adequate protection, dependent families are protected from loss of home and income and business creditors and partners are protected against unexpected changes in the business.

Wealth Accumulation

This is an integral part of financial goal-setting. Wealth accumulation is important for achieving most personal and professional goals, such as buying a new home or a vacation home, funding the education of your children, expanding a business, creating cash reserves, and managing debt. Its importance declines as major life goals are met.

The manner in which wealth is accumulated must be part of an overall investment strategy that focuses on retirement needs, tax strategies, and estate planning. Sample questions in this category are:

- *Are there adequate cash reserves?*
- *Are your goals a house, a second home, education for your children, or business expansion?*

Managing Taxes

Taxes gain importance as wealth accumulates. Important questions are:

- *How can you minimize tax liabilities?*
- *If you own a business, how does it affect your taxes?*

Managing taxes is an ongoing process that requires constant monitoring and new strategies to deal with changes in tax law. Recent tax acts have negatively affected businesses and individuals. Where the intent in the early 1980s was to provide individuals and businesses with more tax-free dollars to invest, the actions since the mid-1980s have consistently closed loopholes, eliminated shelters, and claimed more revenue for the government.

Be aware of tax consequences and changes in tax law

A look at how the Internal Revenue Code has fluctuated in providing a deduction for the consumption of an asset over the last 15 years is a vivid example of why the tax implications of investing and managing a business are important. The Economic Recovery Tax Act of 1981 (ERTA) was a complete overhaul of the depreciation rules of the Internal Revenue Code. Most property placed into service after December 31, 1980 was subject to an Accelerated Cost Recovery System (ACRS). The intent of the act was to stimulate the economy by providing tax incentives to invest (i.e., lower tax liabilities and larger tax write-offs).

The Deficit Reduction Act of 1984 began to undo the depreciation rules of ERTA by stretching the recovery period for real property placed in service after March 15, 1984 from 15 to 18 years. In 1986 the Tax Recovery Act (TRA) further modified ACRS by introducing (MACRS) to expand the classification process of assets and further slow the cost recovery process for the investor. Depreciation was stretched from 18 years to 27.5 years on residential property and from 19 years to 31.5 years on nonresidential property. In 1993 the Revenue Reconciliation Act again acted to slow cost recovery by moving nonresidential property placed into service after May 12, 1993 out to 39 years. *The intent of these acts is to reduce incentives to invest, increase tax liabilities, and maintain government revenues.* An individual needs to work closely

Changes in depreciation (cost recovery) rules have increased tax liabilities

with financial advisors (i.e., accountants, bankers, and planners) to ensure that the tax consequences of investment options are fully reviewed before acting.

Retirement Planning

Start retirement planning from the beginning

A key responsibility of professional life is preparing for retirement. This important category should be emphasized as soon as one begins to earn an income. It is integrally related to wealth accumulation and tax management. An alarming number of Americans arrive at what should be their retirement years with no retirement income other than what Social Security provides.

Putting away for retirement when one is younger is much less expensive than waiting until retirement is imminent, but most professional people have many demands on their financial resources in the early years. The early years of a career are not the prime earning years. This is also the time that people become part of a community, buy and furnish a home, and start preparing for their children's education. All of these demands strain the young professional's budget, leaving little left to fund a retirement that is 40 years down the road.

Important retirement questions are:

- *Will there be adequate income at retirement?*
- *How can you cover medical needs and long term care?*
- *How will you manage distributions from various retirement instruments?*
- *Can business assets be used for retirement?*
- *What are the effects of earlier or later retirement?*

Estate Planning

Although best done before wealth accumulates, this facet gains in importance near the end of one's life. It is important to be able to answer the questions:

- *How can you minimize estate and inheritance taxes?*
- *How can you transfer business and personal assets?*

TYPES AND RISK LEVELS OF INVESTMENTS

Risk

One way of describing investments is by the amount of risk associated with them. For example, Table 18–1 is a model that categorizes investment products according to their risk.

Table 18–1. Risk models.

Risk Level	Description
Highly stable	The principal is not at risk (e.g., government securities are low-risk, low-risk, low-return).
Moderately stable	Possible loss of investment principal (e.g., higher quality municipal or corporate bonds or bond funds).
Moderately aggressive	Moderate risk of principal (e.g., investment grade municipal or corporate bonds or bond funds).
Aggressive	Risk loss of all principal for the chance of greater gain (e.g., growth stock or growth stock funds).

Larger returns on investments generally are achieved by assuming more risk. Individuals must know their risk tolerance before they can decide how to invest their principal. Simple instruments are available from any investment house to help determine one's risk tolerance or risk aversion. Investors need to consider not only the psychology of risk but also their phase of life. As retirement becomes imminent, a more conservative approach to investing is usually prudent.

Types of Investments

Investment risk ranges from *Treasury Bills* (T-Bills) which are often referred to as riskless to *junk bonds* at the opposite end of the spectrum, as illustrated in Figure 18–2. T-Bills are backed by the United States Government. Although they are very safe, they are riskless only in the sense that nominal returns are assured for one period. T-Bills can be purchased in 3-month, 6-month, or 1-year maturities in minimum denominations of $10,000. A portfolio built on T-Bills for income may not produce sufficient income if interest rates decline during the period of investment and maturing funds are reinvested in T-Bills with lower rates. This is called reinvestment rate risk. Because they represent the least amount of risk generally, T-Bills provide the lowest rate of return.

Other Treasury instruments are Treasury Notes and Treasury Bonds. Treasury obligations are backed by the United States Government and are considered safe investments. Their returns are exempt from state taxes but not federal income taxes.

Treasury Notes are intermediate term investments that mature in 1 to 10 years. They are purchased in minimum

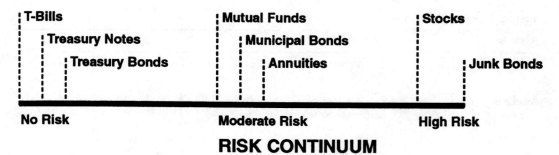

Figure 18–2. Investment vehicles, ranked by degree of risk.

denominations of $1,000. Their rate of return is generally higher than T-Bills because of the greater risk associated with their longer investment period.

Treasury Bonds have the longest investment period, with maturities ranging from 10 to 35 years. They can be purchased in minimum denominations of $1,000. Both Treasury Notes and Treasury Bonds pay interest semi-annually.

Moderate risk investments are securities that are not backed by the United States Government (e.g., *municipal bonds, corporate bonds* or *corporate paper*). They are rated as bank or investment grade by two different rating services. Moody's Investment Services rates bonds as follows:

Aaa—Best quality, little investment risk

Aa—Best quality

A—Higher medium grade

Baa—Lower medium grade (lowest investment grade)

C—Lowest class

Standard and Poor's Corporation rates bonds as follows:

AAA—Prime

AA—High grade

A—Upper medium grade

BBB—Medium grade (lowest investment grade)

C—In default

Mutual funds are considered moderate risk investment vehicles. Mutual funds, such as mutual bond funds and mutual stock funds, provide the average investor with the means of spreading (diversifying) their investments by pooling their resources with those of other investors. In effect, they provide the investor with the means to create a portfolio. This reduces the risk the investor assumes by investing in a single issue of stock or a single industry. The funds are professionally managed and the variety of funds available today allow investors to select funds that match their investment needs and risk tolerances.

Mutual funds dilute risk for individuals

Next in the ascending order of risk is the investment in *stocks*. These equity assets are considered higher risk because the original investment or principal is subject to loss if the fortunes of the market decline. Traditionally, over the long haul investments in stocks provide the investor with excellent opportunities for growth.

The riskiest investments and those that received a great deal of notoriety a few years ago are so-called *"junk bonds."* These are bonds that are rated below investment grade. They pay significant returns to attract investors because there is probable risk that they will default and return to the investor perhaps only pennies on the dollar.

A BALANCED APPROACH TO MONEY MANAGEMENT

To reach financial goals, the investor needs to create a balanced and diversified financial portfolio that simultaneously secures income and generates growth. In a balanced financial portfolio, money must work in four investment categories according to the needs of the individual or business. These four categories are shown in Table 18–2, in terms of their purpose and funding methods.

Cash Reserves and Insurance

Fund cash reserves and insurance first. They provide the dollars for personal or business survival. They combat risk and provide liquidity to take advantage of opportunities without incurring financial liabilities.

Savings accounts and money market funds are examples of cash reserve investments. These investments do not provide growth because their returns are near inflation levels, but they are available immediately when needed. Cash reserves are critical to a balanced approach in all situations. For example, businesses must replace and maintain equip-

Adequate cash reserves are always necessary

Table 18–2. Four investment categories of financial portfolios.

Type	Attributes		Examples
	Primary	**Secondary**	
Cash reserves	Security	Income	Savings accounts and money market funds
Insurance	Security		Insurance for death, disability, elder care, or malpractice.
Fixed assets	Income	Growth	Government bonds or face amount certificates.
Equity assets	Growth	Income	Stocks, your home, mutual funds.

ment, pay suppliers in a timely fashion, and be prepared to survive slow periods or economic reversals. The objective of cash reserves is to meet these business needs without incurring debt. Similarly, adequate personal finances allow for replacing major appliances, repairing a car, taking a vacation, surviving the loss of a job, or starting a business without incurring excessive debt. *As a rule of thumb, individuals should aim to have the equivalent of 6 to 10 months of after-tax salary in cash reserves. Businesses should have at least 3 months of operating expenses.*

As stated before, insurance protects things we cannot afford to lose. Life insurance protects families and businesses in the event of one's death; elder care insurance[1] protects retirement income; disability insurance provides income protection to cover all or part of an owner's salary; "key employee" insurance mitigates the effects of death or disability of an important employee; unemployment insurance covers claims from former employees; office and home insurance protects against fire, theft, vandalism, accidents; malpractice insurance protects against negligence suits.

ASHA offers the following insurance plans to its membership:

■ *Professional Liability Insurance* for employees and those who are self-employed;
■ *Group Life Insurance* for members, spouses, and children ages 14 days to 25 years;
■ *Major Medical Insurance* for members and their families, employees and their families;

---

[1]This type of insurance includes three components: (1) Medicare supplements (i.e., "Medigap" insurance), (2) long-term care (e.g., nursing home policies), and (3) home health care policies, which are an option on long-term care policies.

- *Disability Insurance;*
- *Catastrophe Major Medical Insurance;*
- *Equipment Insurance;*
- *Long-term Care* (nursing home and home health care);
- *Business Overhead Expense Insurance;*
- *Personal Accident Insurance Plan* for members and their families;
- *Group Hospital Money Program*
- *Cancer Care Insurance*

Comprehensive insurance policies should be available through the American Academy of Audiology in 1995. A single policy will include insurance for professional liability, office equipment and furniture, Public Liability, Workers Compensation, Auto and Non-owned Auto, and umbrella coverage.

Consult an insurance agent to be sure that these policies are adequate and that coverage is adjusted as situations change.

Growth Assets

After securing cash reserves and insurance, concentrate on building growth assets. Typically, growth investments are categorized as fixed and equity assets.

Fixed assets have a specified rate of return for a fixed period of time. Government bonds, face amount certificates, or fixed amount annuities are examples of these types of investments. Their sole source of growth is the interest earned. They are good protection against falling interest rates because they are not affected by the market.

Equity assets are the best hedge against inflation. Real estate (commercial or personal) and stocks are examples of equity-type assets. They provide the most growth opportunity because their value is not limited to the contracted rate of return but is set by the marketplace. Equity assets are also riskier investments because the initial investment can be in jeopardy if the market falls.

Tax planning and risk management are factored into the growth assets so that tax liabilities are minimized and risk tolerances are observed. These strategies are discussed in the following section.

INVESTMENT STRATEGIES

The following are general guidelines. Individual investors need to tailor these guidelines to their personal needs.

Obstacles and Barriers

Obstacles and barriers constantly challenge financial plans and goals. Recognizing that these conditions exist can help an individual or business to anticipate and overcome them. Part of successful planning is to take obstacles and barriers into account.

Economic Factors

In the last 15 years, the economy has moved from double-digit inflation in the early 1980s to a recessionary period in the late 1980s and early 1990s. Planning and investment strategies need to anticipate and counter the varying effects of these changing economic conditions.

Taxation

As the individual and the practice become more successful, the government, through taxes, demands a larger portion of the income. Part of financial planning is to develop tax strategies that minimize the effects of taxation.

Diversify to Minimize Risk

Diversification in today's economic environment is best accomplished with observance of the balanced approach and the use of mutual funds. Figure 18–3 summarizes general "rules" discussed in the following paragraphs.

Whenever possible, financial foundations should be laid when people are in their twenties and thirties. In those years, the strategy should emphasize growth investments, with less emphasis on income production and the least emphasis on money market type investments. An investment distribution of 70% in growth or equity assets, 20% in income or fixed assets, and 10% in money market accounts and cash reserves is a common recommendation for this age group.

People usually reach their peak earning years during their forties and fifties. A common recommendation at this stage is to shift investment distributions to 40% growth, 40% income production, and 20% in money market accounts. This distribution is less volatile than the formula used in earlier years but will continue to allow assets to grow.

By retirement, the distribution should shift to about 20% in growth and 80% in income production and capital preservation, keeping 10% of that income production in money markets for cash reserves.

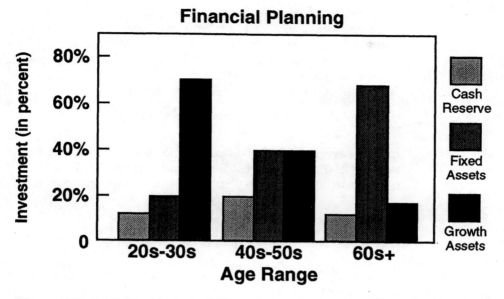

Figure 18–3. Typical balanced investment strategies as a function of age and professional life.

Minimizing Income Taxes

There are enough financial products available in the market place today to address individual diversification needs and provide numerous choices for each level of risk tolerance. The distribution an individual selects in today's environment is probably based more on tax strategy than other factors.

Today's general strategy[2] for individuals who do not own their own businesses is to take advantage of the retirement tax incentives by funding all available retirement vehicles, because they provide the most consistent tax advantages at this time.

If individuals are in high tax brackets (31%, 36%, or 39.6%), their investment portfolios should be heavily weighted in municipal investments.[3] Returns from municipal bonds and municipal bond funds are exempt from Federal Income Tax. If the bonds or bond funds are specific to the state in which the tax payer resides, they also are exempt from state taxes.

---

[2]Specific strategies need to be worked out in consultation with a financial advisor, according to an individual's situation.

[3]Municipal bonds are not for everyone. If an individual is in the 15–28% tax brackets or lives in a state with low state taxes, there is little incentive to search for tax-exempt investments because it is not that difficult to find taxable investments that equal the tax-exempt yield.

To calculate tax equivalent yields, subtract the marginal tax rate from 1 and divide it into the investment yield of the bond. For instance, an individual in the 36% bracket with a municipal bond fund yielding 6.2% can calculate taxable equivalent yield as follows:

$$\frac{.062}{(1 - .36)} \times 100 = 9.68\%$$

In other words, an individual in the 36% tax bracket would need to find regular investments that returned at least 9.68% in order to equal a 6.2% yield for a tax exempt investment.

Retirement Plans for Individuals

A successful retirement plan does three things:

1. Accurately calculates how much money will be needed for retirement.
2. Properly diversifies retirement funding.
3. Takes full advantage of available investment vehicles.

People's retirement incomes should be at least 65–75% of what they made when they were working

As a rule of thumb, individuals should assume that their annual retirement income needs will be about 65 to 75% of their preretirement, after-tax income. If an individual's retirement plan involves a lot of travel or support of family members, a larger percentage should be allowed to meet this demand. Compare the *estimate* of annual retirement income to all available retirement income from all qualified retirement plans and Social Security benefits.[4] The retirement plan is well-funded if current retirement income plus estimated Social Security benefits meet the retirement income need estimate. If current investments are insufficient, the planner and the individual need to determine what is required to achieve the retirement goal and decide on an investment strategy.

Plan life expectancy based on actuarial tables, personal health, and family history

Individuals also must calculate how many years their monies need to last. With today's projected life spans, it is not unreasonable to plan on another 20 years of life if one retires at 65. Based on an estimated rate of return from the retirement plan principal, the investor can calculate how much can be withdrawn each year to make the original

---

[4]To get a current projection of social security beneifts based on individual contributions to date, obtain Form SSA-7004 from the Social Security Administration by calling (800) 771-1213.

principal last twenty years. For example, if 10% a year is removed from an original amount that is earning 5%, the principal will last slightly less than 15 years. But, if 8% were withdrawn in the same situation, the money will last over 20 years.

Retirement investments are typically those with tax-deferred growth. This means the investor does not pay taxes on the income from these investments until funds are withdrawn. Retirement investments commonly outperform inflation, if only because of their tax-deferred status. The most common retirement investments are listed below.

All of the following retirement instruments have similar advantages and restrictions. They all accrue earnings on a tax-deferred basis that is very advantageous to the investor. Their major restriction is that distributions from the plans are subject to a 10% penalty tax as well as normal taxation if taken by investors before they reach a "retirement age" of 59.5 years. For investors who are between 59.5 and 70.5 years of age, distributions can be exercised without incurring any penalties for early withdrawal.

Another restriction of these investments is that distributions must begin in the year the investor reaches 70.5 years. This may force the investor to take distributions when they are not needed and when there may be disadvantages from a taxation standpoint.[5]

IRA

Almost any investment can be declared an IRA (i.e., stock funds, bond funds, money market funds, or certificates of deposit). IRAs are open to everyone. An employed individual can invest up to $2,000 per year in an approved IRA. Married couples with one employed spouse can invest up to $2,250.

The tax ramifications of the initial contribution are determined by three measures:

1. filing status,
2. adjusted gross income, and
3. whether the tax payer is a participant in an employer's qualified pension plan.

These items need to be considered as part of the individual's tax strategy. Employees not covered by another quali-

---

[5]The Internal Revenue Service (IRS) provides some helpful publications on retirement plans from a tax perspective. Form 560, *Self-Employed Retirement Plans*, and Form 590, *Individual Retirement Arrangements (IRAs)*, can be obtained by calling 1 (800) 829-3676.

fied plan can establish their own tax-deductible IRAs, regardless of their adjusted gross income. If the tax payer or spouse is an active participant in another qualified plan, the IRA deduction limitation is phased out proportionately between $40,000 to $50,000 adjusted gross income for couples filing jointly (Hoffman, Smith, & Willis, 1994). For couples filing jointly with adjusted gross incomes of $50,000 or more who participate in another qualified plan, the IRA contribution must be filed as part of their tax return.

SEP/IRA

This is a Simplified Employee Pension/IRA. Under this plan, the employer makes IRA contributions for employees. The employer can contribute up to 15% of an employee's earned income to a maximum of $30,000 annually. In a SEP, the employer must make equivalent contributions for all employees who meets certain age and employment standards. The restrictions are similar to those of many qualified pension plans. The employee may also make elective deferrals under a SEP that are excludable from gross income.

Keogh Plans

These plans are available to the self-employed and owners of small businesses (e.g., sole-proprietorships and partnerships). Keoghs are more generous than SEP/IRAs because they allow contributions equal to 25% of earned income up to a maximum of $30,000. Contributions are tax deductible. Keoghs are more flexible than other listed plans. At retirement they allow for lump sum distributions and 5- and 10-year forward averaging of the distributions.

401K

These are employer-sponsored plans offered by some companies. Invested dollars are put into much the same investments as other retirement instruments. The amount that can be invested varies from year to year and an individual needs to determine the IRS allocation each year.[6] If individuals are employed in organizations that sponsor 401K plans, they should contribute. This is because this plan is particularly advantageous for employees because it would take

---

[6]In 1994 these plans allowed an employee to set aside up to $9,240 of pretax wages on a tax-deferred basis.

more than $15,000 in taxable dollars to equal the 1994 allowable contribution.

Annuities

Some investment companies now offer variable annuities as retirement vehicles. You can have these annuities in addition to other instruments such as IRAs. The earnings on the annuity, like the other retirement instruments, are tax-deferred. These annuities are distinct from other retirement investments because *they do not have the restrictive caps of other vehicles*. However, they also have a distinct drawback: the commissions that one pays to set them up can range from 65% to 165% of the first year's premium depending on the company the investor is dealing with.

SETTING UP QUALIFIED RETIREMENT PLANS FOR SMALL BUSINESSES

Qualified plans are deferred compensation plans in which all contributions are made by the employer for all qualified employees.[7] Qualified plans apply to all business forms, so plans can be incorporated or unincorporated. Refer to Appendix 5-A for types of plans that are applicable to different legal organizations of businesses. The federal government encourages these plans to keep retired people from becoming dependent on the government, in particular on Social Security. Qualified plans offer three major tax advantages:

> In qualified plans, the employer contributes for all qualified employees

- Contributions are immediately deductible by the employer.
- Employees are not taxed until the funds are made available to them.
- Income earned by the plan trust is not subject to tax until it is made available to the employees.

Types of Plans

A wide variety of plans qualify, most notably *pension plans*, *profit sharing*, and *stock bonus plans*.

Qualified Pension Plans

Qualified pension plans provide definitely determinable retirement benefits to employees who meet the requirements

---

[7]In certain circumstances, employees can make additional contributions.

of the plan. Benefits generally are based on factors such as years of service and compensation level. There are two basic kinds of qualified pension plans: defined benefit plans and defined contribution plans. Under a defined benefit plan, the employer must make annual contributions for all participants to a single account, based on actuarial computations.

In a defined contribution plan, separate accounts are maintained for each participant. Benefit is based solely on the amount contributed and the income accrued. Upon retirement, the employee's pension depends on the amount in the individual account. The simplest version of a defined contribution plan is a SEP/IRA created for a small practice consisting of an owner/manager and several employees. Despite of and because of its simplicity, many small businesses shy away from SEP/IRAs: almost any employee who draws a paycheck is soon 100% vested in a SEP/IRA plan. Businesses consisting of a single employee (the owner) that select an SEP/IRA for their qualified plan should consider changing to a profit-sharing plan when they acquire employees.

Profit-Sharing Plans

A profit-sharing plan is established and maintained by the employer to provide for employee participation in company profits. Separate accounts are maintained for each participant. The plan must provide a formula to allow for the allocation of contributions (e.g., tied to compensation, performance, or some other measure). Profit-sharing plans need not emphasize retirement, so benefits to employees may be distributed through lump-sum payouts at any time (but usually when an employee leaves).

Stock Bonus Plans

Stock bonus plans are another form of deferred compensation that can qualify as an incorporated qualified plan. In this case, the employer manages the plan by contributing shares of its stock to the plan in the names of employees. The plan is maintained like a profit sharing plan in that individual accounts are created for each employee. Distribution is made in the form of company stock.

Requirements for Qualified Retirement Plans

To be qualified and receive favorable tax treatment, a plan must meet several requirements. A trust or IRA is created for the exclusive benefit of the employees. The IRS specifies that the trust or IRA meet four investment conditions:

- Cost of investment must not exceed fair market value.
- A fair return must be provided (i.e., the plan portfolio must consist of quality investments).
- Sufficient liquidity must be maintained to meet the terms of the plan.
- The plan must be prudently managed (i.e., the plan portfolio should be sufficiently diversified to minimize risk).

In other words, the manager of the qualified plan has a fiduciary duty to manage the plan with care and competence. Employees have the right to legal action against plan managers or corporations that do not invest responsibly. *This is true even for very small, unincorporated audiology practices using SEP/IRA plans.*

A qualified plan must not discriminate in favor of highly compensated individuals. It must provide eligibility for participation to all employees who are 21 and who have completed 1 year of service. In small businesses where nonkey employees come and go with some frequency, it is especially important to keep track of when employees meet minimum service requirements for vesting.

The plan must provide vesting so that benefits are not lost when an employee is terminated or changes jobs. Under qualified rules, the vesting period is usually 5 years. For SEP/IRAs, qualified employees are vested 100% immediately.

To qualify as a retirement plan, a plan must provide and observe minimum distribution rules. No distributions can be made to employees before they reach 59.5 years of age, and minimum distributions must begin by the time employees are 70.5 years old.

Details on all these requirements are part of the tax code and therefore the specifics of any given requirement should be reviewed with qualified professionals when setting up and administering the plan. According to Chaney (1994a),

> The IRS is actively pursuing 'small plan' audits, and issuing penalties, and so qualified plan administration and reporting must be done by a knowledgeable CPA or lawyer, or pension consulting firm, as IRS penalties for plan non-compliance are very stiff. (pp. 2–8)

Owner/managers of audiology practices must manage their qualified plans wisely or run the risk of employee lawsuits

Tax Consequences of Qualified Plans

As stated earlier, employer contributions to qualified plans are deductible immediately and these amounts are not taxable to the employee until they are distributed. This has immediate tax advantages to the employer and it is a significant tax-deferred advantage to the employee.

The employee has several options when it is time to receive distributions. The employee can elect to roll over the plan to an IRA and be subject to rules of distribution and taxation as applied to IRAs. The employee can, if qualified, elect lump sum distribution for which taxes are often due in the year of distribution. Lump sum distributions *can* be attractive if an individual qualifies for 10-year income averaging, but recent tax changes make this an issue to be reviewed individually with a tax advisor.

Limitations on Qualified Plans

Owner/managers of audiology practices must weigh the expenses of a qualified plan before creating one

When setting up a qualified plan, the owner of a practice needs to be aware that there are limitations on the contributions to qualified plans and on the benefits that can be distributed from these plans. Exceeding either of these limits could disqualify the plan. The limitations are set by the tax code. Section 404 sets the limits of deductibility applicable to the employer. Section 415 sets the limitations on contributions to and benefits from a qualified plan and must be written into the plan. These limitations, coupled with the requirements of nondiscrimination and participation, may force a practice owner to realize that the tax benefits of a qualified plan are not affordable.

ESTATE PLANNING

An individual who actively participates in financial planning will generally leave an estate, unless the objective has been to deplete the estate in his or her lifetime. Financial planning guides the distribution of the estate through normal estate planning vehicles such as wills and trusts. Careful planning minimizes excessive estate settlements and inheritance taxes, and arranges for the distribution or transfer of ownership of personal and business assets. It should not be put off or ignored because it provides the individual an opportunity to provide for those who survive.

Estate planning depends on the state of residence

Estate planning varies from state to state, depending on whether they are common law or community property states. As a general rule of thumb, an older couple with more than $750,000 of net wealth should consider a revocable trust arrangement containing a tax trust provision, and any married couple with net wealth of more than $1,000,000 definitely should consider estate tax planning and instituting an estate tax trust arrangement. During the lifetime of both spouses, the revocable trust may be modified or terminated (Chaney, 1994b).

Life insurance is often used to fund buy/sell agreements to allow for the orderly continuation of a business if an owner dies prematurely. The money from the policy allows another person (usually another shareholder) to purchase the deceased owner's portion of the company. In this way, survivors receive a fair cash settlement, and the business continues uninterrupted. Chaney (1994a) points out a concern for owners of S corporations:

> Transfer of S shares upon death must be handled carefully; only certain type trusts are allowed as an S shareholder. Transfer to an improper shareholder automatically terminates the S election, which may not be remade then for five years by the corporation. (pp. 2–5)

As this brief discussion illustrates, estate planning requires the expertise of professional advisors such as accountants and attorneys, due to the complex areas of state and federal tax law that are involved.

STEPS IN THE FINANCIAL PLANNING PROCESS

The preceding sections have described areas of investment, categories of investment, investment instruments, and investment strategies. They have not, however, informed the reader how to coordinate all of the required activities into a comprehensive plan that maximizes efforts in all areas. That process requires a financial plan, which is developed in a series of definite steps.

The financial planning process is analogous to building a custom home with an architect. Clients give the architect a vision of their dream house and an idea of their financial capabilities. The architect turns the vision into a blueprint, taking into account building codes, ordinances, technology, building trade skills, the building site, the client's financial capabilities, and future build-out plans. The client and the architect review and modify the building plans and blueprint until the client agrees that this is the best solution to the vision. At this point, it is up to the client to initiate action and begin the project.

Similarly, individuals and businesses should use a financial consultant to articulate their financial goals and avoid pitfalls. Documented plans are a financial blueprint by

The financial consultant is the architect that designs the financial plan

Table 18-3. Typical steps in the financial planning process.

Step 1	Set goals
Step 2	Gather information
Step 3	Analyze information in terms of goals
Step 4	Synthesize plans
Step 5	Take action

which a person or business can realize financial goals. If the vision changes in the future, the original plans are available for planning modifications, some of which may have been built into the original plan.

Typical steps in the planning process are listed in Table 18-3, and described below.

Step 1: Set Goals

Start the process by enunciating short- and long-term personal and professional goals. Examples of personal goals are: build adequate cash reserves (short-term) and fund the college education of pre-school age children (long term). Examples of professional goals are: increase salary by 25% this year (short-term) and purchase a building site for investment or future expansion (long-term).

This step also provides the added benefit of articulating potential conflicts between goals in one's personal and professional life.

Step 2: Gather Information

Formulate a financial inventory to determine net worth and develop a clear picture of income and expenses. Use the personal financial statements described earlier in this chapter. Often, the financial consultant will have forms for this purpose and will assist you in completing them.

Step 3: Analysis

The information gathered in step 2 is analyzed in terms of the goals and objectives set forth in step 1. For example, if the goal being worked on is retirement income, then what investments or assets are available to meet that objective? In addition, what type of investments will meet the individual's tolerance for risk and address ongoing tax strategies?

Step 4: Synthesis

Use the analyses to come up with strategic solutions that satisfy as many goals as effectively as possible. Solutions take the form of funding four different plan attributes: cash reserves, insurance, fixed assets, and equity assets. The financial planner develops allocation plans that support the analyses of step 3 and reflect financial realities, individual risk tolerances, and stage of life.

Step 5: Take Action

This step involves commitment on the individual's part to take the steps necessary to follow the financial plan. Too often, people procrastinate and fail to take action on the proposals they have developed on their own or in consultation with a professional planner.

WHY USE A FINANCIAL CONSULTANT?

Financial planning is a complex process because individuals' goals shift, the conditions of the economy change, and the options of the market place are in constant flux. A financial planner's job is to develop strategies and provide advice that help clients reach their goals and objectives. Individuals should utilize financial planners *not* to make financial decisions for them but to sort through all the issues and present the best options for the situation. These options ideally should be a match of the client's personal and professional goals with instruments that reflect financial situations, risk tolerances, and overall tax strategies.

Financial planners should be used in the same manner as one uses accountants, attorneys, bankers, computer consultants, and insurance agents. They are contracted experts paid to maximize the efficient use of time and provide a return to the individual or practice.

Selecting a Financial Consultant

Select a financial planner with the same care you use when selecting any other outside professional. The following is a glossary of professional designations of financial planners that may help in the screening process.

CFP. Certified Financial Planner. The most common professional designation. CFPs generally have 3 years of experience, have met continuing education requirements and have passed a qualifying exam.

PFS. Personal Financial Specialist. PFS is a designation for CPAs. This signifies that beyond being a CPA, they have 3 years of experience and have passed a qualifying exam.

CLU. Chartered Life Underwriter. These planners have a background in insurance. The CLU designation signifies rigorous training and testing to earn the rating.

ChFC. Chartered Financial Consultant. Individuals are closely related to CLUs. Many ChFCs hold both ratings and their training has a little more emphasis on general financial planning and less on insurance.

CFA. Chartered Financial Analyst. These individuals are generally heavily biased toward stocks and may not be the answer for help with estate planning, tax planning, or insurance needs.

IA. Investment Advisor. These individuals usually provide investment advice for a fee. IAs must be licensed by the Securities Exchange Commission; also in some states.

SUMMARY

Financial planning is a complex issue that affects many areas of our personal and professional lives. It requires vision to set goals and objectives. It involves discipline to stop and determine current financial information and translate that information into action plans that address financial goals.

Financial planning addresses areas foreign to most audiologists, such as insurance, taxes, retirement plans, and estate planning. Because the attributes of financial planning often seem obscure, it is wise to enlist experts to help shape the financial planning process. Audiologists need to work closely with their accountants and attorneys on tax, retirement, and estate issues. They should consult regularly with their insurance agents to ensure they have adequate protection. Finally, they should consider consulting a financial planner to help structure comprehensive personal and business financial plans.

REFERENCES

Chaney, D. (1994a). *Closely held business law in Arizona.* Tucson, AZ: Author.

Chaney, D. (1994b). Your estate: *Utilization of a revocable trust.* Tucson, AZ; Author.

Hoffman, W. H., Smith, J. E., & Willis, E. (1994). *West's federal taxation: Individual income taxes.* New York: West Publishing.

Buying and Selling an Audiology Practice

One of the advantages of owning an independent audiology practice is the opportunity to develop equity while generating a respectable income. If the owner(s) has been diligent in maintaining the practice and establishing a defensible valuation of the practice, he or she can eventually sell the practice and end up with a nice reward for years of industry and responsible management.

An advantage of buying an established, viable, audiology practice is that it minimizes the risk inherent in starting one from scratch. Judiciously buying a practice is decidedly lower risk than starting one and going through the dangerous start-up phase. An existing business has already proven its ability to survive and comes with documentation of its past performance and a tangible indication of its future. For an individual who has already attained a fairly comfortable standard of living and/or has family responsibilities, buying is the logical option, because a careful, capitalized purchase of a healthy practice is less likely to disrupt his or her income for an extended period of time. In addition, if the practice that is purchased is well equipped and staffed, and the staff remains, it is less stressful and time-consuming than starting from scratch.

Several complex details need to be negotiated between the parties when a small business changes hands. Both buyer and seller will need different types of protection and face tax issues that warrant competent advice and management. Therefore, even though a buyer and seller may handle preliminary issues independently, it is imperative that both parties independently engage the services of competent and trustworthy professionals (CPAs and attorneys) experienced in the sale of small businesses. Legal and accounting advice will help the prospective seller and buyer avoid unseen obstacles and address tax issues that arise with the sale of the business.

This chapter starts with a discussion of valuing a practice. Valuation is done for a variety of reasons besides selling a practice. These reasons are examined and valuation methods are discussed. The chapter then shifts from valuation to the actual process of selling and buying a practice. It looks at the seller's responsibilities for "grooming" a practice for sale, then at the steps required of a prospective buyer. It concludes with a brief discussion of the negotiation process between a qualified seller and a qualified buyer.

VALUING A PRACTICE

Many people ask themselves "Why do I need to have a business valuation performed?" There are several common reasons for a valuation, only one of which is tied to the direct sale of a practice:

- *Personal financial planning.* As described in Chapter 18, it is essential to have an accurate assessment of personal worth in order to plan and insure one's investments, retirement, and estate distributions.
- *Buy/sell agreements.* As described in Chapter 5 (Appendix 5-B), partnership agreements should include plans for the orderly sale of a partner's interest due to retirement, disability, death, and so on. Buy/sell agreements may be used in any form of business (e.g., sole proprietorship, corporation) to allow another individual to purchase the deceased owner's interest and allow the business to continue without disruption. They are usually funded through life insurance.

Typically, an agreed-on formula is used to establish valuation. Subsequently, the value of the business changes automatically as elements in the formula change value. The formula should be reviewed periodically.

- *Financing.* Accurate valuations are important when seeking capital from lenders.
- *Selling a Practice.* Having a valuation done a year or more prior to the actual sale of a practice—and again when the practice is put on the market—can help present a more positive and realistic picture of an audiology practice.

Clearly, a well-run audiology practice will have been through the valuation process at least once before the owner(s) ever decides to sell the practice. But who should do the valuation and how should it be accomplished? It is one thing to have a "paper" valuation for purposes of financial planning or for estimating life insurance needs. It is something more to have a "working" valuation for selling a practice: that valuation must be acceptable to someone from the outside who is putting up real dollars. The following sections address issues involved in valuing a practice for purposes of selling it.

Who Does The Valuation?

When valuing an audiology practice, it is important to realize the complexity of undertaking such a task and the need to avoid bias. *Valuations should not be performed by the owner of the business, but by an individual who is specifically trained to perform them.*

For example, many people value their businesses based on suggestions given to them by associates. Some of these ways may present a fairly accurate value, but they may also pose some problems. A very important aspect of valuing is being as objective as possible. It is difficult to maintain objectivity when trying to value one's own business. One may arrive at a value felt to be pretty accurate, when in reality it is overvalued, which may lead to a lack of interested buyers. As a result, a practice may be on the market longer than necessary, which may decrease the value because the owner may not be putting as much effort into the practice as before it went on the market. Prospective buyers may wonder why the practice has been on the market so long and assume that something is wrong with it. All of this could happen because the practice was overvalued initially. Usually, when an overpriced practice is eventually sold, the sale price is more in line with fair market value.

As opposed to overvaluing, one can undervalue a practice. This can cost the owner thousands of dollars. Any prospective buyer that has a good business sense will immediately realize when a practice is greatly undervalued and will jump at the opportunity to buy a quality business for a low price. The fact that the practice sold instantly is good for the seller, but the price received for it is not!

The preceding discussion makes it clear why the valuation should not be performed by the owner. However, having the valuation performed by an outside professional is not such an easy task, nor is the result guaranteed to be right. This is because independent audiology practices are relatively new, so no time-tested formulas and few precedents exist for determining the value of individual practices. In this relatively unexplored professional territory, accountants and attorneys struggle to draft documents verifying the value of practices that characteristically:

- are service-intensive;
- equipped with expensive, single-application, technical equipment;
- dependent on professionally licensed and certified staff;
- sell a considerable range of tangible products that vary according to their cost, pricing, taxation, supplier, and inventory; and

■ often have relatively large accounts receivable that may be more complex than those of retail or even other health care practices.

Because of the complexity and uniqueness of our practices and the lack of precedent for practice sales, audiologists operating either as sellers or buyers can be misled by advisors who have little or no experience in the sale of audiology practices. Even though the owner does not do the valuation personally, he or she must monitor the process carefully to ensure against judgment errors.

Valuation Based on Precedent

Hearing aid practices have been around much longer than independent audiology practices and have been sold for many years. But their valuation methods are not adequate for arriving at the value of an audiology practice. Often, an audiology practice will value out somewhat higher than a normal hearing aid practice, even though both have the same annual revenues. There are several reasons for this. First, an audiology practice derives revenues from more than just hearing aids and assistive listening devices. Diagnostic testing helps diversify the revenue base and make the practice less volatile in terms of revenue fluctuations. Because there is virtually no cost of sale with regard to diagnostics, the overall bottom line of a practice is greatly improved by increasing diagnostic revenues. When doing a valuation on a practice, most formula approaches examine adjusted net profit, among other things. The more profit, the more the practice is worth. Second, most audiology practices are better equipped (e.g., sound booths, clinical audiometers, acoustic immittance, real-ear equipment), which increases the valuation.

Eventually, the market place will determine fair purchase or sale prices for independent audiology practices. This will happen after a sufficient number of practices are sold and the buyers and sellers feed back to the market whether or not the sales were mutually remunerative. When that time comes, the negotiators of sale agreements, the financial institutions, attorneys, and accountants will likely value practices in traditional terms, such as multiples of annual gross practice income (Kamara, 1988).

In the meantime, the owners and valuators can use what little precedent there is to try to:

■ compare the practice to other audiology practices in the region,
■ find similar practices that have been sold (outside the region, in many cases),

- compare internal financial information of the practice with analogous information from other practices that have been sold,
- attempt to adjust for the many regional differences that could affect sale price,
- adjust for differences between compared practices, and
- arrive at a "starting number" for the valuation, based on sale prices of comparable practices.

Shortcut Valuation Methods

As we wait for precedent-setting sales of audiology practices to take place, a few rules of thumb may be helpful to sellers and buyers. The legitimacy and usefulness of these will vary according to the individual practice under consideration, and it is not our intent to sanctify them by discussing them in this chapter. Nevertheless, they are practical approaches that can serve as a point of departure for negotiations. Some are easier to calculate than others.

Value Per Active File

A simple way to evaluate a hearing aid dispensing practice is to assign a dollar value to each "active" patient file. For instance, a value of $100.00 per file assumes that future transactions with each active patient will yield a $100.00 profit in a specified time period. Thus, a practice with 2,000 active patients could start with a sale price of $200,000.[1]

In almost every case, this "Active File" approach is a shortcut formula that oversimplifies the process because it ignores such factors as location, lease status, contracts, employees, and equipment. There is also the not inconsequential task of arriving at a mutually acceptable definition of an "active" file.

Most commonly, the Active File approach is one component of the evaluation process. If files are valued and sold as an asset of the business, a list of all active files (by patient name) must be included as an attachment to the sale agreement for tax purposes.

---

[1]It is difficult to put a value on an "active" patient file. An alternative is to structure an "earn out" for the seller. A dollar figure can be assigned to the patient files when and if they return to the practice for services or products. As an example, the buyer could pay $25.00 or more per previous patient who returns for services over the next 3 years.

New Versus Established Practice Annual Returns

This is a more complicated and speculative method, but it merits consideration and offers a useful negotiating point. The question posed is: "How long would it take a new, comparable practice in this community to generate an annual income equivalent to the established practice being sold?"

In this method, the financial history of the established practice is used to generate a growth pattern for the hypothetical new practice. First, develop a year-by-year comparison of the likely income of the "new" practice as it parallels the projected income of the established practice. Next, calculate the difference between the two annual incomes for each year, up to the number of years required for the "new" practice's income to equal that of the established practice. Finally, sum the differences for each year. That total represents the "tilled ground" value of the established practice (Kamara, 1988).

This method is quantitative but subjective. Like the Active File approach, it depends on assumptions of future performance and requires mutual agreement between the seller and buyer on the validity of the assumptions. However, like the Active File approach, the New Versus Established approach does represent a rationale, or at least a cross-check, for the asking price of a practice that is up for sale.

Book Value

Another way to estimate the value of a practice is to calculate its "book value." Recall that, in Chapter 12, owners' equity was defined as assets minus liabilities. Assets were all physical and nonphysical things that had monetary value and were owned by the practice. The *book value* of a practice, then, is the sum of assets (e.g., capital equipment, tools and instruments, consumable supplies, real estate, the quality of the lease, referrals, good will, etc.) less liabilities. The following are some considerations when valuing some of these assets.

■ *Capital Equipment*. Book value of equipment is the amortized value of the equipment on the practice's balance sheet at the time of sale. It is also worthwhile to check the fair market value of each unit with an equipment supplier. It is important that the seller know these values because a buyer would have to pay such prices if he or she were establishing a new practice. The amortized value shown on the balance sheet may not give a true picture of the value of the equipment. In normalized earnings, the only depreciation recognized is economic value; that is, the actual reduction in value over the time being considered. This is consistent with the theoretical definition of straight-line-depreciation: cost less salvage value divided by useful life. However, closely held businesses often use the accelerated depreciation amount as opposed to true economic depreciation. For this reason, the information necessary to calculate depreciation may best be obtained from the professional who is appraising its current value. The equipment valuation should include an estimate of the remaining life of the assets and an estimate of their value at the end of that time.

■ *Tools and Instruments.* In this day of hearing aid dispensing, the audiologist must maintain a much broader array of special instruments and tools than in the predispensing era. A sample list is included in Chapter 9 to highlight this point. A replacement price should be set for each item and added to the book value of the practice.

■ *Consumable Supplies.* Ordinarily, diagnostic and rehabilitation materials are classified as consumable supplies, unless a test is a long-lasting item (e.g., a set of CDs) in which case it is considered a capital expense and amortized as equipment (Kamara, 1988). Office and maintenance supplies are consumable supplies. These items should be inventoried and listed in the sale.

■ *Real Estate.* If the practice is located in a building owned by the practice or an owner of the practice,[2] this constitutes a major sale item. Conventional methods of valuing real estate are the easiest way to calculate this component of the sale. There is a constant market place adjustment which can fine-tune the sale, so if the practice is on the market for an extended time, the price may need adjusting commensurate with real estate fluctuations. In most cases, an audiology practice is located in space leased in a building owned by another party.

---

[2]If the practice has multiple owners and is organized as a corporation or a Limited Liability Company, it is unlikely that the building will be owned by the company. As discussed in Chapters 5 and 7, the owner/employee who owns the building will want to keep it out of the corporation or LLC to protect the asset in the event of a negligence lawsuit brought against the company and one or more of the other owner/employees.

If the practice is in an excellent location and there are few vacancies in the building or surrounding area, the lease value increases. The value also increases if the lease is renewable or long-term, especially if it contains a modest rent escalation clause and other favorable provisions.

■ *Contracts*. The points made about the lease also pertain to contracts for service that belong to the practice. Contracts need to be transferable to the new owner and remunerative. Among other things, their value increases according to how long-term and exclusive they are and the terms of renewal.

■ *Referral Arrangements*. Revenue projections must take into account the effects of a new owner assuming the business. Contracts must be looked at closely to determine when they expire and if they are renewable. Referral sources may have to be treated more delicately, because a majority of the agreements are made verbally and not contractually and physicians and other professionals can refer to whomever they choose.

■ *Goodwill*. The primary worth of most practices is goodwill. Goodwill is an accounting concept for describing the worth of a business. Unfortunately, goodwill is an intangible asset on which it is very difficult to place a value; it also receives poor treatment at the hands of the IRS. When establishing a value for goodwill, it is important to remember that goodwill has value only if it translates into good earnings.

■ *Covenant Not to Compete*. Because the primary worth in most practices is the goodwill generated by the present owner, there is great value in preventing the seller from becoming a prime competitor to the new owner. Hence, the value of a noncompete covenant. Any covenant not to compete must be based upon economic reality, in that the seller must be capable of competing after the sale. If the seller has retired and moved or died, the covenant will not have economic reality.

Valuation by Appraisal

The most accurate method of valuing a practice is to have it appraised. Several hearing aid manufacturers have staff with expertise in appraising dispensing audiology practices. At the time of writing [1994], approaching these companies for help may be the best way to get a good appraisal. The following information is needed to perform an accurate appraisal:

■ **General Information**
History of the practice
Form of ownership
Products/services offered by the practice
Markets targeted by the practice

■ **Physical Facilities**
Office
Equipment

■ **General Outlook for the Practice**
How will the practice prosper without the current owner?
How long will the current owner stay on to help with the transition?
What will happen to the current employees?

■ **Special Situations**
Are there any copyrights or patents?
Is there pending litigation against the current owner or the practice?

■ **Interview of Key Personnel**
Viewpoints from people who are key to the success of the practice
Inquiries to the accountant and attorney

■ **Financial Records**
Tax returns
Financial statements
Accounts receivable

■ **External Information**
Demographics
Local/regional growth trends
Competition survey
General outlook for the industry/profession

With the above information in hand, the appraiser can arrive at a dollar value for the practice. The next step is to make adjustments, largely based on the financial reports.

Adjustments to the Income Statement

These adjustments are made to reflect the costs a prospective buyer would have experienced had they owned the practice. This is sometimes called normalizing the income.

■ *Debt Service.* If financing can be obtained, the amount of money it will take to service the debt on a yearly basis must be factored in. This amount has to be deducted from the net profit, thus affecting the income a person may hope to derive from the practice on a yearly basis.

- *Related Parties.* One area of concern in any closely held corporation is transactions involving owners, their relatives, and related businesses. One of the characteristics of the closely held company is that owners have complete control over the company. Therefore, transactions involving these parties are frequently not at arm's length. For example, salaries, fringe benefits, and perks granted to the owner(s) and related parties need to be carefully examined. The amount that these compensations exceed what a nonowner would be paid to perform the same duties should be added back to the income stream.

- *Payroll Taxes.* If the business is a sole proprietorship or a partnership, the financial statements will not reflect any payroll taxes on owners' salaries. Therefore, when substituting a fair salary to replace owner compensation, payroll taxes should be added to that cost.

- *Benefit Plans.* In businesses with few employers, the owners may have established excellent benefit packages, especially retirement plans. The buyer needs to decide what the level of benefits will be following the purchase, and adjust the expense accordingly.

- *Depreciation.* This has already been discussed above, in the section on Book Value.

- *Rent.* Rent often increases when a lease changes hands. It usually increases when a new lease is negotiated. In the case of ownership of an office or building, tax assessments occur at periodic intervals and when there is a transfer of ownership. In any of these cases, the buyer needs to adjust the monthly cost to reflect increased rent or taxes.

- *Nonrecurring Items.* In normalizing income, the buyer is attempting to adjust the income stream to what is considered normal. Therefore, the buyer needs to examine unusual items included in the income statement (e.g., discontinued business operations, gains or losses on major asset dispositions). However, it is important not to overdo such adjustments. In typical business life, nonrecurring items will continue to crop up, and each instance will be different from the one before. Before adjusting these items, the buyer should be certain that failing to do so will materially distort the true value of the practice.

Adjustments to the Balance Sheet

As pointed out in Chapter 12, the balance sheet does not show how much a business is worth because it uses a cost basis for valuing assets. For sale purposes, it was suggested that balance sheets can be constructed that show assets at current appraised values. In either case, cash will be valued at face value.

The following are possible adjustments that may need to be made to the balance sheet. There may be other areas that need adjusting as well.

- *Accounts Receivable.* An inquiry should be made into the collectibility, age, and nature of the accounts in order to make a reasonable estimate of the uncollectibles that offset the balance.
- *Equipment, Furniture, and Fixtures.* The fastest way to estimate the value of equipment is to use the depreciation schedules and adjust the depreciation to straight-line and a reasonable useful life.
- *Plant Assets.* Plant assets should be adjusted to their fair market value; that is, what it would cost to replace the existing assets with similar assets of the same capacity, age, and condition that are installed and operational?
- *Nonoperating Assets.* These are assets that are not a part of the operating function of the business. They may range from investments in stocks and bonds to cash accounts (other than temporary excesses in working capital) to real estate or other ventures. These assets should be valued outside the primary business valuation, if they are to be sold with the business; otherwise, they should be eliminated for the purpose of the evaluation.

"SPADE WORK" FOR THE SELLER

Once a practice owner makes the decision to sell, there is much he or she can do before spending any more money on professional services. The first thing is to establish a clear understanding of why the practice is going up for sale. There are obvious and acceptable reasons (e.g., retirement, poor health), but other reasons may raise suspicion in the mind of a prospective buyer (e.g., relocation, change of pace). A buyer wants to know why the practice is for sale, and the seller needs to have a consistent, honest, and direct answer.

Another important consideration for a prospective seller is the timing for the announcement of the intent to sell. Good timing helps to maintain the confidence and morale of staff members, as well as patients. It is unfortunate when the sale of a practice comes as a shock to staff, and patients receive no transition or announcement of the transfer of the ownership and personnel. Timing also affects the value of the practice. It is natural for a prospective seller to loose impetus and allow the practice to start withering, once the decision is made to leave or sell the practice. This is very detrimental to the health of the practice and ultimately affects the sale price. The owner of a practice must maintain a steady pace until the time of sale. Stated differently, if the financial records show a steady decline, it gives a prospective buyer a false signal of the potential of the practice and may result in a lower bid for the practice.

This precautionary advice does not preclude the possibility of a prospective seller operating a practice on a part-time basis in later years. If this is the case, it is imperative that the seller maintain time records and calculate the productivity of the practice if operated full-time, projected from the part-time activity. Stated more simply, if a seller has been generating "x" amount of income working 75% time for the past 3 years, it is legitimate and important to show what the practice could generate at full-time by adding 25% to the existing figure.

The more tangible the information and documentation the seller can assemble, the better. A display of this information in an organized, indexed portfolio can be impressive and provide a positive first impression to a prospective buyer and/or broker. The contents of such a piece should include, but not be limited to the items described in Table 19–1. Note that many of these items should be forthcoming if the owner(s) has gone through the steps required for a practice appraisal, as described earlier in the chapter.

This seems like a lot of work, and it can be, depending on the modus operandi of the practice. If the practice is computerized, much of the information cited above is easily retrievable; otherwise, it may take many hours to collect the data. However, the information is well worth knowing and collecting, as it is very helpful in management of the practice (i.e., updating the business plan) and can be extremely effective in facilitating a sale.

Audiologists who are still some time away from selling should start compiling documents and materials for present and future use. Ideally, from the day a practice opens it is

Table 19–1. Portfolio categories and information prepared by the buyer.

Type of Documentation	Method of Documentation
Descriptive Statistics	
Demographics	Number of people in target market area, according to age, income, marital status, etc.
Local/regional growth trends	Percent change in population by census tract, according to age, income, etc.
	Home sales
	Percent change in number of businesses and description of types of businesses in the area
Competition survey	All sites, broken down according to location, services offered, number and qualifications of staff, target markets, financial statistics, fees, reputation
	Additional analysis of hospital, clinic, agency, university, and government sites: offering or likely to offer services? Salary or contract?
Special situations	Local and state regulatory activities (e.g., state licensure)
	Third party insurance regional reimbursement policies and rates for audiologists
	Managed care groups' arrangements for audiology services
General outlook for independent audiology practice	Highlights and summarizes above information, concluding with owner's subjective impressions, in the form of present and future SWOT[a] analyses
Practice Documentation	
Mission and philosophy	Copy of Mission Statement
	Copy of Practice Philosophy
	List of short- and long-term practice goals
Physical premises	Square footage
	Photos and floor plans of the building and practice
	Photos of exterior and interior signages
	Owned or leased, length of lease, assignable lease?
	Copy of deed or lease
Products and services	List of services and fees
	List of tangible products and pricing structure

[a]SWOT: Strengths, weaknesses, opportunities, threats. For example of SWOT analysis, see Chapter 4.

Table 19–1. *(continued)*

Type of Documentation	Method of Documentation
Practice Documentation *(continued)*	
Target markets	Computer printout of active patient base (e.g., patients served within the past 12, 18, or 24 months)
	Computer printout of inactive patient base (e.g., patients who have not been served within the specified time frame, have a disconnected phone number, no forwarding address, etc.)
Profile of patient population	Central tendency statistics (range, average, mode) for age, needs, etc. (e.g., "on the average, 50% of new patients require hearing aids, but the range varies from only 25% in June/July to 75% in January.")
	Percent of total patients that are new patients
	Average number patients/day
	Annual percentage increase in total patients
	Average reimbursement per patient
	Average number of encounters per patient per year
Referral sources	List of sources, including a breakdown of the sources of new patients (e.g., word of mouth, promotions, physician referrals, contractual arrangements, etc.)
Promotional materials	Compilation of materials, including (but not limited to) waiting room brochures; newsletters; direct mailing; referral program materials; ad copies (yellow pages, newspapers, radio/tv, etc.); practice brochure, staff biographies, etc.
Practice Forms and Documentation	
Office and audiology forms	Test forms
	Sample referral letters and other referral correspondence forms
	Insurance and private pay billing forms
	Patient information forms (e.g., insurance billing procedures and policies; product return policies; etc.)
	Product order forms
	Product sales agreements
	Product repair agreements
	Inventory control forms

(continued)

Table 19–1. Portfolio categories and information prepared by the buyer. *(continued)*

Type of Documentation	Method of Documentation
Practice Forms and Documentation *(continued)*	
Licenses, Credentials, and Registration	Copy of state business registration and any local forms that apply
	Verification of legal business entity (e.g., IRS approval of S election; state corporate registration, etc.)
	Copies of audiology certification/licenses and hearing aid licenses held by owner(s) and/or employees of the practice
Insurance	List of insurances held by the practice for owner(s) and/or employees: malpractice, office, workers' compensation, disability, life, health
Equipment and Supplies	
Equipment	Inventory list of major equipment showing date of purchase, serial number, supplier, purchase price, and maintenance record
	A list of leased equipment, with rate and age of lease
Furniture and fixtures	Inventory list showing date of purchase and purchase price
Instruments and tools	List showing quantity and cost of each
Audiology and hearing aid supplies	Listed with date of inventory
Consumable office supplies	Listed with date of inventory
Financial Information and Trend Analyses	
Pension or profit sharing plan	Report of current status of the plan, including percent vesting of each employee
Tax returns	Copies of last 3 years' business returns
Financial Statements	Annual income statements for last 3 years with the CPA's signed cover letters included
	Interim income statement to present date
	Pro forma income statement for next 3 years
	Current balance sheet
Accounts Receivable	Listed according to aging of accounts
Accounts Payable	Show according to due date
Trend Analyses	Quarterly sales volume for last 3 years
	Annual profit for last 3 years
	Percentage of owner(s)' net income to gross receipts for last 3 years
	Percentage of cost of sales for last 3 years

wise for the owner(s) to think about selling it one day. Records should be maintained as though the practice were to be put up for sale tomorrow. Ongoing management decisions about purchasing, record keeping, data collection, filing, and an array of other matters can someday contribute to the value and sale of the practice.

Presenting the Practice

It is essential that a seller present the practice in a favorable light. This is obvious, but it is worth mentioning because a positive and well-considered approach is always better than one that has several qualifications and "ifs" attached. In putting the practice on the market, the seller may rely solely on word of mouth, advertise the sale in the trade journals, or hire a broker.[3]

As stated earlier, the buyer should have compiled an attractive portfolio, and this should be readily available with documented financial records to demonstrate the security of the practice. The documents should also provide a profile of the patient population served by the practice.

A description of the advantages of the practice's location and a copy of the lease should be part of the documentation. A good office site and a well-written, favorable lease can be very significant assets in the valuation of the practice.

The prospective seller should have a clear idea of the practice's potential for growth, based on measurable statistics in the practice (e.g., average reimbursement per patient, annual percentage increase in total patients, managed care contracts, etc.) and outside the practice (e.g., percentage increases in target markets, growth of managed care groups, new businesses to the area, etc).

Regarding the "looks" of the day-to-day practice, the staff should be informed of the seller's plans and, to the extent it is possible, advised of the stability of their positions in the event of a sale. In this way, the seller can present the staff in a positive manner to the prospective buyer. All equipment and instruments need to be in good working order and supported with proper calibration documentation and manuals. The physical plant should be clean and refurbished as much as possible to present attractively. In this regard, selling an audiology practice is much like selling a house.

---

[3]A few brokers sell hearing aid dispensing practices, as evidenced by their classified advertisements in the hearing aid journals. Brokers' fees are usually based on a percentage of the sale price—as much as 15%. The broker fee usually comes out of the seller's pocket as an up-front cost of the sale.

"SPADE WORK" FOR THE BUYER

The burden of the sale of a practice does not rest solely with the seller. The buyer also must do homework if he or she expects to get the serious attention of a seller or broker.

Personal Planning

Like the seller, the buyer needs to have a clear understanding of why he or she wants to buy an audiology practice and what kind of practice is desirable. Chapter 3 in this handbook addresses these issues. If a prospective buyer feels comfortable with the messages in that chapter, then he or she can proceed with some preliminary homework for a purchase.

Prospective buyers should establish as firmly as possible the kinds of practices they are seeking to purchase. That is, is it a practice that involves primarily a pediatric population, a practice that is heavily involved in diagnostic testing, a practice that primarily dispenses hearing aids, a practice that relies on industrial hearing conservation contracts, and so on.

Buyers should establish some time lines for seeking out and negotiating to purchase a practice. Simply "looking around" can extend indefinitely and get nowhere. The buyer should study carefully Chapters 7, 8, 9, and 18 in this handbook before setting out to search for a practice.

Preliminary Steps

Once a clear picture emerges of what the buyer is seeking and the time frame designated for the search, the buyer needs to do the following homework (refer to Chapter 18 for details on financial preparations):

- Prepare a statement of net worth. This is simply a listing of all assets minus all liabilities.
- Compose a biographical sketch or curriculum vita outlining financial and professional qualifications.
- Do a preliminary investigation to determine approximately how much capital is available to get a realistic idea of the price range for a practice. That is, if a prospective buyer can raise a maximum of $25,000, it probably makes little sense to get interested in a practice that has a market value of $500,000.
- Decide whether to use a broker or do a self-search.

Finding a Practice to Buy

There are various ways to look for a practice to buy. The ideal is to sign on as an employee with an option to buy. This scenario provides both the buyer and the seller an opportunity to evaluate each other's worth. The prospective buyer gets to learn the true value and potential of the practice, while the seller has the opportunity to appraise the competence, integrity, and potential of the prospective buyer.

Another version of this scenario is for two audiologists who have known one another for some time to enter into negotiations for a sale or partnership. Presumably, a rapport has already been established and the negotiations can move forward in a productive and mutually agreeable manner.

Other ways of identifying a practice for sale are: (a) check the classified section of audiology and hearing aid periodicals, (b) word-of-mouth, and (c) hire a broker. The broker approach is largely unexplored at the time of writing (1994) because few audiology practices have been sold by brokers. Although a broker's assistance in finding an appropriate practice may be highly desirable in some situations, it is also possible for audiologists to do better on their own, due to most brokers' inexperience in our field. The situation may change in the future as sales of audiology practices become more commonplace and brokers take more of an interest in the transactions. Whether a broker "brokers" the entire deal, he or she may prove useful in some aspects of a sale (e.g., locating financing, advising on tax considerations, etc.).

The prospective buyer should not limit the search only to practices that are openly for sale. A particular practice need not be for sale for the right prospective buyer to ultimately convince the owner to sell. For example, an audiologist may have a good practice in a searcher's geographic area of interest. Although the owner may have no thoughts of selling, that thinking may be swayed by persuasive reasoning and an enticing offer on the part of the prospective buyer.

Buyers who are free to relocate to other parts of the country have more opportunities to find good practices; however, there are more unknowns in such ventures than there are when purchasing a practice in one's own community. When a potential purchase is considered in another community, the prospective buyer needs to gather the following information about the area in which the practice is located:

■ Population demographics
■ Economy of the community

- ■ Competition
- ■ Community support
- ■ Transportation

Audiology is a small and relatively close-knit profession and word-of-mouth is an effective means of advertising. Simply telling some colleagues that a practice is for sale may elicit one or more prospective buyers. Likewise, a seller may identify an audiologist who is employed in the community who may have dreamed of owning a practice, but has never actively searched for one. In this case, the prospective seller can point out the advantages of having a private practice and indicate a willingness to work with the audiologist to facilitate the purchase.

EVALUATING THE PRACTICE

A prospective buyer should reread Chapters 7, 8, and 9 and analyze the location, lease, physical plant, and competition of any practice of interest that may be for sale.

The buyer should always "kick the tires" to see if there are any hidden agendas or flaws in the business (e.g., disgruntled employees or patients, potentially negative changes on the horizon, financial problems). A prospective buyer kicks the tires by:

- ■ interviewing staff members,
- ■ checking major inventory items to ensure that they are in good working condition and well maintained, and
- ■ working in the office for a reasonable amount of time.

It is important to inspect a random sample of the patient records to see: (a) their general condition, (b) how patients are managed, (c) how encounters are noted in the charts, (d) how evaluations are performed and documented, (e) how carefully product sales and warranties are recorded, and (f) how current they are.

A prospective buyer should study the history of the practice as it is presented by the seller and talk with audiologists and other professionals in the community who may be cited in the history. If none are cited, the buyer should seek out the opinions of colleagues in the community to obtain their opinions on the conduct and health of the practice in question. If the practice uses only a few hearing aid manufacturers or suppliers, the buyer should attempt to get an appraisal of the practice from these manufacturers.

Finally, a buyer should never buy a practice without a clear understanding of the lease and contract arrangements. Assuming the lease is transferable, it is a significant asset to the value of a practice in some circumstances. Referral contracts are often the very fiscal heart of a practice, so their transferability is an obvious asset.

If the buyer's evaluation of the practice suggests that it is a solid and honestly run business, the next step is to put the financial projections through a "capitalization of earnings" analysis. Simply put, this analysis sets a specific return on investment (ROI)—say 8%—that the buyer could expect to get over a specified period of years from putting the purchase money into standard investments. It then asks whether the same amount of money put into the practice will yield the same or better ROI in the same number of years. If the ROI from the business is less than or equal to 8%, purchasing the practice is usually not a good investment.

NEGOTIATING THE SALE

As in the case of most items of this nature, there will be a negotiation process leading to an agreement. Those who have bought or sold a home can appreciate this point. The asking price is not necessarily the selling price.

Knowing when to "qualify" a potential buyer and introduce confidential information about the practice (e.g., tax records) is critical to the negotiation process. Negotiations need to proceed in good faith, but the seller should not spend too much time or give out too much information unless the prospective buyer can show serious intent, financial capability, and professional and managerial competence.

The buyer is likely to make legitimate adjustments to the practice's balance sheet and income statement, which may reduce the sale price. As an example, the buyer may acknowledge the importance of existing contracts or referral sources to the practice, but express concerns about the fragility of the relationships. As a compromise, the buyer make offer to pay the seller a percentage of fees generated by the contracts or referral sources for a set number of years. In this way, the final purchase price will remain high if the referral sources are maintained, but be reduced if contracts are not renewed or referral sources cease to refer.

If the buyer and seller each have conducted research on the value of the practice, there should be mutual agreement on the selling price and a sales contract can be drafted based upon the research.

Legal counsel is necessary at this stage, as well as in other aspects of the negotiation. It is important to use attorneys with expertise in tax law who have arranged sales of small businesses, especially if they have arranged sales of medical or dental practices. Both the potential buyer and seller should scrutinize very carefully the recommendations of legal counsel and not hesitate to obtain second opinions.

Allocating the Assets: Tax Implications

Once an agreement is reached regarding the purchase price, the purchase price must be allocated (broken down into individual assets). It is important to remember that the buyer should be purchasing the assets of a practice, not the business entity itself. Purchasing the business itself exposes the new owner to the inherent liabilities (patient- and tax-related) of the original business. A prospective buyer can never know what the seller may have run through their corporate tax returns in the past. Purchasing only the assets ensures that the buyer will never have to find out!

Allocation must follow relatively strict rules, as described in Section 1060 of the Internal Revenue Code. The buyer will desire allocation to items that allow the quickest tax write-off (e.g., equipment), whereas the seller usually will try to allocate to items that receive capital gain treatment (e.g., patient files). Chaney (1994) summarizes federal tax rules on allocations of a sale as follows:

> For asset sales after August of 1993, the required allocation to intangibles allows the buyer a 15 year amortization write-off . . . . Such intangibles include information sources, customer-related information, a covenant not to compete, goodwill, a franchise, a trademark as well as a trade name. While the write-off period for all those items to the buyer is 15 years, the seller may recognize capital gain for the allocation to information sources, customer related information and goodwill, but the allocation to covenant not to compete will be treated as ordinary income to the seller. (p. 34)

In addition to federal taxes, some states charge substantial sales tax on the sale of business assets.

Financing the Sale

In most situations, a large part of the purchase price must be carried by the seller. This is particularly the case for audiology practices in today's (1994) financial environment, especially if a large portion of the sale is allocated to goodwill. It is extremely difficult to get financing from traditional lending institutions which usually demand hard assets to collateralize a loan. In the past, hearing aid manufacturers have stepped in, either to guarantee a loan or to provide cash for a buyout. With decreasing sales in the industry for the last several years, most manufacturers have either stopped financing transactions or are being very selective and conservative. As a result, most sales today involve the buyer putting a downpayment on the practice and the owner carrying the balance on a note (which sometimes will be guaranteed by a hearing aid manufacturer).

Because the seller is carrying the loan, an agreement must be reached regarding the size of the downpayment. In most cases, the seller should require a substantial downpayment from the buyer, not only to protect the sale, but to cover tax events associated with the sale. Tax law requires that the seller recognize any depreciation recapture in the year of the sale, regardless of the amount of downpayment made by the buyer.

The agreement must also stipulate the length of the payoff period and the interest rate. The IRS also requires that a minimum interest rate must be charged. The terms of the agreement determine what the buyer's monthly payment will be. In small business sales, it is a fact that many buyers default, leaving the seller with no choice but to foreclose. For this reason, the seller must be very careful to agree to a monthly payment that leaves the buyer able to meet other business overhead and personal expenses.

Once the agreement is made, the sale can be recorded through a title company, which can also collect the monthly payments for the seller. The cost of using a title company is minimal, and psychologically it creates a more business-like atmosphere for future relations between the seller and the buyer.

Protective Provisions

To protect the seller, Chaney (1994) suggests that the contract contain clauses stipulating:

■ the seller is provided financial statements and tax returns to monitor the business;

■ the buyer cannot remove money from the practice for personal purposes which would lower the business cash balance below a set amount (e.g., 1 month's overhead);

■ assets are sold "as is";

■ a due-on-sale provision accelerates the note if the buyer resells the business;

- default triggering remedies (e.g., failure to pay on the note, failure to make payroll or sales tax payments, failure to pay rent, etc.);
- remedies in the event of default (e.g., right to retake and resell; right to regain the company name, logo, telephone numbers; termination of a covenant not to compete; "reverse" covenant against the defaulting buyer; right to a deficiency judgment on the unpaid note; etc.).

On the buyer's side, Chaney (1994) suggests different clauses in the contract:

- a warranty of good working order of equipment, usable supplies and sellable inventory (as opposed to the "as is" clause desired by the seller);
- representation that assets are sold free and clear;
- seller verification that accounting information and tax returns provided in the negotiations are reasonably accurate;
- a grace period and written notice before default remedies go into effect.

Contingencies on the Sale

The sale contract needs to contain contingencies that must be met before the sale can close. As examples:

- The buyer must secure a loan.
- The seller may demand extra security. Because of the real threat of buyer default in business purchases, the seller may require that the buyer provide a personal guarantee by other family members (e.g., parents) or put up equity in real estate that is owned by someone other than the buyer.
- The buyer must make a downpayment.
- The business premises lease must be assigned to the buyer.
- Equipment leases must be assigned to the buyer.
- Contracts must be transferred to the buyer.
- The seller must send out "comfort letters" to patients and referral sources. These should be one-page letters that: (a) inform the reader of the sale and the reason for the sale; (b) provide assurances that important characteristics of the practice (e.g., services, prices, employees) will remain the same, at least for awhile; (c) introduce the buyer ("hand-picked" by the seller);

(d) let the reader know that the seller will be on the premises for a certain length of time; and (e) perhaps give the reader the seller's home telephone number, in case of serious questions.

■ The buyer must take adequate legal steps to reorganize the business. Buyers must remember that they are purchasing the assets of a business, not the business itself. Therefore, as soon as the buyer signs the final note, he or she must "go back to the beginning" (in this case, Chapter 5) and create a new, legal business entity.

SUMMARY

Converting an audiology practice into cash is a complex operation that should be contemplated carefully from the day the practice opens its doors. For a variety of reasons, the owner(s) should establish a value for the practice and update the valuation periodically. Whenever possible, the valuation should be performed by an outside expert with the owner monitoring the process at every stage.

When the owner(s) decides to sell the audiology practice, the valuation should be performed through a formal appraisal process. That process looks at external and internal factors affecting the practice's value, as well as the financial statements and adjustments to those statements. The owner(s) should compile a portfolio documenting the information used in the appraisal process. This should present the practice in its best light to prospective buyers, stressing its strong points.

Those wishing to purchase a practice must also prepare a portfolio. The portfolio needs to document their professional and financial credentials, thus "qualifying" them as prospective buyers. Prospective buyers must evaluate practices for sale carefully and critically. They should always use an accountant and attorney when putting together an offer.

Negotiating the sale involves agreeing to a purchase price, an allocation of assets of the sale, and a contract with protective clauses and contingencies. Usually, it also involves the parties agreeing for the seller to carry a note for a large portion of the purchase price, with the interest rate and payoff period stipulated. All negotiations at this stage should be carried out with both parties represented by competent tax attorneys. The final agreement needs to contain protective contingencies for both buyer and seller. Finally, the buyer must be prepared to start the business organization process again, immediately on completion of the sale.

REFERENCES

Chaney, A. D. (1994). *Closely held business law in Arizona: Business owner guide and attorney/CPA desk reference*. Tucson, AZ: Author.

Kamara, C. A. (1988). Buying and selling a private practice. *Asha, 30*(1), 35–36.

SUGGESTED READINGS

Horn, T. W. (1985). *The business valuation manual*. Lancaster, PA: Charter Oak Press.

Libby, E.R. (1991). How to value a hearing instrument dispensing practice. *Hearing Instruments, 42*(10), 18–19.

Appendix 19-A

Sample Sale Agreement

AGREEMENT OF PURCHASE AND SALE OF ASSETS

between

Cardinal Hearing Services, Inc.

a [State] Corporation

and

Dr. A

and

ABC Corporation

In this case, a [State] Corporation

INDEX

SECTION TEN
   10.1 Before and After Closing—Risk of Loss

SECTION ELEVEN
   11.1 Confidential Nature of Sale

SECTION TWELVE
   12.1 Change of Name

SECTION THIRTEEN
   13.1 Adjustments

SECTION FOURTEEN
   14.1 Service Plan—Liabilities to Third Parties

SECTION FIFTEEN
   15.1 Debt on Automobile—Assumption of Debt

SECTION SIXTEEN
   16.1 Signage Installation or Credit

SECTION SEVENTEEN
   17.1 Accounts Payable and Receivable—Obligations

SECTION EIGHTEEN
   18.1 Notices
   18.2 Agreement, Modification, Waiver
   18.3 Headings
   18.4 Exhibits
   18.5 Successors and Assigns
   18.6 Governing Laws
   18.7 Parties of Interest
   18.8 Counterpart
   18.9 Inseverability
   18.10 Acknowledgment of Reading and Receipt

SECTION NINETEEN
   19.1 Change in Office Supplies

SECTION TWENTY
   20.1 Lease Rights

PURCHASE AGREEMENT

THIS PURCHASE AGREEMENT is made and entered into this_____ day of _____, 19__ by and between CARDINAL HEARING SERVICES, INC., a [State] Corporation (hereinafter referred to as "CHS") and Dr._____ (hereinafter referred to as Dr. A) and ABC Corporation (hereinafter referred to as "ABC").

RECITALS

1. CHS is a [State] corporation solely owned by Dr. A. CHS currently operates an audiology practice from an office at Physicians' Medical Plaza, Suite____, Central City, [State] (hereinafter referred to as the "Office").

2. CHS has a lease on the Office dated the 1st day of January, 1995. A copy of the Lease Agreement is attached to this Agreement and marked as Exhibit "A," and is hereinafter referred to in this agreement as the "Lease."

3. ABC is a [State] corporation of 1234 Hearing Aid Road, Central City, [State], and is desirous of acquiring and purchasing certain assets of CHS and of becoming the assignee of the Lease.

4. CHS is desirous of terminating its business at the Office; of assigning its interest in the Lease to ABC; of selling certain of its assets to ABC; Dr. A is willing to enter into a Covenant Not to Compete with ABC and a Consulting Agreement with ABC.

5. CHS is willing to change its name and to permit ABC to change its Articles of Incorporation to adopt the name CHS in the conduct of the business by ABC.

6. CHS has sold certain coupon books and certain service plans to patients. CHS and ABC are desirous of entering into an agreement with respect to the performance of those service plans in the future.

To accomplish the above recited intentions, the parties do contract and agree with each other as follows:

NOW, THEREFORE, in consideration of the premises, warranties, conditions and mutual covenants contained in this Agreement, the parties hereto agree as follows:

SECTION ONE

Actions at Closing

Subject to the terms and conditions of this Agreement, and in exchange for the consideration hereinafter set forth, the parties to this Agreement agree to consummate the following transaction at the closing to be held as set forth in Section 2.0 of this Agreement.

    1.1 <u>Transfer of Assets of CHS</u>. ABC agrees to purchase from CHS, and CHS agrees to sell, transfer, assign, and convey to ABC, by such documents as are reasonable, appropriate, and necessary, as hereinafter set forth, the following assets of CHS existing at time of closing.

A. <u>Equipment</u>: Certain equipment owned by CHS on the Closing Date, the items of which are set forth on Exhibit "B," a copy of which is attached hereto and is by reference made a part hereof. The [brand name] audiometers will be calibrated with current certificate.

B. <u>Supplies</u>. Supplies owned by CHS on the Closing Date, listed on Exhibit "C," a copy of which is attached hereto and is by reference made part hereof. (See Section 21)

C. <u>Patient Files</u>. All patient files in the possession of CHS being approximately 2,500 in number, including all information in possession of CHS, in connection with those patients.

D. <u>Automobile</u>. One 19__ Sable Mercury Station Wagon.

E. <u>Assignment of all Rights of the Lessee</u> under the Lease described herein and attached as Exhibit "A."

1.2 <u>Consulting Agreement</u>. Dr. A and ABC agree at time of closing to enter into a Consulting Agreement whereby Dr. A will prepare for ABC:

A. Two newsletters;

B. Letters of introduction to referral sources and clients.

In addition, Dr. A will be at the Office for an average of three days per week, 8 hours per day, performing clinical orientation duties until April 1, 19__. In addition, Dr. A will spend 6 days (8 hours per day) of Open Houses to promote the profession practice of ABC, to be accomplished within 18 months from Date of Closing at times mutually agreed upon between Dr. A and ABC. In addition, Dr. A will promote and attend a social open house for referral sources, some clients, and tenants of the building, held during the first 60 days after the date of Closing, at a time mutually agreeable.

1.3 <u>Covenant Not to Compete</u>. It is recognized that Dr. A's knowledge, information, and relationship with the suppliers and patients of CHS, and the knowledge of the business methods, systems, plans, and policies of CHS which she has heretofore received or obtained as the owner of CHS are valuable and unique to the business of CHS. Dr. A and CHS agree that for a period of 36 months after the Closing Date, neither of them will, from or at any location within a 10 mile radius of Physicians' Medical Plaza, Central City, [State], (i) directly or indirectly, by ownership or securities or otherwise, engage in the retail sale of hearing aids or receive fees for services to persons with hearing loss or engage in any business competitive with the business of CHS or become associated with or render services, other than the consulting services set forth in this Agreement, to any person, firm, corporation, or other entity so engaged, or (ii) disclose or use, directly or indirectly, any confidential or nonpublic proprietary knowledge or information pertaining to the now business of CHS, its management, financial condition, patient lists, sources of supply, business, personnel, policies, or prospects, to any person, firm, corporation, or other entity, for any reason or purpose whatsoever. Recognizing that damages at law would be inadequate in the circumstances, Dr. A and CHS consent and agree that if they or either of them violates any of the noncompetition or nondisclosure provisions set forth herein, ABC would sustain irreparable harm and, therefore, in addition to any other remedies which ABC may have under this Agreement or otherwise, ABC shall be entitled to the injunctive relief of restraining Dr. A and/or CHS from committing or continuing any such violation and neither of them shall object to any application for such relief made by ABC to any court of competent jurisdiction.

SECTION TWO

Closing

2.1 <u>Date of Closing</u>. The date of closing shall occur on January 2, 19__.
2.2 <u>Location of Closing</u>. The location of closing shall be by mutual agreement of Dr. A and ABC.

SECTION THREE

Notices Prior to Closing

3.1 <u>Notices to Patients</u>. All notices to patients, whether before or at closing or after closing, shall contain information as shall be mutually agreeable to Dr. A and ABC. Neither Dr. A nor ABC or CHS will distribute any information to patients concerning this transaction without the consent of Dr. A and ABC.
3.2 <u>Notice to Landlord</u>. CHS shall provide at time of closing assignment and transfer of its lease interest to ABC in the Office, and all requisite consents from Landlord as required in Paragraph 15 of said Lease. Landlord will void in writing Paragraph 3 of the rider to that Lease and ABC will agree with that action.
3.3 CHS <u>Liability Insurance</u>. CHS will carry professional liability insurance until termination of the consulting period with ABC.

SECTION FOUR

ABC Name Change

4.1 CHS agrees to delivery at time of Closing a properly executed corporate resolution changing its name and to execute any documentation as may be reasonably requested by ABC giving permission and consent by ABC to change its corporate name to CHS.

SECTION FIVE

Purchase Price

5.1 <u>Total Purchase Price.</u> Total purchase price shall be the sum of _____ thousand dollars ($_____) plus assumption of debt on the Sable Mercury Station Wagon, not to exceed the sum of _____ thousand dollars ($_____).

5.2 <u>Payment at Closing</u>. The amount payable at Closing shall be _____ thousand dollars ($_____) together with Promissory Note in the sum of _____ thousand dollars ($_____). With respect to the cash paid at time of closing, _____ thousand dollars ($_____) of the cash will be allocated to the Consulting Agreement. The _____ thousand dollars ($_____) owed under the aforesaid Promissory Note shall be for and in consideration of the Consulting Agreement. Said _____ thousand dollars shall be paid in full on the first day of April, 19__, with the understanding that the due date can be extended for the period up to thirty (30) days at the option of ABC by paying _____% interest on a per annum basis on the unpaid balance for the number of days after April 1, 19___ to the date of payment. Any partial payment shall be credited first to interest and balance to the reduction of principal.

5.3 <u>Payment of Adjustment Items</u>. Adjustment items as described in Section Thirteen shall be payable in cash at Closing.

SECTION SIX

Purchase Price Allocation

6.1 The Purchase Price shall be allocated among the assets as follows:
  A. For the automobile—$_____, plus the unpaid debt assumed, not exceeding the sum of $_____.
  B. For the Equipment, the sum of $_____.
  C. For the Supplies the sum of $_____.
  D. For the Patient Files, the sum of $_____.
  E. For the Consulting Agreement, the sum of $_____.
  F. For the Covenant Not to Compete, the sum of $_____.
  G. For the Leasehold Improvements, the sum of $_____.

The parties, by execution of this Agreement, state that this Agreement was made by "an arm's length negotiation," and the Total Purchase Price, together with the valuation placed on the various assets, represent a negotiated value between the parties, based upon the parties' best judgment. Neither of the parties shall take a position contrary to this allocation with respect to reporting for Federal or State Income Tax purposes.

SECTION SEVEN

Financing Contingency

7.1 <u>ABC Option to Rescind</u>. In the event that ABC cannot borrow the sum of _____ thousand dollars ($_____) from either [hearing aid company] or from any bank, involving a guarantee of the borrowing by [hearing aid company], then and in that event ABC shall have the option of rescinding this transaction.

SECTION EIGHT

The Representations and Warranties of CHS and Dr. A

As of the date of this Agreement, and as of the Closing Date, ABC and Dr. A represent and warrant as follows:

8.1 <u>Absence of Undisclosed Liabilities</u>. CHS and Dr. A shall not be obligated for, nor any of the assets sold hereunder, subject to any liability or obligation, with the exception of a debt on the said Mercury Station Wagon not to exceed the sum of $_____.

8.2 <u>Marketable Title</u>. CHS now has, and will have at Closing Date, good and marketable title to all of its assets being sold hereby free and clear of all conditions and liens and mortgages and charges and encumbrances.

8.3 <u>Absence of Default in Lease</u>. There shall be no default in any obligation of CHS in said Lease existing at time of Closing.

8.4 <u>Consent Not Necessary</u>. No consents or waivers of or by any third parties are necessary in order to permit the transfer of assets or the assignment of the Lease or the Covenant Not to Compete or the Consulting Agreement herein contemplated.

8.5 <u>Conduct of Practice of CHS until Date of Closing</u>. CHS will continue until the Closing Date to carry on its audiology practice in the normal course. Nothing has or will be done by CHS, or by Dr. A, which will in any way materially adversely affect the value of the CHS audiology practice, or the value of any of the assets of CHS, other than in the normal course of said business.

8.6 <u>Warranty Regarding Condition</u>. As of the Closing Date, all of the tangible personal assets being sold hereunder by CHS shall be in good working order and in a good state of repair, and certain equipment shall be calibrated as set forth in Section 1.1(A) on page 2 hereof.

8.7 <u>Warranty Regarding Financial Statements and Taxes</u>. The financial statements of CHS for 19___, 19___, 19___ and the first 9 months of 1991 (all of which are attached hereto as Exhibit D and hereby made a part hereof) represent in each instance, fairly and accurately the financial condition and performance of CHS for the respective period stated, and there are no known liabilities or claims pending against CHS not reflected in said financial statements. All state and federal taxes of CHS have been fully paid when due and there are no unresolved state or federal tax matters of CHS which would give rise to any lien or claim against the assets of CHS being transferred hereby.

SECTION NINE

Conditions Precedent to ABC Obligations to Close

The obligations of ABC hereunder to consummate this Agreement is expressly subject to the satisfaction on or prior to the Closing Date of the following conditions, compliance with which or the occurrence or non-occurrence of which may be waived, in whole or in part by ABC in writing.

9.1 <u>Representations, Warranties of Dr. A and CHS</u>. All representatives, warranties, and covenants of Dr. A and CHS contained in this Agreement shall be true and correct as of the Closing Date and Dr. A and CHS shall have performed and satisfied all of the covenants and conditions required in this Agreement to be performed and satisfied by either, on or prior to the Closing Date. ABC shall obtain from CHS such Bills of Sale and instruments of transfer as ABC shall reasonably request, all of which shall be satisfactory in all respects to legal counsel for ABC.

9.2 <u>Absence of Litigation</u>. No action or proceeding shall have been instituted prior to or at the Closing Date before any Court, or other governmental body or authority, pertaining to the transaction to be consummated hereunder, the result of which would prevent or make illegal the consummation of such transaction.

9.3 <u>Financing</u>. That ABC shall be able to borrow the sum of $_____ as is set forth in Section Seven above.

9.4 <u>Conduct of Audiology Business.</u> The audiology business of CHS complies with all laws and rules and regulations of all jurisdictions having lawful authority to regulate this profession of CHS, so as not to place the audiology practice of CHS in violation of any laws or rules and regulations or ordinances.

SECTION TEN

Risk of Loss

10.1 <u>Before and After Closing</u>. All risk of loss to the assets of CHS, whether the same be by fire or other hazard, shall, until the Closing Date, be that of CHS. All risk of loss to the assets of CHS after the date of Closing shall be that of ABC.

SECTION ELEVEN

Restrictions on Disclosure by ABC

11.1 <u>Confidential Nature of Sale</u>. It is understood and agreed between CHS and ABC that as a result of said sale of the said patient files to ABC, ABC shall be obtaining medical information of a confidential nature. ABC shall maintain the confidentiality of all information or knowledge so obtained. ABC shall not disclose any such information or knowledge to any third party, without the express permission of the patient. ABC shall hold CHS and Dr. A harmless from an liability as a result of any disclosure by ABC in breach of this Agreement.

SECTION TWELVE

CHS Name Use

12.1 <u>Change of Name</u>. CHS shall execute a proper amendment to the Articles of its corporation, changing its name as registered with the Secretary of State of the State of [State] and deliver executed copies of that Resolution to ABC on the Closing Date, and shall execute any other document as may reasonably be required by ABC, which would allow ABC to change its name to CHS, or any facsimile thereof.

SECTION THIRTEEN

Adjustments

13.1 <u>Adjustments</u>. If there exist at time of Closing any prepaid rent under the Lease, or any prepaid utilities, or any prepaid payroll or any prepaid advertising, an amount equal to the amounts so prepaid shall be repaid by ABC to CHS. ABC shall pay to the Lessor such damage deposits as may be required by the Lessor.

SECTION FOURTEEN

Service Plan

14.1 <u>Liabilities to Third Parties</u>. CHS has sold and/or distributed to various patients or potential patients certain coupon books and service plans which give patients holding such coupon books and service plans the right to receive from CHS hearing aid batteries and to receive from CHS, at no cost to the patient, hearing tests and hearing aid checks and office visits. With respect to any service plans and coupon books delivered to ABC after date of Closing, CHS will deliver to ABC at no cost to ABC, hearing aid batteries in an equal amount to the hearing aid batteries which ABC may distribute to the patients who have presented to him the coupon book service plan. ABC in this regard agrees to honor all coupon book service plans that request the delivery of hearing aid batteries, with the understanding that the hearing aid batteries will be reimbursed to ABC by CHS for a period of 3 years from Closing Date. With respect to any requests of ABC for hearing tests or hearing aid checks or office visits as a result of the coupon book service plan, ABC will perform such functions as may be required of ABC as disclosed in the coupon book service plan and agrees to hold harmless and indemnify CHS from any liability or obligation which CHS might have to third parties to provide hearing tests or hearing aid checks or office visits as a result of any coupon book service plan issued by CHS.

SECTION FIFTEEN

Debt on Automobile

15.1 <u>Assumption of Debt</u>. At time of Closing, there shall be a bank debt on the automobile described in Section One in an amount not to exceed the sum of $1,500.00. Payments on the automobile shall be current. Payments due after the date of Closing shall be made by ABC and ABC shall indemnify CHS from any loss or liability, should ABC fail to make those payments when due.

SECTION SIXTEEN

Signage

16.1 <u>Signage Installation or Credit</u>. CHS is currently working with other tenants of the building wherein the office is part, for the joint construction of signage on the exterior of the building. CHS shall use its best efforts to have the signage completed and paid for by the time of Closing. The signage will display as one of the tenants in the building CHS. In the event that the signage is not completed at time of Closing and in the event that CHS has not paid for any installation of the signage, then and in that event CHS shall pay ABC at the time of Closing the sum of $_____. If no sign is installed with 12 months, ABC shall refund to CHS said $_____.

SECTION SEVENTEEN

Accounts Payable and Receivable of CHS

17.1 <u>Accounts Payable and Receivable—Obligations</u>. Accounts Receivable of CHS are not involved in this transaction and shall remain, in all respects, the property of CHS after the date of Closing. Accounts Payable by CHS and all other liabilities of CHS (except those payable on the automobile) are not assumed by ABC and shall be the sole obligation of CHS after the date of Closing. CHS shall indemnify and save harmless ABC from any liability or obligation with respect to the business of CHS unpaid or unsatisfied as of the date of Closing. After the date of Closing, ABC shall deliver to CHS all mail which is directed to CHS at the Office address, including, but not limited to, all payments made to CHS for professional services rendered by CHS to patients prior to the date of Closing.

SECTION EIGHTEEN

Miscellaneous

18.1 <u>Notices</u>. All notices, requests, demands, and other communications required or permitted by this Agreement shall be in writing and shall be deemed to have been given at the time when mailed at any general or branch United States post office, registered or certified mail and postage prepaid, return receipt requested, to the address as stated below, which address may be amended in writing from time to time in the manner herein provided for notices:

As to CHS or Dr. A: 1234 W. Main St.
                    Central City, [State]
As to ABC: 1234 Hearing Aid Rd.
             Central City, [State]

18.2 <u>Agreement. Modification, Waiver</u>. This Agreement constitutes the entire agreement between the parties hereto pertaining to the subject matter hereof and supersedes all prior agreements, understandings, negotiations, and discussions, whether oral or written, of the parties, and there are no warranties, representations or agreements between the parties in connection with the subject matter hereof, except as set forth or referred to herein. No supplement, modification or waiver or termination of this Agreement, or any provision hereof, shall be binding unless executed in writing by the parties to be bound. No waiver of any provision of this Agreement shall constitute a waiver of any other provision, nor shall such waiver constitute a continuing waiver unless otherwise expressly provided.

18.3 <u>Headings</u>. Sections and subsection headings are not to be considered part of this Agreement and are included solely for convenience and are not intended to be full or accurate descriptions of the contents hereof.

18.4 <u>Exhibits</u>. Exhibits referred to in this Agreement are an integral part of this Agreement and are hereby incorporated by reference into this Agreement.

18.5 <u>Successors and Assigns</u>. This Agreement is not assignable or transferable by either party. If Mr. B, who is the sole stockholder of ABC shall die prior to Closing, this agreement shall be null and void. This Agreement shall inure to the benefit of and be binding upon the parties hereto and their permitted respective successors and assigns. All representations of both parties shall survive the Closing.

18.6 <u>Governing Laws</u>. The parties hereby agree that this Agreement has been executed in the State of [State] and shall be governed by the laws of the State of [State].

18.7 <u>Parties of Interest</u>. Nothing in this Agreement is intended to confer upon any person other than CHS and Dr. A and ABC any right or remedies under or by reason of this Agreement, nor is anything in this Agreement intended to relieve or discharge the liability of any other party, nor shall any provision hereof give any entity any right of subrogation against or action against any party to this Agreement.

18.8 <u>Counterpart</u>. This Agreement may be executed in one or more counterparts, each of which shall be deemed an original, but all of which separately shall constitute one and the same Agreement.

18.9 <u>Inserverability</u>. The provisions of this Agreement are intended to be inseverable. The invalidity or unenforceability of any provision, or portion of any provision in this Agreement, shall render the entire Agreement null and void and unenforceable.

18.10 <u>Acknowledgment of Reading and Receipt</u>. The parties, by the signing of this Agreement, state that this Agreement has been read and that they hereto agree to each and every provision of this Agreement and do hereby acknowledge receipt of a copy of this Agreement.

SECTION NINETEEN

Office Supplies

19.1 <u>Change in Office Supplies</u>. A part of Exhibit "C" is a list entitled "Office Supplies." After the date of this Agreement, CHS shall use and replenish such supplies in the ordinary course of doing business. Office supplies on hand at time of closing shall be the office supplies sold under this Agreement and such supplies may be greater than, or less than, those supplies shown under "Office Supplies" of Exhibit "C."

SECTION TWENTY

Copier Lease

20.1 <u>Lease Rights</u>. At time of closing, CHS, without any additional payment from ABC, shall transfer to ABC all of its Lease rights in a certain [manufacturer's name] Copier (Model #_____).

IN WITNESS WHEREOF, the parties have executed this Agreement this _____ date of _____, 19_____.

By_____
   Dr. A

CARDINAL HEARING SERVICES, INC., a [State] Corporation

By_____
   Dr. A, Its President

ABC Corporation, a [State] Corporation

By_____
   Mr. B, Its President

PERSONAL GUARANTEE

Mr. B, being the owner of all, or the majority of the stock of ABC Corporation, for valuable consideration, the receipt and sufficiency of which is hereby acknowledged, does hereby agree to personally guarantee all of the undertakings of ABC Corporation herein contained, including those undertakings which survive or may survive the Closing of the transaction contemplated hereby.

     _____
     Mr. B.

THIS AGREEMENT PREPARED BY:

_____, Attorney for
Dr. A and Cardinal Hearing Services, Inc.
[attorney's address and telephone number]

20

Audiologists as Managers

> *To survive in today's evolving business environment, audiologists must adopt modern management skills*

As the 21st century approaches, the scope of management is changing dramatically, not only in business but also in other facets of modern society such as health care service delivery. The focus is on how to manage in increasingly competitive and global environments where expanding technology is being offset by a contracting work force. Political, economic, social, and technological (PEST) influences in these environments must be used in innovative ways that reduce costs while encouraging individual contributions and enhancing overall quality. The challenge for today's employees and managers is to adopt and promote new leadership skills and flexible organizations as the foundations of success.

Audiologists typically have not viewed themselves as operating in the mainstream of American business

The successful audiologist of the 1990s and beyond needs to grasp the significance of the changing work place and adopt successful management skills and strategies to survive and flourish. Audiologists, whether running their own practices or as employees in a larger organization, must prepare to accept larger roles in adapting the work place to meet the desires or needs of the customer or patient. The guiding principle is that the business process starts with the customer. This principle seems obvious and has been recognized for many years in other service industries (Firnstahl, 1989). But the concept of managing for the customer is only now beginning to be addressed in a sophisticated manner in the areas of communication disorders (Harrison, 1994; Singleton-Filio, 1993).

Modern management is a natural development of the Industrial Revolution

THE EVOLUTION OF MANAGEMENT

The turmoil facing society and businesses today is not unlike that which remade the agrarian societies of the early 19th century. It was called the Industrial Revolution because it changed the very fabric of society. Individuals, families, communities, and the culture itself were forever altered by the forces of this phenomenon. Today, we are embarking on some of the most significant societal and economic changes that have occurred in the last two centuries. The step into the 21st century is presenting numerous indications that there will be major restructuring in the work place as well as society. As industries such as health care become more global in nature, the ability of enterprises to compete will be enhanced by the talents and skills of its managers and people. To survive, organizations and the individuals comprising them will have to constantly strive to reinvent themselves to stay viable (Peters, 1993).

The industrial age was preceded by the era of the craftsman and his apprentices. Guilds and apprenticeships were one of the earliest forms of management. Skilled individuals such as carpenters, tailors, shoemakers, blacksmiths, and others were very familiar with their customers. They knew them by name and were able to tailor their goods and services to the individual consumer's requirements. They could not, however, produce the volume of goods and services demanded by a rapidly expanding industrial society. Soon more modern manufacturing processes began to dominate, and the personal relationship between the craftsman and the end consumer began to disappear. The age of the Industrial Revolution was upon society (Scherkenbach, 1991).

Management is more than keeping track of money, production, and people—it is a professional discipline with a history

The concept of customer primacy was lost to modern business for many years

Modern management was a natural development of the Industrial Revolution. As society moved from an agrarian culture to an urban environment and as the demands for goods and services escalated, new skills and techniques were required to run the factories and direct the expanded work force. The evolution of these skills became the basis of modern management. Over time, different schools of management developed to address the growing and changing needs of industrial-based societies. As in most human endeavors, a lot of trial and error was involved in the evolution of management training. The early schools focused on process solutions and organizational structure, to the exclusion of human variables. Later schools of thought began to recognize an equation in which human factors interacted with productivity and organizational structure.

Classical School

The earliest school of management thought was the *Classical School.* The Classical School is generally broken into two segments: The *Scientific Management* approach concentrated on increasing productivity of the facility and the work force; the *Organizational Theory* concentrated on how to manage these new organizations (Stoner & Wankel, 1986).

Scientific management was key in addressing the system or process side of the management equation. Scientific management developed several concepts that improved efficiency:

■ the division of labor, which became the foundation for the concept of the assembly line,
■ time motion studies, which were used to speed up manufacturing by increasing efficiency, and
■ systems such as Gantt Charts to improve production scheduling (Stoner & Wankel, 1986).

The weakness or limitation of this approach was that it did not distinguish workers as unique from machines or other technical parts of the process, believing that management could be defined solely by quantitative measures.

Classical Organizational Theory used large organizational work forces such as the military as models for systematizing management. This theory defined many of the principles of management we are familiar with today, such as division of labor, hierarchical "vertical" organizations, centralization, discipline, subordination of individual interest, stability, and

The concept of the assembly line emerged from the classical school

authority. As their name implies, organizational theorists were interested in structure. They believed management could be diagramed, measured, and built by controlling all variables. Educationally, they believed that management could and should be taught; they called for the introduction of management training in schools (Stoner & Wankel, 1986). Most current schools of business owe their inception to this theory of management.

Many of the principles of Classical Organizational Theory are being challenged and eliminated in the downsizing corporations of today. Current business texts describe a new world of dynamic work teams and new corporate structures that will be required to survive and succeed in the new global economies (Boyett & Conn, 1991). But well before today's demands, managers realized that they had been addressing only one side of the management equation by tailoring systems and structures. The question arose of how to improve and motivate the human component.

Behaviorism

The *Behavioral School* was a response to the failure of the classical approaches to completely resolve issues of work place efficiency and harmony (Stoner & Wankel, 1986). The behaviorists were the first to address the people side of the management equation. They concentrated on determining what motivated employees and using their insights on human motivation to build a better work force. Many corporations today use behaviorist concepts in management training and procedures. One of the best examples of human motivation came from Elton Mayo's Hawthorne Experiments from which the *Hawthorne Effect* was derived (Hersey & Blanchard, 1982). Initial results in these management experiments were confusing. As predicted, worker productivity increased when the experimenters introduced environmental improvements (e.g. better lighting). The unexpected and unexplained finding, however, was that worker productivity also improved when the same factory environments were degraded (e.g. poorer lighting). In short, workers responded to management initiative whether it was positive or negative. The key was that management was taking action and the researchers finally concluded that employees worked harder if they believed management was concerned about them (Hersey & Blanchard, 1982).

The behaviorists recognize that motivation varies with the individual. Their approaches demand that managers tailor their communication to each individual and accept the premise that as a rule all workers are willing workers.

> Behavioralists recognized that people were part of the production equation

Practitioners of Behaviorism concentrate on motivating employees to produce within the boundaries of the business system. As the 1990s come to a close, the demands of the work place are that employees become "self-starters," assuming responsibility for creating and maintaining their own motivation in the work place.

Management Science

The *Management Science* approach to management was born out of necessity during World War II in response to the shortage of manpower and huge production demands that prevailed. Management science is generally used as a problem-solving approach for large organizations. Here, specialists from key disciplines are brought together to create a mathematical model of a problem and provide management with rational bases for decision making (Stoner & Wankel, 1982). Although management science uses a traditional quantitative systems-oriented approach, it is also the first theory to break away from hierarchically structured organizations and advocate problem-oriented, flexible working teams. Also, as organizations continue to downsize in today's economic environment, it may have a rebirth as more use is made of computerized modeling for decision making.

Management Science created work teams for mathematical problem solving

Systems Management

The *systems approach* to management evolved from work teams made up of employee experts. This modern approach advocates breaking down organizational barriers and allowing a freer flow of information and procedures, thus creating a continual improvement process through team work and feedback (Scherkenbach, 1991). In systems management, work teams are flexible and transient, with their composition and life span dictated by the problem they address. For example, a team might consist of contracted members who report to a corporate representative for the life of the project. At the end of the project, the team is then broken up and eliminated. When a new project is started, a new team is formed. This is a situation analogous to a movie company making a movie. Actors, producers, directors, technicians and others are all brought together as a team for the project of making a movie. When the movie is completed, the team is broken up and members go off and sign up on another project with different players.

Systems Management uses transient teams of experts, based on changing needs

A very current example of the systems approach was the design and development of the 1994 Mustang by *"Team*

Mustang." The team completed the remake of the car 25% faster and with 30% less cost than comparable new car programs. Team Mustang did it by breaking down the paradigms of traditional production teams and bringing diverse groups, even suppliers, together under one roof to develop and bring to market the best car in the most efficient manner and at the lowest cost (White & Oscar, 1993).

A current example in the hearing aid industry is the total team approach adopted by Oticon, where stationary desks were replaced in 1991 with employee carts that move with employees to different project teams as ideas and problems arise. All communications, including mail which is optically scanned, goes through a computer workstation network that makes the entire plant a paperless operation. This systems approach allowed Oticon to bring the Multifocus programmable hearing aid to market in half the usual time, resulting in a significant increase in market share and profits. The management change was as dramatic as the effect on profits: To quote Lars Kolind, chief of Oticon,

> We removed the entire formal organization. We took away all departments. We took away all managers' titles. And with them went the red tape. There are no secretaries to protect us. (Peters, 1994, p. B4)

Contingency Management

Contingency management addresses new management needs brought about by the system theory. It advocates allowing management to tailor management techniques to the situation. The philosophy of this theory is that as situations change, the management technique applied should also change (Stoner, 1982). For flexible work teams to be effective, management teams that have diverse sets of skills must also be constructed. Managers cannot be solely bound to one set of procedures for arriving at solutions. They need to be adept in recognizing the contributing factors in different situations and then bring the right skills and techniques to bear.

Contingency Management requires flexible, adaptive management styles with different teams of workers

In the future, individuals and organizations that adopt combinations of systems and contingency styles will have a better chance of success. This is because their approach will be incorporating earlier approaches in a much more adaptive manner.

THE JOB OF MANAGEMENT

In any industry or profession the primary job of management is to define the business. It begins by determining

Audiology must define itself in the eyes of its patients and customers

"Who is the customer?" because the business process starts with the customer. What product the business provides is not determined by the producer but by what the customer or consumer buys (Peters, 1991).

The first steps in defining the business are to determine who the customer is, how to reach the customer, and what the customer considers of value (Drucker, 1986). Once it is determined what the business will be, then management can tailor itself to what the business should be through constant contact with its customers. Not paying attention to these basic first steps has dire consequences. Many a business has failed, even though everyone performed with dedication and devotion, because it produced the wrong product or service.

The need to define the business is as true for audiologists as it is for any other business or profession. Audiology as part of the health care service industry must define itself in the eyes of its patients or consumers. Who are our patients? How can we reach them? How do they perceive us and our service in relation to other health care providers? And what is it that they consider of value?

In addition to the primary consumer or patient, audiologists have numerous secondary customers or suppliers to be considered in defining the business. What are the needs and expectations of the different referral services? Are you providing service to third party payers? What does the patient's family expect? How do the patients friends and acquaintances perceive the effects of your services? Are you following FDA guidelines? These and many more customers need to be considered in defining the practice (Singleton-Filio, 1993).

Once the business is defined, the next step for the manager is to develop a vision of what the future should or could be. This vision forms the basis for developing the plan for achieving the results of the vision. From the vision we determine the objectives and build the strategies and action plans to achieve the vision. Such philosophical efforts may seem ethereal and of little practical (i.e., immediate) value to new practitioners. A carefully enunciated vision, however, forms the cornerstone on which a business stands and flourishes. Without that cornerstone, the business is sure to founder eventually.

A mission statement defines the purpose of the audiology practice

When a new business entity begins or redefines its direction, it must determine its basic goals and philosophies. A common vehicle to achieve this is what is called a *mission statement*. The statement is one of attitude, outlook, and orientation. Its objectives are to ensure purpose, a basis for motivation, and establish an organizational climate. It basically defines the purpose of the business, what the business does, and where the business operates.

For an audiology practice, a mission statement might define who the primary and secondary customers are, what products and services are provided, what geographic locations are serviced, what types of technologies are employed, what the philosophy of operation is, how the audiologists see themselves in relation to the health care community, and what the audiologists' concerns for the public are (Pearce & Robinson, 1991). The mission statement needs to be put in writing, explained and discussed with all employees, posted for customers to read, and periodically reviewed and revised.

With the mission defined, a business needs to define its objectives or goals and put them in writing. It is wise to base these objectives on an analysis of the operating environment in which the business functions. In the case of the audiologist, what are the strengths and weaknesses of the practice? Do employees have special areas of expertise or lack expertise in areas for which there is consumer demand? Does the practice have a large physician referral base or does it relying on self-referrals? What opportunities or threats does the practice face? Are they building a new clinic next door to your private practice? Is a well-established provider moving into your traditional territory? Your objectives need to relate to your stated mission and perceived situation.

Goals and objectives need to exhibit several qualities. They should be specific. Unlike the mission statement, goals and objectives are precise, and they are measurable. They also must be motivating. Objectives should be aggressive in nature with specific time frames that can be realistically achieved with extended effort.

Make goals and objectives specific and concise

Once the goals and objectives are defined and documented, the practice needs to set strategies and action plans to achieve them. The strategies are used to outline how the practice proposes to achieve its strategic goals, and the action plans identify what must be done by whom and when to meet the objectives. The key to the action plans is the assigning of responsibilities, setting deadlines and implementing checks and balances. Again, the action plans must be in writing. Scenario 20–1 looks at management considerations when goals are not well understood by an employee and an objective is not met.

SCENARIO 20-1

Every quarter the staff of Cardinal Hearing Services (CHS) gets together to review the last quarter's performance to objectives, analyze any areas that fell below objectives, and set the objectives for the next quarter. Often this activity results in additional staff work to be shared by all members of the staff.

For example, one activity is to contact patients who fall into the inactive category, meaning that they have not been seen or contacted for some predetermined period of time. This helps CHS weed out truly inactive files and bring a certain percentage of patients back into the practice. The work is divided up among Dr. A and the rest of the staff and a target date for completion is set.

Mr. B is one of the senior employees. He fails to make any effort to complete his part of the assignment. At the target completion date, very few patients in Mr. B's group have been contacted. Other staff members have done better, but none have brought their assignment to completion.

Analysis:

This is a situation where management thought there was consensus and commitment and there was not. It is also a situation where an experienced and senior employee adopts a passive but insubordinate position that does not support the direction of the practice and in effect undermines the authority of management and the morale of the rest of the staff. The staff is always well aware when these contests of wills are being played out. Management needs to address and resolve the situation directly.

Question 1: Everyone was slow to start and the target date was missed. What is your response as manager?

Suggested Answer: With everyone slow to get started, it is obvious that there was not the commitment you assumed at the start of the project. In the future, you will need to ensure that the commitment is firm. Use project management techniques such as Gantt charts to clearly identify to the staff when phases of a project are to be completed. In the situation at hand, the manager needs to go back to the staff, individually or as a group, and reestablish the objectives. Failure to follow up sends a message to the staff that passive resistance is an effective strategy to avoid doing unpopular activities.

Question 2: The majority of the staff is actively completing their assignments, and the practice is seeing an influx patient contacts as a result of this activity. Is it important that Mr. B has not started yet?

Suggested Answer: It is very important that Mr. B has not really started yet. In fact Mr. B's lack of participation may be part of the reason no one started or finished on time. Mr. B, as one of the senior employees, is a role model; and if his response is at best to ignore the activity and at worse to subvert the activity, it is very important that his behavior be challenged and modified.

Question 3: The value of this activity is plainly apparent. It has resulted in a dramatic increase in patient contacts and revenues for the practice. Should you ignore the issue with Mr. B for now and divide up his portion among the rest of the staff to get the contacts completed?

Suggested Answer: You should only divide up Mr. B's assignment if you get rid of Mr. B. Failure to step up to the issue of insubordination and then expecting other staff members to carry the load will create a major management and leadership issue down the road.

Question 4: Mr. B is a real nice guy and he has been very adroitly putting you off on his progress. You're very busy and do not need the hassle at this time. Should you just write this off as one of Mr. B's eccentricities and get on with your other activities?

Suggested Answer: As owner/manager you cannot afford to opt for the path of least resistance no matter how busy the rest of your schedule is. It is important that a leadership position be established with Mr. B and for the rest of the staff. Failure by a manager to establish and maintain his or her position of leadership leads to an eventual crisis situation for any business. A practice without a course of direction and a firm hand guiding it will soon founder. The art of management often involves addressing uncomfortable situations. The manager has a responsibility to the practice to develop and enhance his or her leadership qualities. Failure to do so will be to the extreme detriment of the practice. Certain core qualities and skills are required to get any organization through challenging periods, and leadership is one of them.

THE CHANGING BUSINESS ENVIRONMENT

It is important to say again that there is a new climate of business today. This changing climate affects the traditional role and scope of the job of management. Companies are downsizing to keep costs in check and increase their competitive edge. Downsizing means fewer employees to manage, resulting in a "flattening" of hierarchies and bringing workers closer to the decision-making point.

Flatter hierarchies bring audiologists closer to the product

Audiologists have an opportunity to take advantage of the effects of downsizing in the health care services industry by positioning the profession as the entry point for consumers with hearing loss into the health care system. Ninety percent or more of hearing losses in the adult population are not amenable to medical treatment (Grahl, 1993), and many health care dollars would be saved if medical referrals to specialists were based on audiologic findings (Yaremchuk, Schmidt, & Dickson, 1990). Audiologists advocating this position can point out that it results in fewer levels of "management," lowers health care costs, and improves the quality of hearing health care services. But our apparently unassailable position is supportable only if audiologists become effective, *modern* managers.

Audiologists must assume responsibility for the satisfaction and concerns of their patients and customers

The scope of the manager's job traditionally has been to control and monitor the business process. Outside of strategic planning, in the past, managers ran businesses by looking backward at how they did. They implemented company policy and directed, monitored and evaluated employee performance. Now, managers are being asked to be more proactive in running businesses. They are being called upon to develop employees and empower individuals to take responsibility for their own performance and the customer's satisfaction for the goods or service that are being delivered (DePree, 1989). For the audiology model, that means that the patient's service provider is responsible for the satisfaction of the patient and is expected to take the steps necessary to address concerns of the patient and related customers. This can and often does mean following up with the referring or primary care provider, counselling with family members, resolving issues with insurance providers, acting as a liaison to suppliers of devices or instruments, and familiarizing potential customers with the goals and "products" of the practice.

Flatter Hierarchies Mean Audiologists Are:

- *Closer to the product*
- *Responsible for customer satisfaction*

Flatter hierarchies mean that everyone is "closer to the product." Organizations are leaner, and everyone makes more than one contribution to the operation. Few companies today can afford people who can only type or file or use the computer. Everyone has to be able to stretch. The employed audiologist may be very much like the entrepreneurial audiologist in that emptying the trash, filing patient records, and using the computer for managing the office are tasks that are very much within the scope of the job.

Flatter hierarchies also mean that responsibility for the patient's satisfaction resides with the care provider. Managers in this environment need to provide employees with the training, confidence, support, and authority to make the decisions necessary to satisfy the customer. For management, this means providing guidelines and clear communications on what the goals and philosophies of the business are. This puts a sizable burden on audiologists to learn to motivate, train, communicate and lead by example. We conclude this chapter with the following scenario, which looks at management decisions that are needed when customer satisfaction is critical and employee responsibility is lacking.

Scenario 20–2

Mr. B is the senior audiologist in CHS's second office. He has wonderful talents and an imposing knowledge in the field. However, Dr. A finds that Mr. B is occupying an inordinate amount of her time because she get a disproportionate number of complaints about his manner. Dr. A has also noticed that some of CHS's patients have switched to other providers without explanation.

Besides the complaints, the situation has manifested itself in several other troubling formats that range from patients storming out of examination rooms, improper fittings of hearing aids, and patients showing up without appointments.

Today, one of CHS's best patients (who has been with CHS since it first opened 5 years ago) came in to pick up new hearing aids. The aids she is expected are a second set of CIC aids that she intends to use as back-up while on a 2-month tour of China. She is leaving in 3 days on the tour. The patient saw Mr. B 1 week ago. He assured her there would be no problem getting in the instruments fitted before her trip. There are no entries in her file, no indication that any aids have

(continued)

Scenario 20–2 *(continued)*

been ordered, and no unaccounted for aids have been received in either of CHS's two offices.

Analysis:

On the strength of Dr. A's interpersonal skills, the situation may be salvageable. If everything goes as planned, the patient will appreciate CHS's responsiveness. This is one more time, though, that Dr. A has had to recover one of Mr. B's fumbles. Mr. B's brusque manner and hurried approach have been a constant theme throughout his periodic reviews and a disruptive influence on the rest of the staff and the operation of the practice in general.

Questions and Management Direction for Dr. A:

Question 1. First and foremost, how do you handle the patient right now?

Suggested Answer: Apologize to the patient for the obvious disorganization. Prevail upon her graciousness to allow you time to unravel things. Give her assurances that every effort will be made to get her off to China with her new hearing aids. Tell her you will get back to her within the hour with a plan of action.

Question 2. Mr. B confirms the patient encounter, but cannot recall what happened with the impressions. How do you handle this initial encounter with Mr. B?

Suggested Answer: Your initial response needs to focus on solving the patient's problem and recovering her goodwill and continued patronage. Slowly walk Mr. B through the encounter, updating the patient's files as required, and determine what exactly happened. Having an emotional angry outburst with Mr. B will not help resolve the patient's problem. It may or may not feel good, but it resolves nothing and will probably create other problems just when you do not need them.

Question 3. Or, Mr. B apologizes for not documenting the patient encounter but insists that he sent the impressions to the manufacturer. A call to the manufacturer reveals that they did receive some impressions on the day in question, but they were not accompanied by an audiogram, order form, name, or account number. They have been waiting for someone to call looking for delinquent hearing aids! If CHS faxes them an audiogram before noon, they guarantee hearing aid delivery by 10:00 a.m. tomorrow. How do you handle the call to your patient?

Suggested Answer: Once the facts are known and you have developed a course of action, honesty is the best policy with the patient. Without naming names, explain the situation and the alternatives that you can provide. You will need to be receptive to the patient's suggestions or desires, and if all that works out, you will need to recover the patient's goodwill. That may mean a deep "goodwill" discount on the instruments on top of bending over backward to be responsive.

Question 4: The audiogram has been faxed to the manufacturer. The patient is amenable to rearranging her schedule and coming in tomorrow morning. What is your approach with Mr. B?

Suggested Answer: When all the dust has settled, Mr. B's on-the-job performance must be addressed. Most of us dislike the confrontation of dealing with a difficult personnel issue, but in this instance, the life of the practice may very well be in jeopardy.

Patients perceive Mr. B to be rude because he seldom slows down long enough to find out why they are there. They do not perceive a caring and consultative approach. Misdiagnosis or misprescription occurs sometimes because there is a failure to probe for patient history or complaints. In those cases, it usually takes an additional visit and a third party (whoever gets the patient the next time) to determine the patient's original complaint. Patients show up without appointments because Mr. B is too busy to enter appointments into the schedule. This causes confusion and anger on the part of the patient, embarrassment for the rest of the staff, and juggling of resources to accommodate the patient. For the practice though, the worst event is the patients who eventually take their business elsewhere. They vote with their feet as they walk out of your practice and into someone else's. This begins a chain reaction of events that has numerous negative impacts on the practice.

When patients quietly leave the effects are lingering. First, it is a while before the practice realizes they are gone. When any service organization fails to *promptly* rectify an unhappy encounter, the relationship is broken. The patient is not so reticent with others outside your practice. They have surely shared their experiences with friends and relatives, destroying one of the most rewarding aspects of autonomous endeavors, self-generating referrals. Also, the practice can be sure they have shared their feelings with their new provider and their original referral source. This sends a negative message about your practice to your peers and referral sources in the community.

If you been a good manager and kept well-documented periodic performance reviews on all your employees, now is the time to clearly inform Mr. B he is being fired and for what reasons. If you have not been doing a good job in the human resources area, it is now time to start. Clearly, inform Mr. B as to what is happening now and what will happen if things do not change.

SUMMARY

To survive in today's evolving business environment, audiologists need to grasp the significance of the changing health care environment. They must adopt modern management skills and strategies to survive and thrive in the market place. The concept of the primacy of the customer is key to this survival.

Modern management has evolved since the Industrial Revolution. The first school of management was the *Classical School*. It had two branches: *Scientific Management* focused on process control, such as assembly lines to improve production; *Organizational Theory* developed many of our traditional business concepts, such as division of labor and vertical organization.

The classicists were followed by the *behaviorists*. The Behavioralist School addressed the shortcomings of classical approaches by evaluating factors that affected employee motivation. By concentrating on the human aspect, a management equation began to emerge, combining the classicist's concern for production control with the behaviorist's concern for human motivation.

World War II prompted the *Management Science* approach, which attempted to solve complex problems mathematically for large organizations with limited manpower. *Systems management* is a modern management approach in which flexible work teams from diverse groups are brought together to handle specific problems and tasks. *Contingency management* advocates different management styles depending on the situation at hand.

The primary job of management is to *define* the business. This is as true of audiology as any other business. The key to defining the practice is to determine who the customers are. Having defined the practice, audiologists need to set the *vision*, set the *objectives*, build the *strategies*, and establish *action plans*.

Today's business environment is characterized by a downsizing of work forces and a flattening of management hierarchies. The old-fashioned scope of management to control and monitor is being replaced with new requirements to motivate, train, support, and lead. As audiologists learn and implement modern management concepts, the profession has an opportunity to improve the level of service to patients and become a more vigorous entry point into the health care system.

REFERENCES

Boyett, J., & Conn, H. (1992). *Workplace 2000*. New York: Plume.

Depree, M. (1989). *Leadership is an art*. New York: Dell.

Drucker, P. (1986). *The practice of management*. New York: Harper & Row.

Grahl, C. (1993). Hearing care reform: Changing access, changing reimbursement. *Hearing Instruments, 44*(8), 8–15.

Harrison, M. (Ed.). (1994). Total quality management: Application to audiology. *Seminars in Hearing, 15*(4), 259–330.

Hersey, P., & Blanchard, K. (1982). *Management of organizational behavior.* Englewood Cliffs, NJ: Prentice-Hall.

Pearce, J. A., II, & Robinson, R. B., Jr. (1991). *Formulation, implementation and control of competitive strategy* (4th ed.). Homewood, IL: Irwin.

Peters, T. (1991, September 17). Concern for quality is dandy, but the customer is still No. 1. *The Arizona Daily Star,* p. A6.

Peters, T. (1993, September 14). Economic race is likely to go to the curious, slightly mad. *The Arizona Daily Star,* p. B4.

Peters, T. (1993, September 21). Biggies must invent a new game or lose out to discounters. *The Arizona Daily Star,* p. B4.

Peters, T. (1994, August 9). It's all or nothing when changing culture of your firm. *The Arizona Daily Star,* p. B4.

Scherkenbach, W. (1991). *The Deming route to quality and productivity.* Rockville, MD: Mercury Press.

Singleton-Filio, K. (1993, Summer). Starting with a commitment to quality: The creation of an organization. *Quality Improvement Digest,* pp. 1–6.

Stoner, J., & Wankel, C. (1986). *Management* (3rd ed.). Englewood Cliffs, NJ: Prentice-Hall.

White, J., & Oscar, S. (1993, September 21). How a "skunk works" kept the mustang alive—on a tight budget. *The Wall Street Journal,* p. A1.

Yaremchuk, K., Schmidt, J., & Dickson, L. (1990). Entry of the hearing impaired into the health care system. *Henry Ford Hospital Medical Journal, 38*(1), 13–15.

APPENDIX I

Record Keeping

This Appendix contains information on record keeping, much of it in the fashion of sample forms used in different audiology practices. It is divided into four sections:

Section A. Registering the business

Section B. Professional communications with physicians

Section C. Patient forms

      1. General information
      2. History and testing
      3. Hearing aids
      4. Patient satisfaction

The potpourri of forms in Sections B and C is meant to convey a few ways in which different audiologists have approached their markets and acknowledged state and federal regulations. By including these samples, we are in no way advocating their use by other audiologists, although they may provide helpful guidelines. Audiologists should develop their own forms that: (1) characterize their own, unique practices; (2) best target their particular target markets; and (3) conform to contemporary rules and regulations.

Section A. Registering the Practice

The following are federal forms that apply regardless of the state in which the practice is located. Use Form SS-4 to obtain an Employer Identification Number (EIN), as discussed in Chapter 5. Use Form 2553 if the practice is to be incorporated with an S election (also discussed in Chapter 5).

In the course of doing business, audiologists can expect to receive W-9s if they have received income from another company that did not withhold federal taxes or social security contributions (e.g., third party reimbursements directly to the audiology provider; honoraria).

There are many other forms that a practice must obtain and complete, but these vary from state to state. Consult a local accountant to find out which forms are required in the state of practice.

Form **SS-4**
(Rev. April 1991)
Department of the Treasury
Internal Revenue Service

Application for Employer Identification Number

(For use by employers and others. Please read the attached instructions before completing this form.)

EIN

OMB No. 1545-0003
Expires 4-30-94

Please type or print clearly.

1 Name of applicant (True legal name) (See instructions.)

2 Trade name of business, if different from name in line 1

3 Executor, trustee, "care of" name

4a Mailing address (street address) (room, apt., or suite no.)

5a Address of business (See instructions.)

4b City, state, and ZIP code

5b City, state, and ZIP code

6 County and state where principal business is located

7 Name of principal officer, grantor, or general partner (See instructions.) ▶

8a Type of entity (Check only one box.) (See instructions.)

☐ Individual SSN _____
☐ REMIC   ☐ Personal service corp.
☐ State/local government   ☐ National guard
☐ Other nonprofit organization (specify) _____
☐ Other (specify) ▶ _____

☐ Estate
☐ Plan administrator SSN _____
☐ Other corporation (specify) _____
☐ Federal government/military   ☐ Church or church controlled organization
                    If nonprofit organization enter GEN (if applicable) _____

☐ Trust
☐ Partnership
☐ Farmers' cooperative

8b If a corporation, give name of foreign country (if applicable) or state in the U.S. where incorporated ▶

Foreign country

State

9 Reason for applying (Check only one box.)
☐ Started new business
☐ Hired employees
☐ Created a pension plan (specify type) ▶ _____
☐ Banking purpose (specify) ▶

☐ Changed type of organization (specify) ▶ _____
☐ Purchased going business
☐ Created a trust (specify) ▶ _____
☐ Other (specify) ▶

10 Date business started or acquired (Mo., day, year) (See instructions.)

11 Enter closing month of accounting year. (See instructions.)

12 First date wages or annuities were paid or will be paid (Mo., day, year). Note: If applicant is a withholding agent, enter date income will first be paid to nonresident alien. (Mo., day, year) . . . . ▶

13 Enter highest number of employees expected in the next 12 months. Note: If the applicant does not expect to have any employees during the period, enter "0." . . . . ▶

Nonagricultural	Agricultural	Household

14 Principal activity (See instructions.) ▶

15 Is the principal business activity manufacturing?
If "Yes," principal product and raw material used ▶

☐ Yes   ☐ No

16 To whom are most of the products or services sold? Please check the appropriate box.
☐ Public (retail)   ☐ Other (specify) ▶

☐ Business (wholesale)

☐ N/A

17a Has the applicant ever applied for an identification number for this or any other business? . . . . ☐ Yes   ☐ No
Note: If "Yes," please complete lines 17b and 17c.

17b If you checked the "Yes" box in line 17a, give applicant's true name and trade name, if different than name shown on prior application.

True name ▶   Trade name ▶

17c Enter approximate date, city, and state where the application was filed and the previous employer identification number if known.

Approximate date when filed (Mo., day, year) | City and state where filed

Previous EIN

Under penalties of perjury, I declare that I have examined this application, and to the best of my knowledge and belief, it is true, correct, and complete.

Telephone number (include area code)

Name and title (Please type or print clearly.) ▶

Signature ▶

Date ▶

Note: Do not write below this line.   For official use only.

Please leave blank ▶	Geo.	Ind.	Class	Size	Reason for applying

For Paperwork Reduction Act Notice, see attached Instructions.

Cat. No. 16055N

Form **SS-4** (Rev. 4-91)

Election by a Small Business Corporation

(Under section 1362 of the Internal Revenue Code)

▶ For Paperwork Reduction Act Notice, see page 1 of instructions.

▶ See separate instructions.

OMB No. 1545-0146

Expires 8-31-96

Notes: 1. *This election, to be an "S corporation," can be accepted only if all the tests are met under Who May Elect on page 1 of the instructions; all signatures in Parts I and III are originals (no photocopies); and the exact name and address of the corporation and other required form information are provided.*

2. *Do not file Form 1120S, U.S. Income Tax Return for an S Corporation, until you are notified that your election is accepted.*

Part I	Election Information

Please Type or Print

Name of corporation (see instructions)	A Employer identification number (EIN)
Number, street, and room or suite no. (If a P.O. box, see instructions.)	B Date incorporated
City or town, state, and ZIP code	C State of incorporation

D Election is to be effective for tax year beginning (month, day, year) . . . . ▶ / /

E Name and title of officer or legal representative who the IRS may call for more information | **F** Telephone number of officer or legal representative ( )

G If the corporation changed its name or address after applying for the EIN shown in A, check this box . . . . ▶ ☐

H If this election takes effect for the first tax year the corporation exists, enter month, day, and year of the **earliest** of the following: (1) date the corporation first had shareholders, (2) date the corporation first had assets, or (3) date the corporation began doing business . . . . ▶ / /

I Selected tax year: Annual return will be filed for tax year ending (month and day) ▶ ....

If the tax year ends on any date other than December 31, except for an automatic 52-53-week tax year ending with reference to the month of December, you must complete Part II on the back. If the date you enter is the ending date of an automatic 52-53-week tax year, write "52-53-week year" to the right of the date. See Temporary Regulations section 1.441-2T(e)(3).

J Name and address of each shareholder, shareholder's spouse having a community property interest in the corporation's stock, and each tenant in common, joint tenant, and tenant by the entirety. (A husband and wife (and their estates) are counted as one shareholder in determining the number of shareholders without regard to the manner in which the stock is owned.)	K Shareholders' Consent Statement. Under penalties of perjury, we declare that we consent to the election of the above-named corporation to be an "S corporation" under section 1362(a) and that we have examined this consent statement, including accompanying schedules and statements, and to the best of our knowledge and belief, it is true, correct, and complete. (Shareholders sign and date below.)*		L Stock owned		M Social security number or employer identification number (see instructions)	N Shareholder's tax year ends (month and day)
	Signature	Date	Number of shares	Dates acquired		

*For this election to be valid, the consent of each shareholder, shareholder's spouse having a community property interest in the corporation's stock, and each tenant in common, joint tenant, and tenant by the entirety must either appear above or be attached to this form. (See instructions for Column K if a continuation sheet or a separate consent statement is needed.)

Under penalties of perjury, I declare that I have examined this election, including accompanying schedules and statements, and to the best of my knowledge and belief, it is true, correct, and complete.

Signature of officer ▶   Title ▶   Date ▶

See Parts II and III on back.   Cat. No. 18629R   Form **2553** (Rev. 9-93)

486

Part II   Selection of Fiscal Tax Year (All corporations using this part must complete item O and one of items P, Q, or R.)

O   Check the applicable box below to indicate whether the corporation is:

1. ☐   A new corporation adopting the tax year entered in item I, Part I.

2. ☐   An existing corporation retaining the tax year entered in item I, Part I.

3. ☐   An existing corporation changing to the tax year entered in item I, Part I.

P   Complete item P if the corporation is using the expeditious approval provisions of Revenue Procedure 87-32, 1987-2 C.B. 396, to request: (1) a natural business year (as defined in section 4.01(1) of Rev. Proc. 87-32), or (2) a year that satisfies the ownership tax year test in section 4.01(2) of Rev. Proc. 87-32. Check the applicable box below to indicate the representation statement the corporation is making as required under section 4 of Rev. Proc. 87-32.

1. Natural Business Year ▶ ☐ I represent that the corporation is retaining or changing to a tax year that coincides with its natural business year as defined in section 4.01(1) of Rev. Proc. 87-32 and as verified by its satisfaction of the requirements of section 4.02(1) of Rev. Proc. 87-32. In addition, if the corporation is changing to a natural business year as defined in section 4.01(1), I further represent that such tax year results in less deferral of income to the owners than the corporation's present tax year. I also represent that the corporation is not described in section 3.01(2) of Rev. Proc. 87-32. (See instructions for additional information that must be attached.)

2. Ownership Tax Year ▶ ☐ I represent that shareholders holding more than half of the shares of the stock (as of the first day of the tax year to which the request relates) of the corporation have the same tax year or are concurrently changing to the tax year that the corporation adopts, retains, or changes to per item I, Part I. I also represent that the corporation is not described in section 3.01(2) of Rev. Proc. 87-32.

Note: If you do not use item P and the corporation wants a fiscal tax year, complete either item Q or R below. Item Q is used to request a fiscal tax year based on a business purpose and to make a back-up section 444 election. Item R is used to make a regular section 444 election.

Q   Business Purpose—To request a fiscal tax year based on a business purpose, you must check box Q1 and pay a user fee. See instructions for details. You may also check box Q2 and/or box Q3.

1. Check here ▶ ☐ if the fiscal year entered in item I, Part I, is requested under the provisions of section 6.03 of Rev. Proc. 87-32. Attach to Form 2553 a statement showing the business purpose for the requested fiscal year. See instructions for additional information that must be attached.

2. Check here ▶ ☐ to show that the corporation intends to make a back-up section 444 election in the event the corporation's business purpose request is not approved by the IRS. (See instructions for more information.)

3. Check here ▶ ☐ to show that the corporation agrees to adopt or change to a tax year ending December 31 if necessary for the IRS to accept this election for S corporation status in the event: (1) the corporation's business purpose request is not approved and the corporation makes a back-up section 444 election, but is ultimately not qualified to make a section 444 election, or (2) the corporation's business purpose request is not approved and the corporation did not make a back-up section 444 election.

R   Section 444 Election—To make a section 444 election, you must check box R1 and you may also check box R2.

1. Check here ▶ ☐ to show the corporation will make, if qualified, a section 444 election to have the fiscal tax year shown in item I, Part I. To make the election, you must complete Form 8716, Election To Have a Tax Year Other Than a Required Tax Year, and either attach it to Form 2553 or file it separately.

2. Check here ▶ ☐ to show that the corporation agrees to adopt or change to a tax year ending December 31 if necessary for the IRS to accept this election for S corporation status in the event the corporation is ultimately not qualified to make a section 444 election.

Part III   Qualified Subchapter S Trust (QSST) Election Under Section 1361(d)(2)**

Income beneficiary's name and address	Social security number
Trust's name and address	Employer identification number

Date on which stock of the corporation was transferred to the trust (month, day, year) . . . . ▶   /   /

In order for the trust named above to be a QSST and thus a qualifying shareholder of the S corporation for which this Form 2553 is filed, I hereby make the election under section 1361(d)(2). Under penalties of perjury, I certify that the trust meets the definitional requirements of section 1361(d)(3) and that all other information provided in Part III is true, correct, and complete.

_____   _____
Signature of income beneficiary or signature and title of legal representative or other qualified person making the election   Date

**Use of Part III to make the QSST election may be made only if stock of the corporation has been transferred to the trust on or before the date on which the corporation makes its election to be an S corporation. The QSST election must be made and filed separately if stock of the corporation is transferred to the trust after the date on which the corporation makes the S election.

♲ *Printed on recycled paper*

487

| Form **W-9**
(Rev. December 1987)
Department of the Treasury
Internal Revenue Service | **Request for Taxpayer
Identification Number and Certification** | Give this form
to the requester. Do
NOT send to IRS. |

Please print or type

Name (If joint names, list first and circle the name of the person or entity whose number you enter in Part I below. See instructions if your name has changed.)

Address

City, state, and ZIP code

List account number(s)
here (optional) ▶

Part I **Taxpayer Identification Number**	**Part II** **For Payees Exempt From Backup Withholding (See Instructions)**
Enter your taxpayer identification number in the appropriate box. For individuals and sole proprietors, this is your social security number. For other entities, it is your employer identification number. If you do not have a number, see *How To Obtain a TIN*, below. **Note:** *If the account is in more than one name, see the chart on page 2 for guidelines on whose number to enter.*	**Social security number** | | | + | | + | | | | **OR** **Employer identification number** | | + | | | | | |	
		Requester's name and address (optional)

Certification.—Under penalties of perjury, I certify that:

(1) The number shown on this form is my correct taxpayer identification number (or I am waiting for a number to be issued to me), **and**

(2) I am not subject to backup withholding either because I have not been notified by the Internal Revenue Service (IRS) that I am subject to backup withholding as a result of a failure to report all interest or dividends, or the IRS has notified me that I am no longer subject to backup withholding (does not apply to real estate transactions, mortgage interest paid, the acquisition or abandonment of secured property, contributions to an individual retirement arrangement (IRA), and payments other than interest and dividends).

Certification Instructions.—You must cross out item (2) above if you have been notified by IRS that you are currently subject to backup withholding because of underreporting interest or dividends on your tax return. (Also see *Signing the Certification* under *Specific Instructions*, later.)

Please Sign Here Signature ▶   Date ▶

Instructions

(Section references are to the Internal Revenue Code.)

Purpose of Form.—A person who is required to file an information return with IRS must obtain your correct taxpayer identification number (TIN) to report income paid to you, real estate transactions, mortgage interest you paid, the acquisition or abandonment of secured property, or contributions you made to an individual retirement arrangement (IRA). Use Form W-9 to furnish your correct TIN to the requester (the person asking you to furnish your TIN), and, when applicable, (1) to certify that the TIN you are furnishing is correct, (2) to certify that you are not subject to backup withholding, and (3) to claim exemption from backup withholding if you are an exempt payee. Furnishing your correct TIN and making the appropriate certifications will prevent certain payments from being subject to the 20% backup withholding.

Note: *If a requester gives you a form other than a W-9 to request your TIN, you must use the requester's form.*

How To Obtain a TIN.—If you do not have a TIN, you should apply for one immediately. To apply for the number, obtain Form SS-5, Application for a Social Security Number Card (for individuals), or Form SS-4, Application for Employer Identification Number (for businesses and all other entities), at your local office of the Social Security Administration or the Internal Revenue Service. Complete and file the appropriate form according to its instructions.

To complete Form W-9 if you do not have a TIN, write "Applied For" in the space for the TIN in Part I, sign and date the form, and give it to the requester. For payments that could be subject to backup withholding, you will then have 60 days to obtain a TIN and furnish it to the requester.

During the 60-day period, the payments you receive will not be subject to the 20% backup withholding, unless you make a withdrawal. However, if the requester does not receive your TIN from you within 60 days, backup withholding, if applicable, will begin and continue until you furnish your TIN to the requester.

Note: *Writing "Applied For" on the form means that you have already applied for a TIN OR that you intend to apply for one in the near future.*

As soon as you receive your TIN, complete another Form W-9, include your new TIN, sign and date the form, and give it to the requester.

What Is Backup Withholding?—Persons making certain payments to you are required to withhold and pay to IRS 20% of such payments under certain conditions. This is called "backup withholding." Payments that could be subject to backup withholding include interest, dividends, broker and barter exchange transactions, rents, royalties, nonemployee compensation, and certain payments from fishing boat operators, but do not include real estate transactions.

If you give the requester your correct TIN, make the appropriate certifications, and report all your taxable interest and dividends on your tax return, your payments will not be subject to backup withholding. Payments you receive will be subject to backup withholding if:

(1) You do not furnish your TIN to the requester, or

(2) IRS notifies the requester that you furnished an incorrect TIN, or

(3) You are notified by IRS that you are subject to backup withholding because you failed to report all your interest and dividends on your tax return (for interest and dividend accounts only), or

(4) You fail to certify to the requester that you are not subject to backup withholding under (3) above (for interest and dividend accounts opened after 1983 only). or

(5) You fail to certify your TIN. This applies only to interest, dividend, broker, or barter exchange accounts opened after 1983, or broker accounts considered inactive in 1983.

For other payments, you are subject to backup withholding only if (1) or (2) above applies.

Certain payees and payments are exempt from backup withholding and information reporting. See *Payees and Payments Exempt From Backup Withholding*, below, and *Exempt Payees and Payments* under *Specific Instructions*, on page 2, if you are an exempt payee.

Payees and Payments Exempt From Backup Withholding.—The following lists payees that are exempt from backup withholding and information reporting. For interest and dividends, all listed payees are exempt except item (9). For broker transactions, payees listed in (1) through (13), and a person registered under the Investment Advisers Act of 1940 who regularly acts as a broker are exempt. Payments subject to reporting under sections 6041 and 6041A are generally exempt from backup withholding only if made to payees described in items (1) through (7), except that a corporation that provides medical and health care services or bills and collects payments for such services is not exempt from backup withholding or information reporting. Only payees described in items (2) through (6) are exempt from backup withholding for barter exchange transactions, patronage dividends, and payments by certain fishing boat operators.

(1) A corporation.

(2) An organization exempt from tax under section 501(a), or an individual retirement plan (IRA), or a custodial account under 403(b)(7).

(3) The United States or any agency or instrumentality thereof.

Form **W-9** (Rev. 12-87)

Section B. Professional Communications with Physicians

In almost all cases, independent audiologists communicate with physicians by sending letters or reports that summarize test results and recommendations on patients. In addition, audiologists must find ways of establishing initial contact with physicians, obtain referrals from those physicians, and comply with FDA regulations for medical clearance for hearing aid fittings. The following are a few samples of ways in which audiologists communicate with physicians.

Sample Marketing Letter to Existing Physician Referral Sources

CARDINAL HEARING SERVICES, INC.
Medical Arts Building, Suite 100
Medical Drive
Central City, [State]

January 1, 19--

John Smith, M.D.
1 Pharmacy Lane
Central City, [State]

Dear Dr. Smith:

We have just completed our ____ year of practice here in Central City, and want to take this opportunity to thank you for the confidence you have placed in us when referring your patients to our office.

We also would like to update you on some of the services we now offer, as well as make it easier and more efficient to refer patients that may benefit from our services. Enclosed you will find a Rolodex card, referral slips, and a copy of our recent newsletter.

I hope you can find the time to read the newsletter, as it not only describes some of the services we offer, but also gives an indication of our practice philosophy. We try to offer total hearing health care, and feel that people should consult with their primary care physician if they are experiencing hearing or balance problems. As you know, some causes of hearing loss (otitis media, wax impaction) often can be treated in your office and many causes of dizziness will resolve in a few days. We are available when you feel additional testing or treatment is indicated.

Over the past ___ years we have seen too many people that paid more attention to T.V. ads and offers for "free" hearing tests, than to their physicians. As you might expect, many of these people receive less than satisfactory service at more than reasonable prices.

We hope that you will encourage your patients to discuss hearing and balance problems with you, so that they may get appropriate care if indicated. We want to make it easier for you to counsel your patients regarding hearing and balance problems. My office will be contacting your staff within the next few weeks to see if you would like additional copies of our newsletter to hand out to interested patients. Also, we will be happy to provide you with a hearing screening device, a pocket otoscope, and additional literature regarding hearing and balance problems. If you think you would make use of these items, simply let your office manager or head nurse know. We will ask for him/her when we call.

If you have any questions, feel free to call me at _____.

Cordially,

_____

Dr. A

CARDINAL HEARING SERVICES, INC.
Medical Arts Building, Suite 100
Central City, [State] [Zip]
[Area code and phone number]

Date _____

Referring Physician _____

This will introduce my patient

_____

For: ☐ Diagnosis Only   ☐ Diagnosis and Treatment

Regarding: ☐ Hearing Problem
            ☐ Balance Problem
            ☐ Tinnitus
            ☐ Speech Problem
            ☐ Middle Ear Problem
            ☐ Other _____

Remarks: _____

_____

_____

_____

                  ☐   ☐   ☐   ☐   ☐
Appointment: Mon.   Tues.   Wed.   Thurs.   Fri.
              at _____ a.m.
                               p.m.   (map on back)

For record keeping and marketing purposes, it is important to give physicians a simple means of referring patients; also to inform patients of whom they are to see, the purpose of the visit, and the location of the appointment. This form and the map on the back (see next page) are one means of accomplishing these goals. This form could be put on NCR paper with copies for the physician, patient, and audiologist.

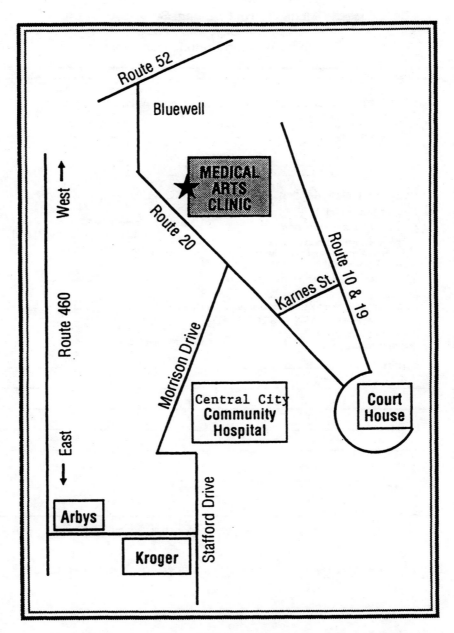

Note: This map is a good illustration of the use of Psychological Mapping discussed in Chapter 7.

CARDINAL HEARING SERVICES, INC.
Medical Arts Building, Suite 100
Central City, [State] [Zip]
[Area code and phone number]

Patient's Name _____ Date _____

Address _____ Phone _____

REFERRAL FOR EVALUATION

☐ Comprehensive Hearing Evaluation
☐ Hearing Evaluation
☐ Pediatric Hearing Evaluation
☐ Diagnostic Site of Lesion Testing
   (Special auditory tests for cochlear vs.
   eighth nerve lesion)
☐ Brain Stem Evoked Response Audiometry
☐ Diagnostic Central Auditory Testing
   (Tests for brain stem and cortical lesion,
   and central auditory processing problems)
☐ Electronystagmography
   (Balance testing)

☐ Electrocochleography
   (ECOG)
☐ Acoustic Impedance Tests
   (Tympanometry and Acoustic Reflex)
☐ Hearing Aid Evaluation
☐ Swim Plugs
☐ Pediatric Auditory Rehabilitation
☐ Earmolds
☐ Personal Hearing Protection Plugs
☐ Tinnitis Masker
☐ Otoacustic Emissions

Comments: _____
_____
_____
_____
_____

_____   _____ M.D.
Referring Agency   Referring Physician

WHITE—PHYSICIAN   CANARY—AUDIOLOGIST   PINK—PATIENT COPY

Another example of a referral form that is placed in physicians' offices.

TO: CARDINAL HEARING SERVICES, INC.

FROM:

I am referring
for a diagnostic hearing evaluation.

_____   _____
Physician's Signature   **Date**

Another example of a referral form that is placed in physician's offices. This one has much less information than the previous two examples, but is distinguished by being printed on a brightly colored light cardboard material, making it readily identifiable to the staff members and difficult to overlook.

CARDINAL HEARING SERVICES, INC.
Medical Arts Building, Suite 100
Central City, [State]
[Area code and phone number]

Patient Name: _____
Date: _____
Audiologist: _____
Reliability: _____

HEARING SCREEN

Which is your worst ear?　☐ Right　☐ Left　　　Ear Inspection:　Right_____　Left_____

	E	OU	A	I	K	T	P	S	Th
	125	250	500	750	1000	1500	2000	3000	4000	6000	8000

Ability to understand speech

-10

NORMAL

0

No significant difficulty with faint speech

10

MILD

20

Difficulty only with faint speech

30

MODERATE

40

Frequent difficulty with normal speech

50

Loss in Decibels

60

Frequent difficulty with loud speech

70

SERIOUS

80

Can understand only shouted or amplified speech

90

Usually cannot understand even amplified speech

100

PROFOUND

110

AREA OF CRITICAL SPEECH UNDERSTANDING

Middle C on piano (256 Hz)

COMPLAINT:

INTERPRETATION: _____

Dear Dr._____:

I recommend a comprehensive hearing evaluation for this patient, based on the above screening results. Please sign and return the enclosed referral form if you concur with this recommendation. Your patient's Medicare benefits may cover diagnostic audiometry if physician referred.

_____

Dr. A, Ph.D., CCC-A
Certified Clinical Audiologist

Example of a referral request form associated with hearing screening activities in a Senior population.

Acquainting physicians, agencies hospitals, and their staffs with audiology providers is a good positioning strategy for the product (hearing care) and the market (your practice). One method is to provide brief biographies of all professional staff members. These can also be given to new patients at the time of registration.

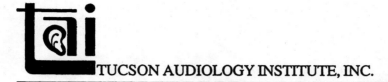

TUCSON AUDIOLOGY INSTITUTE, INC.

Mr. B, M.A., CCC-A

Mr. B is a Certified Clinical Audiologist and a licensed hearing aid dispenser in the state of [State]. He is a member of the American Speech-Language-Hearing Association, and the American Academy of Audiology. In addition, he is a licensed educational audiologist in the state of [State].

Mr. B's interest in audiology stems from his experience in psychology. During his bachelor's degree program at the University of Northern [State], he became interested in audiology during a short term auditory memory recall experiment that he was involved with. Shortly thereafter, he enrolled in the master's program at [State] University in communication disorders and audiology. While at [State] University, Mr. B taught human anatomy and physiology and received a U.S. Department of Education grant. He graduated number one in his class. Currently he is a pursuing his doctoral degree at the University of [State] and receives a doctoral fellowship. His area of interest is physiological measures of hearing and hearing aids.

Prior to moving to Central City, Mr. B was involved as a contract audiologist for the U.S. Public Health Service in [city], [state] and subsequently as the Chief of Audiology for the U.S. Public Health Service, Indian Health Service in [city], [state].

Mr. B is currently building his own home in Central City and his hobbies include sailing, travel, windsurfing, snowboarding, skiing, scuba diving and other recreational pursuits. Mr. B has traveled extensively including three around the world trips to Europe, Asia, Africa, the Middle East, and South America.

CARDINAL HEARING SERVICES, INC.
Medical Arts Building, Suite 100
Central City, [State] [Zip]
[Area code and phone number]

Date

_____, M.D.
[Street]
[City], [State] [Zip]

Dear Dr. _____:

Primary care physicians and audiologists are a natural team for providing high quality hearing care services at lower cost.

Close to 90% of adult hearing losses are not medically treatable. Dr. David Kessler, FDA Commissioner, recently testified to the Senate Committee on Aging that a comprehensive hearing evaluation is needed to fit hearing aids properly and "audiologists are exquisitely trained to provide this service."

Cardinal Hearing Services, Inc., has a long track record of working hand-in-glove with primary care doctors. Our Mission Statement, formulated in 1988, states that our company is:

> ". . . . dedicated to improving the hearing and quality of life of patients with hearing loss by working closely with the patients' physicians to provide timely services that are excellent, complete, cost-effective, and tailored to the individual."

Eighty percent of our patients are referred by physicians, most of them Internists or Family Practitioners. Our approach has been so successful that we were invited to describe it in the October issue of the Bulletin of the American Academy of Audiology. A reprint is enclosed.

We would like to work with you and help your patients who have hearing problems. We have enclosed "get acquainted" information about our practice and hope that you will consider us when hearing problems come up!

Cordially,

_____
Dr. A, Ph.D. CCC-A

Sample marketing letter to potential physician referral sources.

Section C. Patient Forms

A variety of information is available on record keeping. Refer to Chapter 17 on this topic. Other references in the literature are:

Paul-Brown, D. (1994). Clinical record keeping in audiology and speech-language pathology. *Asha, 36*(5), 40–42.
Rao, P. (1991, Fall). The Policy and procedure manual: Managing "by the book." *Quality Improvement Digest*, pp. 1–7. (Available from American Speech-Language-Hearing Association, Rockville Pike, MD)

1. General Information

Newsletters, brochures, and handouts are important means of educating the public and potential referral sources about the audiology profession. The following are examples of newsletters from three different independent audiology practices. Each newsletter aims to educate and attract customers by using articles and layouts that reflect the image and philosophy of their individual audiology practice.

HEAD LINES

The Newsletter For Hearing
Volume 7, Number 7, Fall 1993

Desert Life Medical Plaza
2001 W. Orange Grove Rd., Suite 510 • (602) 575-0870

2506 North Alvernon
(602) 325-2547

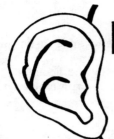

Holly Hosford-Dunn, Ph. D., CCC-A
Tucson Audiology Institute (TAI)--NW Office

In This Issue

- Audiologists and Hearing Aid Regulations

- Hearing in the Computer Age

- Hearing Aid Updates

- Health Beat

- Staff News

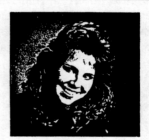

Sharon K. Hopkins, M.A., CCC-A
Tucson Audiology Institute (TAI)--Alvernon Office

Hearing Aids And Consumer Protection--Who Knows Best?
by Holly Hosford-Dunn, Ph.D., Clinical Audiologist

The Senate Committee on Aging recently asked "Is the consumer adequately protected in the hearing aid marketplace?" The FDA intends to strengthen hearing aid rules. The FDA has also threatened regulatory action against hearing aid manufacturers who make "misleading claims about their products." Not since the 1970's has there been such regulatory activity surrounding the making and fitting of hearing aids.

News reports on these activities are confusing and often alarming to the public, not to mention hearing health care workers! But, just as in the 70's, audiologists are emerging as the clear victors as the committees and agencies hear testimony and collect data.

Dr. David Kessler, FDA Commissioner, stated to the Senate Committee that a major problem for consumers was that they were not getting proper diagnostic hearing evaluations prior to hearing aid purchase. Kessler stated that a comprehensive hearing evaluation is what is needed and that

audiologists are "exquisitely trained" to provide this service.

The Senate Committee also received testimony from the AARP's new consumer report on hearing aids. That report stated "**Audiologists generally are the most knowledgeable of the practitioners that evaluate and fit hearing aids. They also conduct the most thorough evaluations.**" The President of Self Help for Hard of Hearing People (SHHH) testified that "**Consumers should have audiological diagnostic evaluations...We feel that the present FDA law preempts the critical role audiologists play in the rehabilitation process.**"

The present, inadequate FDA law--that Dr. Kessler, AARP and SHHH want to change--requires that patients have a medical examination (or sign a waiver) before being fit with a hearing aid. But it does **not** require an examination by an audiologist! Based on testimony to the Senate Committee, it seems likely that revised FDA regulations will require audiology testing

prior to hearing aid fitting, with a medical examination required only if "red flags" are noted (e.g., sudden hearing loss, draining ear). At the Senate Committee meeting, even the Association of Otolaryngologists (ENT doctors) went along with the idea that a medical exam could be waived when "red flags" are absent, as is the case in most adult-onset nerve type hearing losses.

Recognition of audiologists as the "entry-point" in the hearing care system has important ramifications. 90% of adult hearing losses are not medically treatable, so hearing health care costs would be reduced considerably if the medical examination was ordered judiciously rather than across the board. As the American Academy of Audiology stated to the President's Task Force on Health Care Reform: "**Audiologists are qualified ...to provide hearing care services. Delivery of hearing care services by audiologists can result in lowered cost and increased accessibility without sacrifice of quality.**"

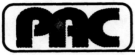 **Princeton Audiology Clinic, Inc.**

Alan L. Desmond, M.S., CCC-A

Celebrating 10 Years in Princeton

DEALING WITH DIZZINESS

**By Alan L. Desmond,
Audiologist, M.S., CCC-A**

We all know that we hear with our ears; what many people don't know is that the ear is also primarily responsible for balance. Along with the eyes, central nervous system and sense of touch, the inner ear makes up a complex system to provide us with information about balance, gravity, speed, and spatial orientation. If a problem with any part of this system occurs, the result will be a feeling of dizziness or vertigo. This can occur when there are mixed signals from the balance system, and any breakdown of this complex system can contribute to dizziness.

The balance system usually works so well that we don't pay much attention to it. A good demonstration as to the speed and efficiency of a healthy balance system can be done while reading this article. Hold this newsletter about 18

(See Dealing with Dizziness *on Page 4)*

EAR INFECTIONS AND HEARING LOSS IN CHILDREN

**by Alan Desmond, M.S., CCC-A
Clinical Audiologist**

Most young children suffer from "ear infections" at one time or another. It is one of the most commonly diagnosed and treated conditions in the offices of most pediatricians and primary care physicians. It's important, then, for parents to know what causes these common middle ear problems - known as otitis media - the various forms of treatment and the long-term effects of untreated otitis media.

Otitis media refers to a build-up of fluid behind the eardrum. It is usually a result of a malfunction of the Eustachian tube. The Eustachian tube travels from the back of the mouth and nose and connects to a cavity behind the eardrum that is normally filled with air. In this cavity lie the three little bones of hearing: the hammer, anvil and stirrup. Normal hearing relies on the eardrum and three bones vibrating freely in response to sound entering the ear canal. If for any reason the movement of the eardrum, or ossicle, is restricted, hearing loss will follow.

Now, back to the Eustachian tube. Most of us have experienced the sensation of a stuffy feeling in our ear as we travel up or down a mountain or fly in a plane. This is caused by a change in atmospheric pressure as we change elevation. Air gets trapped in the middle ear cavity and creates a sensation of pressure and decreased hearing. When we swallow, yawn or stretch our jaw, the Eustachian tube opens and allows the trapped air to escape. We then notice a release of pressure and improved hearing.

(See Ear Infections *on Page 3)*

HEARING AIDS:
IT'S BETTER TO GET THEM FITTED RIGHT THE FIRST TIME

**By ALAN L. DESMOND
and HOLLY HOSFORD-DUNN**

More than 20 million people in the United States suffer from hearing loss and need hearing aids. Only about 3 million have hearing aids, and not all of those are worn.

Hearing aids have gotten a tarnished reputation over the years, justifiably in some instances. Anyone needing help with their hearing would be wise to develop a little healthy skepticism when seeking help.

Here are a few facts and common tips to help you decide what to do if you have a hearing problem. The single most important consideration is the qualifications of the person that you choose to trust with your hearing. There is a wide range of quality to choose from, and it usually doesn't cost any more to see a qualified professional than it does to see a poorly trained hearing aid salesperson. In fact, it may cost less since insurance companies usually cover professional test fees, but rarely those of hearing aid salespersons.

The most qualified person to test hearing and fit hearing aids is a certified clinical audiologist. These people go to college at least six years before starting out in private practice. In almost all cases, they work closely with physicians to insure that your hearing loss is not due to active disease processes, or other medically-treatable conditions.

A certified clinical audiologist is identified by the letters CCC-A after their name. Audiologists should not be confused with a "certified hearing aid audiologist." That term has been ruled "deceptive to persons with hearing loss"

(See Hearing Aids *on Page 2)*

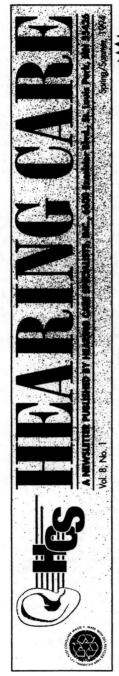

HEARING CARE

A NEWSLETTER PUBLISHED BY Hearing Care Consultants, Inc., 2400 Emerson Blvd. N, St. Louis Park, MN 55426

Spring 1994

Vol. 8; No. 1

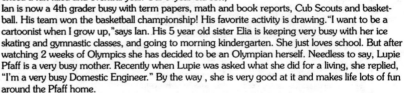
SPECIAL:
The
Sounds
of
Spring
insert enclosed

Think Spring.

WOW! 1993 was quite a year and one we won't soon forget. I hope you all weathered the recent severe cold winter. I'm sure you are as anxious as we are to hear *The Sounds of Spring*, which are right around the corner.

1993 was eventful and memorable for the Hearing Health Care system too. The Food And Drug Administration (FDA) has taken a renewed and over-due interest in the regulation of the Hearing Aid Industry. It has finally decided to flex its muscle and curb the misleading advertising and substandard prac-tices by providers of hearing aids. It's about time! The Minnesota Department of Health has also taken steps to ensure that all dispensers of hearing aids in the state meet certain minimal qualification requirements. This too, I applaud. I'll discuss these important topics in more detail later in this newsletter.

On a personal side, the Pfaff family also experi-enced a fun filled and eventful year. Our 9 year old son, Ian is now a 4th grader busy with term papers, math and book reports, Cub Scouts and basket-ball. His team won the basketball championship! His favorite activity is drawing. "I want to be a cartoonist when I grow up," says Ian. His 5 year old sister Elia is keeping very busy with her ice skating and gymnastic classes, and going to morning kindergarten. She just loves school. But after watching 2 weeks of Olympics she has decided to be an Olympian herself. Needless to say, Lupie Pfaff is a very busy mother. Recently when Lupie was asked what she did for a living, she replied, "I'm a very busy Domestic Engineer." By the way , she is very good at it and makes life lots of fun around the Pfaff home.

I made a personal commitment many years ago to helping people with a hearing problem and I am dedicated to offering you the best in hearing health care. Please read on to learn about the changes in our profession and how you may benefit. Read about the exciting new diagnostic procedures, technologies and products we have available for your benefit.

HAVEN'T YOU HEARD?... WE CAN HELP!

Sincerely,

HEARING AIDS AND THE FDA

Hearing aids and related fitting issues were newsworthy topics in 1993. In August, the FDA issued an industry-wide warning about advertising practices. The FDA stated it would not allow the use of certain claims in the adver-tising and promotion of hearing aids. Any and all claims that are used must be substantiated by clinical research data that is submitted to and approved by the FDA.

In addition to curbing unethical advertis-ing, Dr. David Kessler, Commissioner of the FDA, is looking towards a complete review and possible revision of the 1977 federal hearing aid

cont.'d pg. 2

500

2. History, Billing, and Reminders

The following are examples of forms for use with patients.

History forms need to elicit information to document patients' (a) primary and secondary complaints, (b) general health, (c) historical factors that may have affected their auditory or vestibular function, and (d) subjective impressions of handicap. Different history forms may be appropriate, depending on the nature of the encounter.

Anticipate and deter billing and collection problems by providing patients with explanations of office billing procedures, and by using billing forms that are acceptable to the insurer.

Establish office procedures for tracking patients for whom follow-up is recommended. Use letters, cards, or telephone calls to remind patients when they are due for follow-up.

FU APPT DATE: _____

CARDINAL HEARING SERVICES, INC.
Medical Arts Building, Suite 100
Central City, [State] [Zip]
[Area code and phone number]

Name: _____ Phone:_____ Birthdate: ___ / / ___
City:_____ State:_____ Zip Code:_____

ASSESSMENT OF COMMUNICATION PROBLEMS

Please check the box which best describes your answer for each question below.

		YES	**SOMETIMES**	**NO**
1.	Has a spouse or friend ever told you that you don't hear well?	☐	☐	☐
2.	Do you hear people speaking but have difficulty understanding the words?	☐	☐	☐
3.	Do you hear some people better than others? If yes describe: _____	☐	☐	☐
4.	Do you have difficulty understanding in large crowds?	☐	☐	☐
	in restaurants?	☐	☐	☐
	in small groups?	☐	☐	☐
5.	Do you have difficulty understanding on the telephone?	☐	☐	☐
	Which ear do you use on the phone most often? ☐ Right ☐ Left			
6.	Can you hear the phone ring?	☐	☐	☐
7.	Any problems when listening to a sermon in church or a lecture in a large hall?	☐	☐	☐
8.	Must others raise their voice or come closer to make you hear them?	☐	☐	☐
9.	Have you ever avoided a social situation you enjoy because of a hearing problem?	☐	☐	☐
10.	Do you concentrate so much to listen that you become tired of it?	☐	☐	☐
11.	Can you hear car horns, sirens or other warning signals when they occur?	☐	☐	☐
12.	Have you ever worked in a noisy place? If yes, describe _____	☐	☐	☐
13.	Are you exposed to noise in any of your pastimes? If yes, describe _____	☐	☐	☐
14.	Do you have any ringing or buzzing in your ears?	☐	☐	☐

15. How long ago did you notice difficulty with your hearing? _____
16. What do you miss hearing the most? _____
17. If we find through the evaluation that you can be helped, are you ready for that help? _____

(The Audiologist will review your questionnaire with you prior to the screening)

Audiologist to Complete below this line

Date: _____
Notes and Recommendations: _____

Example of a simple history of communication problems, used with hearing screenings.

[Patient Name]
[Patient address]
[City], [State] [Zip]
[Patient phone number]
Referral: _____, M.D.

CARDINAL HEARING SERVICES, INC.
Medical Arts Building, Suite 100
Central City, [State] [zip]
[Area code and phone number]

COMPLAINT:

	Yes	No
Do you have any problems hearing?	☐	☐
How long? _____ Which ear? ☐ Right ☐ Left ☐ Both		
Have you had a hearing test here before?	☐	☐
What year? _____		
Does your family or friends complain about your hearing?	☐	☐
Do you keep the TV volume high?	☐	☐
Do you hear noises (tinnitus) in your ear or head?	☐	☐
Which ear? ☐ Right ☐ Left ☐ Both		
How often? ☐ Constantly ☐ Unsure ☐ Occasionally		
Do you have dizziness, ear pain, or headaches? (Circle one)	☐	☐
Have you ever worn a hearing aid?	☐	☐
How long? _____ Which ear? ☐ Right ☐ Left ☐ Both		

HISTORY:

Does anyone in your family, including cousins, have a hearing loss?	☐	☐
Who? _____		
Have you ever had a skull fracture or concussion?	☐	☐
Have you ever had any ear surgery?	☐	☐
Which ear? ☐ Right ☐ Left ☐ Both		
Have you ever had any ear infections	☐	☐
Which ear? ☐ Right ☐ Left ☐ Both		
Have you ever been exposed regularly to loud noises?	☐	☐
If yes, where? _____ How long? _____		
Do you take any medications regularly?_____	☐	☐
If yes, for what conditions? _____		
_____		
Have you ever been given drugs that you were told might affect your hearing or balance?	☐	☐
What were the drugs? _____		

Check the illnesses that you have had:

☐ Meningitis	☐ Malaria	☐ Mumps	☐ Scarlet Fever
☐ Diabetes	☐ Heart Trouble	☐ High Blood Pressure	☐ Asthma
☐ Lung Trouble			

503

CARDINAL HEARING SERVICES, INC.
Medical Arts Building, Suite 100
Central City, [State] [Zip]
[Area code and phone number]

MEDICARE REIMBURSEMENT INFORMATION

We are billing Medicare electronically for your hearing services today. This means that in the next 24 hours Medicare will receive your claim, review it for errors, and insure that any updates or corrections are made. That way, no time is lost and reimbursement is made in a matter of days.

We accept assignment on your claim. This means that Medicare will "assign" a value to our services that is somewhat less than the total of our bill. We agree to accept that assigned value as payment in full.

If you have met your deductible, Medicare will send us a check for 80% of the assigned amount within a few weeks. Otherwise, it will apply the amount, or some portion of it, to meet your deductible. In either case, you will receive an "explanation of benefits" (EOB) that you may send to your supplementary insurance for additional reimbursement. In some circumstances, Medicare will do this automatically for you.

You are responsible to pay us for any deductible that has not been met, as well as the 20% that Medicare does not pay on the assigned amount. If you have a secondary insurer that covers the 20%, they will reimburse directly to you.

Example of explanation to patients about how their Medicare insurance will be billed electronically.

APPROVED OMB-0938-0008

CARRIER

PICA

HEALTH INSURANCE CLAIM FORM

PICA

MEDICARE	MEDICAID	CHAMPUS	CHAMPVA	GROUP HEALTH PLAN (SSN or ID)	FECA BLK LUNG (SSN)	OTHER	1a. INSURED'S I.D. NUMBER	(FOR PROGRAM IN ITEM 1)
☐ (Medicare #)	☐ (Medicaid #)	☐ (Sponsor's SSN)	☐ (VA File #)	☐	☐	☐ (ID)		

2. PATIENT'S NAME (Last Name, First Name, Middle Initial)

3. PATIENT'S BIRTH DATE MM DD YY   SEX   M ☐ F ☐

4. INSURED'S NAME (Last Name, First Name, Middle Initial)

5. PATIENT'S ADDRESS (No., Street)

6. PATIENT RELATIONSHIP TO INSURED   Self ☐ Spouse ☐ Child ☐ Other ☐

7. INSURED'S ADDRESS (No., Street)

CITY   STATE

8. PATIENT STATUS   Single ☐ Married ☐ Other ☐

CITY   STATE

ZIP CODE   TELEPHONE (Include Area Code) ( )

Employed ☐ Full-Time Student ☐ Part-Time Student ☐

ZIP CODE   TELEPHONE (INCLUDE AREA CODE) ( )

9. OTHER INSURED'S NAME (Last Name, First Name, Middle Initial)

10. IS PATIENT'S CONDITION RELATED TO:

11. INSURED'S POLICY GROUP OR FECA NUMBER

OTHER INSURED'S POLICY OR GROUP NUMBER

a. EMPLOYMENT? (CURRENT OR PREVIOUS)   ☐ YES ☐ NO

a. INSURED'S DATE OF BIRTH MM DD YY   SEX   M ☐ F ☐

OTHER INSURED'S DATE OF BIRTH MM DD YY   SEX   M ☐ F ☐

b. AUTO ACCIDENT?   PLACE (State)   ☐ YES ☐ NO

b. EMPLOYER'S NAME OR SCHOOL NAME

EMPLOYER'S NAME OR SCHOOL NAME

c. OTHER ACCIDENT?   ☐ YES ☐ NO

c. INSURANCE PLAN NAME OR PROGRAM NAME

INSURANCE PLAN NAME OR PROGRAM NAME

10d. RESERVED FOR LOCAL USE

d. IS THERE ANOTHER HEALTH BENEFIT PLAN?   ☐ YES ☐ NO   If yes, return to and complete item 9 a-d.

READ BACK OF FORM BEFORE COMPLETING & SIGNING THIS FORM.

12. PATIENT'S OR AUTHORIZED PERSON'S SIGNATURE I authorize the release of any medical or other information necessary to process this claim. I also request payment of government benefits either to myself or to the party who accepts assignment below.

SIGNED _____   DATE _____

13. INSURED'S OR AUTHORIZED PERSON'S SIGNATURE I authorize payment of medical benefits to the undersigned physician or supplier for services described below.

SIGNED _____

14. DATE OF CURRENT. MM DD YY ◄ ILLNESS (First symptom) OR INJURY (Accident) OR PREGNANCY(LMP)

15. IF PATIENT HAS HAD SAME OR SIMILAR ILLNESS. GIVE FIRST DATE MM DD YY

16. DATES PATIENT UNABLE TO WORK IN CURRENT OCCUPATION MM DD YY   FROM _____ TO _____

17. NAME OF REFERRING PHYSICIAN OR OTHER SOURCE

17a. I.D. NUMBER OF REFERRING PHYSICIAN

18. HOSPITALIZATION DATES RELATED TO CURRENT SERVICES MM DD YY   FROM _____ TO _____

19. RESERVED FOR LOCAL USE

20. OUTSIDE LAB?   ☐ YES ☐ NO $ CHARGES

21. DIAGNOSIS OR NATURE OF ILLNESS OR INJURY. (RELATE ITEMS 1,2,3 OR 4 TO ITEM 24E BY LINE)

1. ___ . ___   3. ___ . ___
2. ___ . ___   4. ___ . ___

22. MEDICAID RESUBMISSION CODE   ORIGINAL REF. NO.

23. PRIOR AUTHORIZATION NUMBER

A DATE(S) OF SERVICE From To 24. MM DD YY MM DD YY	B Place of Service	C Type of Service	D PROCEDURES, SERVICES, OR SUPPLIES (Explain Unusual Circumstances) CPT/HCPCS MODIFIER	E DIAGNOSIS CODE	F $ CHARGES	G DAYS OR UNITS	H EPSDT Family Plan	I EMG	J COB	K RESERVED FOR LOCAL USE

25. FEDERAL TAX I.D. NUMBER   SSN ☐ EIN ☐

860588256

26. PATIENT'S ACCOUNT NO.

27. ACCEPT ASSIGNMENT? (For govt. claims, see back)   ☐ YES ☐ NO

28. TOTAL CHARGE $

29. AMOUNT PAID $

30. BALANCE DUE $

31. SIGNATURE OF PHYSICIAN OR SUPPLIER INCLUDING DEGREES OR CREDENTIALS I certify that the statements on the reverse apply to this bill and are made a part thereof.)

SIGNED _____   DATE _____

32. NAME AND ADDRESS OF FACILITY WHERE SERVICES WERE RENDERED (If other than home or office)

33. PHYSICIAN'S, SUPPLIER'S BILLING NAME, ADDRESS, ZIP CODE & PHONE #

PIN#   GRP#

PLEASE PRINT OR TYPE

FORM HCFA-1500 (12-90)
FORM OWCP-1500   FORM RRB-1500

PATIENT AND INSURED INFORMATION

PHYSICIAN OR SUPPLIER INFORMATION

This HCFA-1500 form is used by many offices to submit insurance that is not billed electronically.

JUST A REMINDER!

☐ It has been nearly 1 year since your last hearing evaluation. In the best interest of your hearing health, please schedule an appointment for a hearing re-check.

☐ It has been 11 months since you purchased your hearing aid(s). It would be advisable that you make an appointment for a hearing check within the next few weeks. We will be glad to advise you of your options for warranty extension at this time.

Call for an appointment.

Haven't You Heard? We Can Help!

This is an example of a reminder notice to an established patient.

3. Hearing Aids

Documentation and record keeping are extremely important when dealing with hearing aids sales, and the paperwork requirements vary from state to state. The following pages give reasons for and examples of different kinds of documentation that can help practices maintain good relations with customers and authorities.

TIPS FROM TERRY

Documentation: a 10-step survival guide

TERRY S. GRIFFING

Like it or not, the recent FDA warning about industry marketing and programs like Dateline, with its indictment of dispensers, mean that it is time to accentuate the positive in this industry. This recent publicity, and other stories scheduled to appear, such as the upcoming one from AARP, suggest that dispensers should go as far as possible to avoid problems by documentation. Put as much in writing as possible. Here are a few ideas, some new, some previously mentioned, about what to do. They will help you present a more professional picture and clarify expectations for your clients.

1 Know the FDA's red flag requirements that you must ask prospects about. These are listed in Fig. 1, and they are essential. I suggest that dispensers have clients review the answers they give, then sign and date them. This avoids any debate at some future date.

Dispensers should advise prospective hearing aid wearers to consult with a licensed physician (preferably an ear specialist) before dispensing hearing aids if any of the responses are affirmative.

2 Upgrade your testing and evaluation equipment as soon as possible within your budget so you can finetune, and document, your fitting techniques. Here are some useful tools for doing this:
   a. video otoscope
   b. new audiometer
   c. computer record keeping and client management system
   d. sound room
   e. real ear measurement equipment

3 Take no shortcuts in testing, reporting and recording all information.

4 Post copies of cancellation and refund laws conspicuously. In states where required or perhaps as a voluntary procedure, have clients read, date and sign such documents.

5 Post and provide in writing all of your practice's warranties and guarantees.

6 Post and provide a 4-point information sheet each client must read, date and sign that says:
   • *The use of hearing instruments cannot retard the progression of sensorineural hearing loss.*
   • *The use of hearing instruments cannot restore hearing to normal levels.*
   • *Hearing instruments cannot distinguish between speech sounds and undesirable noises.*
   • *Speech recognition will vary based upon the severity and duration of the hearing problem. Therefore, not all persons using hearing instruments will ben-*efit equally.

7 Create a form to make every hearing aid wearer and prospect well informed about the benefits of monaural vs. binaural hearing.

8 Review very carefully the sales contract you now use; is it current, is it precisely correct and does it conform to all existing rules and regulations?

9 Have a written repair consent agreement designed to avoid any possible misunderstanding about terms, conditions, prices and length of warranty.

10 Offer service contracts that carefully outline all the services you will provide during the first year warranty period. This should be in written form, with both the dispenser and the wearer signing it.

Compliance and perhaps a touch of overresponding might serve you exceptionally well both in the present and the long-term. Complete documentation will always be the best insurance. Make sure every client is fully informed to eliminate later debatable issues. ◻

Address inquiries to: Terry S. Griffing, national sales director, Starkey Labs, 6700 Washington Ave. South, Eden Prairie, MN, 55344, 612-941-6401.

NO	YES		
◻	◻		Acute or chronic dizziness.
	Right Left		
ASKED			
◻	◻	◻	Pain or discomfort in the ear.
◻	◻	◻	History of sudden or rapidly progressive hearing loss within the previous 90 days.
◻	◻	◻	Unilateral hearing loss of sudden or recent onset within the previous 90 days.
◻	◻	◻	History of active drainage from the ear within the previous 90 days.
OBSERVED			
◻	◻	◻	Active drainage from the ear.
◻	◻	◻	Visible congenital or traumatic deformity of the ear.
◻	◻	◻	Visible evidence of significant cerumen accumulation.
TESTED			
◻	◻	◻	Audiometric air-bone gaps equal to or greater than 15 dB at 500 Hz, 1000 Hz and 2000 Hz.

Fig. 1. Federal regulations require that dispensers ask clients the above questions before fitting.

[1]We have reprinted Terry Griffing's article in full here because it clearly points out the reasons for documentation and provides ideas for good record keeping and improved quality of care.

[2]Reprinted from "Documentation: A 10-Step Survival Guide" by T. S. Griffing, 1993, p. 18. *Hearing Instruments, 44*(9), with permission.

CARDINAL HEARING SERVICES, INC.
Medical Arts Building, Suite 100
Central City, [State] [Zip]
[Area code and phone number]

PURCHASE AGREEMENT

Date: _____

DESCRIPTION

⊐ HEARING AID(S)	$
⊐ INSTRUMENTS ARE: NEW ☐ USED ☐ BEING USED ON TRIAL ☐ RENTAL ☐	
⊐ EARMOLD(S) RIGHT ☐ LEFT ☐ STYLE:	
⊐ BATTERIES QUANTITY _____ pkgs. SIZE 312 675 230 13	
⊐ EXTRA ACCESSORIES	
⊐ FULL SERVICE PLAN	
⊐ WARRANTY	
⊐ WARRANTY EXTENSIONS: 1 YEAR ☐ 2 YEARS ☐ 3 YEARS ☐	
⊐ OTHER	

TERMS		
	NET CASH PRICE	$
	Less Deposit	
	BALANCE DUE	$
		$
	Property belongs to seller until paid in full.	

"The undersigned Seller agrees to sell and the undersigned Buyer agrees to purchase the hearing aid(s) and accessories, according to the terms set forth below;

I have been advised by Cardinal Hearing Services that my best hearing health interest would be served if I had a medical evaluation by a physician specializing in disorders of the ear (or by a duly licensed physician if no such ear specialist is available) before I purchase a hearing aid.

A. The purchaser was advised that the Seller is not a physician licensed to practice medicine; and

B. No examination or representation made by the Seller should be regarded as a medical examination. opinion. or advice.

A. Is the person being fitted under 18? _____ If the person being fitted is under eighteen years of age, has that person been examined by an otolaryngologist for recommendation within six months prior to fitting? YES_____ NO_____ . No person under eighteen years of age may be fitted without our receipt of such a recommendation.

B. If the person being fitted is eighteen years of age or older he or she should be examined and obtain and provide to us a written statement by a licensed physician stating that the hearing loss has been medically evaluated within the preceding six months and that he/she may be a candidate for a hearing aid(s). Patient has provided statement suggested above. YES_____ NO_____ .

C. Persons age eighteen or older who do not provide a physician's statement must sign below. "I have been advised to obtain a written statement by a licensed physician stating that my hearing loss has been medically evaluated within the preceding six months and that I may be a candidate for a hearing aid(s). I have elected not to obtain such a statement notwithstanding the audiologist's recommendation that I do so. The audiologist's recommendation that I do so. The audiologist has not encouraged me to waive the medical examination and it is my own decision."

_____
(Patient's Signature)

[State]'. STATE LAW GIVES THE BUYER THE RIGHT TO CANCEL THIS PURCHASE FOR ANY REASON ANY TIME PRIOR TO MIDNIGHT OF THE 30TH CALENDAR DAY AFTER RECEIPT OF THE HEARING AID(S). THIS CANCELLATION MUST BE IN WRITING AND MUST BE GIVEN OR MAILED TO THE SELLER. IF THE BUYER DECIDES TO RETURN THE HEARING AID(S) WITHIN THIS 30-DAY PERIOD, THE BUYER WILL RECEIVE A REFUND OF $_____ .

I have been advised that I am entitled to a 30-day trial period with the above hearing aid(s). I understand that full payment of the Purchase Price is due upon delivery. I have been further advised that 10% of the total purchase price is NON-REFUNDABLE. This fee covers the materials and services necessary for the ordering and fitting of hearing instruments. Testing fees prior to the order of this/these instruments are also NON-REFUNDABLE.

30-Day Period Starts _____ and ends _____

"I have received a copy of the MDH brochure about purchasing a hearing aid." _____ (buyers initial)

PURCHASER'S NAME:

ADDRESS:

_____
(Signature of Purchaser)

[State] Permit Number_____

Dr. A, Ph.D. CCC-A

Example of a hearing aid purchase agreement in a state where the law requires a 30-day trial period and sets a limit to the non-refundable amount.

CARDINAL HEARING SERVICES, INC.
Medical Arts Building, Suite 100
Central City, [State] [Zip]
[Area code and phone number]

[State] PERMIT # _____

HEARING AID DISPENSING, PRODUCT PURCHASE, and REPAIR

NAME: DATE:
ADDRESS:

QTY	PRODUCT DESCRIPTION	$ PER UNIT	TOTAL AMT

INSURANCE/DELIVERY

PURCHASE PRICE

BALANCE DUE AT TIME OF FITTING

POLICY RELATING TO THE PURCHASE AND DISPENSING OF HEARING AID/S

[State]   STATE LAW GIVES THE BUYER THE RIGHT TO CANCEL THIS PURCHASE FOR ANY REASON ANY TIME PRIOR TO MIDNIGHT OF THE 30TH CALENDAR DAY AFTER RECEIPT OF THE HEARING AID(S). THIS CANCELLATION MUST BE IN WRITING AND MUST BE GIVEN OR MAILED TO THE SELLER. IF THE BUYER DECIDES TO RETURN THE HEARING AID(S) WITHIN THIS 30 DAY PERIOD, THE BUYER WILL RECEIVE A REFUND OF $_____(WHICH IS___% OF THE PURCHASE PRICE.)

The price of the hearing aid(s) includes the fees for dispensing and fitting services. The price also includes professional and technical follow-up pertaining directly to the fitting and use of the hearing aids for 3 months starting from the date of fitting.

THE COST OF THE PRODUCT DOES NOT INCLUDE PROFESSIONAL SERVICES PRIOR TO THE PRESCRIPTION OF THE HEARING AID/S.

Example of a transaction for a hearing aid purchase. (**Note:** Laws regarding trial periods and refundable portions vary by state.)

Example of an information form/disclaimer form for patients who elect to be fitted monaurally, despite a recommendation for a binaural fitting.

CARDINAL HEARING SERVICES, INC.
Medical Arts Building, Suite 100
Central City, [State] [Zip]
[Area code and phone number]

BINAURAL VS. MONAURAL

When a hearing aid dispenser makes a recommendation for two hearing aids for a patient, there is often a question in the mind of the patient as to the reasons behind this recommendation.

For several reasons, not the least important of which is the additional expense of the second aid, the question is a reasonable one. It is best answered with an outline of some relevant facts about binaural hearing aids that have been proven by research and clinical experience:

1. Two hearing aids can allow better reception of quiet sounds and soft spoken works. With many patients, the inability to hear soft spoken or environmental sounds is one of their major complaints. To approximate the performance of two aids, a single aid may have to be worn with volume at a higher level than it would be when two aids are worn. The higher volume setting puts the patient closer to the point beyond which an increase in sound level becomes uncomfortable or painful. The addition of the second aid can have the effect of increasing the range of sound pressure that the patient can comfortably hear.

2. Two hearing aids can help the patient better understand speech in the presence of unwanted noise. Even a person who has one normal ear and one non-functioning ear has trouble with understanding speech in the presence of noise. In order for the central nervous system to "sort out" speech from noise, input from both sides of the head is required.

3. Reception of sound from both sides of the head is possible with two hearing aids. The addition of a second hearing aid reduces the need of rotating the head around to face the speaker, making communication easier and more comfortable.

4. The ability to locate the source of a sound is improved with two hearing aids. The ability to localize the origin of a sound allows a person to react more appropriately to his environment.

Two hearing aids are not recommended for all patients evaluated. When the recommendation is made, it is because the Audiologist feels that the communicative abilities of the patient will be significantly improved by wearing two hearing aids instead of one.

I have been advised by _____ that my best interest would be served by being fitted with Binaural (2) Hearing Instruments for Environmental Safety and Proper Acoustic Balance. At this time I wish to be fitted only with a Monaural (1) Hearing Instrument. I understand that by only wearing one I may not be receiving the full benefits of amplification.

Signature_____ Date_____

WAIVER OF MEDICAL EVALUATION FOR HEARING

I have been advised by: _____
Dispenser's Name

a representative of:

CARDINAL HEARING SERVICES, INC.
Medical Arts Building, Suite 100
Central City, [State] [Zip]
[Area code and phone number]

that the Food and Drug Administration has determined that my best health interest would be served if I had a medical evaluation by a licensed physician (preferably a physician who specializes in diseases of the ear) before purchasing a hearing aid. I do not wish a medical evaluation before purchasing a hearing aid.

_____   _____
Date   Signature of User

Certificate of Clinical Competence
AUDIOLOGIST
CCC
* ASHA *
American
Speech-Language-Hearing
Association

Example of a medical waiver.

CARDINAL HEARING SERVICES, INC.
Medical Arts Building, Suite 100
Central City, [State] [Zip]
[Area code and phone number]

October 15, 1993

title   *name*
street
city   *state•   *zip*

Dear *title*   *last name*,

In just a few weeks, your hearing aids will be five years old and they will no longer be covered by Starkey's comprehensive warranty plan. The average replacement age for hearing aids is less than five years, according to national surveys. So, you have already gotten more than the average use from your instruments by taking good care of them. In order to keep them functioning correctly in the future, it's more important than ever to bring them in periodically for free cleaning.

But, before the warranty expires, you should schedule an appointment to have them checked at no charge. If the aids have problems, we can correct them one last time under warranty. It's a good idea to have an annual screening. The usual $25.00 charge will be waived for you, our valued customers.

When you come in, we can also answer questions you have about upgrades in hearing aids, especially about the new computerized, programmable aids. There have been dramatic improvements in "noise control" with these new instruments which we're sure you'll want to know about.

Very truly yours,

_____
Dr. A, Ph.D. CCC-A

Example of a follow-up letter to established patients regarding hearing aid warranties, using computer-generated fields in a patient data base.

4. Patient Satisfaction

As we have stressed throughout the book, all audiology practices must continually monitor and improve patient satisfaction if they hope to survive in the evolving health care marketplace. Needs assessment surveys are one facet of this process. Practices are likely to want to develop their own needs assessment forms (cf. Lacap, 1994). In addition, the newly revised Consumer Satisfaction Measure forms included in the following pages can be ordered from the American Speech-Language-Hearing Association.

REFERENCE

Lacap, M. K. (1994). Knowing your customer: Designing a survey. In M. Harrison (Ed.), *Total Quality Management: Application to audiology* (chap. 6, pp. 312–318). *Seminars in Hearing.* New York: Thieme.

CODE [   ]

• •

Dear Client/Patient:

    Two weeks ago we sent you a form requesting some information about the services you received at our facility. Please complete and return the form so we can evaluate our services to better serve you. Your input is important to us and will be kept confidential.

                                      Thank you for your assistance,

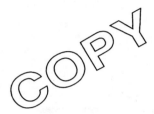

• •

Dear Client/Patient:

    Your feedback is important in helping us evaluate the quality of the services you received recently at our center. Please take a few minutes to answer these items, and then return the form within two weeks. This form may be completed by you or by another family member or caretaker. Your responses will be kept anonymous.

                                      Thank you for your assistance,

    Example of two choices of contact cards to accompany a customer satisfaction survey (see page 516) of evaluation services. This survey along with three other survey products were developed by the American Speech-Language-Hearing Association for use in audiology and speech-language pathology practice. Reprinted with permission from ASHA.

    The four products, ASHA-QA Consumer Satisfaction Measure/Speech-Language Pathology or Audiology—Evaluation, Limited Visits item #0111909 and ASHA-QA Consumer Satisfaction Measure/Speech-Language Pathology or Audiology—Treatment, Multiple Visits item #0111910, ASHA-QA Consumer Satisfaction Measure/Rehabilitative Services—Evaluation, Limited Visits item #0111911, and ASHA-QA Consumer Satisfaction Measure/Rehabilitative Services—Treatment, Multiple Visits item #0111912 can be purchased from ASHA Fulfillment Operations at 301-897-5700 x218 9:15 a.m.–5:15 p.m. E.S.T.

Speech-Language Pathology and/or Audiology Services— Evaluation

• •

Consumer Satisfaction Measure

After answering all items, detach here and return

READ each item carefully and CIRCLE the one answer that is best for you.

SA = Strongly Agree   **N** = Neutral   **SD** = Strongly Disagree

A = Agree   **D** = Disagree   **NA** = Not Applicable

1. **It is important that we see you in a timely manner.**
   - A. My appointment was scheduled in a reasonable period of time.   SA   A   N   D   SD   NA
   - B. I was seen on time for my scheduled appointment.   SA   A   N   D   SD   NA

2. **It is important that you benefit from Speech-Language Pathology and /or Audiology Services.**
   - A. I feel I gained valuable information from my visit.   SA   A   N   D   SD   NA
   - B. I feel I benefited from this appointment.   SA   A   N   D   SD   NA

3. **Your are important to us; we are here to work with you.**
   - A. The support staff (e.g., secretary, transporter, receptionist, assistant) who served me were courteous and pleasant.   SA   A   N   D   SD   NA
   - B. The clinician was experienced and knowledgeable.   SA   A   N   D   SD   NA

4. **Our Speech-Language Pathology and Audiology staff are highly trained and qualified to serve you.**
   - A. My clinician was prepared and organized.   SA   A   N   D   SD   NA
   - B. The procedures were explained to me in a way that I could understand.   SA   A   N   D   SD   NA
   - C. My clinician was experienced and knowledgeable.   SA   A   N   D   SD   NA

5. **It is important that our environment is secure, comfortable, attractive, distraction-free, and easy to reach.**
   - A. Health and safety precautions were taken when serving me.   SA   A   N   D   SD   NA
   - B. The environment was clean and pleasant..   SA   A   N   D   SD   NA
   - C. The environment was quiet and free of distractions.   SA   A   N   D   SD   NA
   - D. The building and treatment areas were easy to get to.   SA   A   N   D   SD   NA

6. **It is important that we provide you with efficient and comprehensive services.**
   - A. I feel that the purpose and nature of the procedures used were explained clearly.   SA   A   N   D   SD   NA
   - B. I feel that my clinician planned ahead and provided sufficient instruction.   SA   A   N   D   SD   NA
   - C. I feel that the services I receive at your center are appropriately coordinated with other services I need (i.e., teachers, dentist, nursing staff, physician).   SA   A   N   D   SD   NA

7. **We respect and value your comments.**
   - A. Overall, the program services were satisfactory.   SA   A   N   D   SD   NA
   - B. I would seek your services again if needed.   SA   A   N   D   SD   NA
   - C. I would recommend your services to others.   SA   A   N   D   SD   NA
   - D. Check the services you received.   ❏ Speech-Language Pathology   ❏ Audiology

Comments_____

_____

Thank you for your time.

American Speech-Language-Hearing Association Quality Assurance

CODE [   ] Please staple /seal the questionnaire so that the Center's address is on the outside and return it to us.

AMERICAN SPEECH-LANGUAGE-HEARING ASSOCIATION

SLP/Aud. Serv.—Evaluation

#0111909 © 1994

APPENDIX II

Handling Difficult Patients

We have reprinted the following excellent, chapter in its entirety here because: (1) it gives a variety of illustrations on the importance of good record keeping when working with patients who fail at compliance for one reason or another, or who practice provider abuse, (2) it does not "fit" anywhere else in this book, and (3) the book it is in is no longer in print, yet the information in the chapter remains contemporary.

We appreciate the authors and publisher giving us permission to reprint "How to Recognize (and Handle) the Troublesome Client" by H. F. McCollom, Jr. and J. M. Mynders (1984). In *Hearing Aid Dispensing Practice*, Chapter 17, pp. 115–131. Copyright 1984 Interstate Printers and Publishers

How to Recognize (and Handle) the Troublesome Client

I've been an audiologist since 1958. In all those years the nearest thing I've seen to an admission in the profession that there even are such things as troublesome clients was a few journal articles about malingering or a note that testing children can tax your patience and ingenuity. It's as though there simply are no problem people out there. If someone has such a client, he or she apparently never admits it. Since there are no courses in audiology on this matter, to my profession, the problem doesn't exist.

Well, I must have been doing a lot of things wrong, but in the last five years with a private dispensing practice, I've found 12 basic types of problem behaviors clustered into three severity groups. The three groups may be defined as light-weight, middle-weight and heavy-weight problems. Within each of these three groups I've found four behavior types. They are listed in the order of increasing problem to the dispenser.

PEOPLE WHO CAUSE LIGHT-WEIGHT PROBLEMS

1. The Complainer
2. The Know-It-All
3. The Shrewd Operator
4. The Shopper

PEOPLE WHO CAUSE MIDDLE-WEIGHT PROBLEMS

5. The Careless
6. The Hermit
7. The Impatient
8. The Liar

PEOPLE WHO CAUSE HEAVY-WEIGHT PROBLEMS

9. The Pressured
10. The I'll-Show-You'er
11. The Thief
12. The Disturbed

In truth, I never had much experience with the above 12 behaviors until I began to dispense hearing aids. While I don't believe these client behaviors are unique to a dispensing practice, I do believe that the providing of a costly (relative to size) prosthesis to an essentially naive (electro-acoustically speaking) public is a fertile ground in which such behaviors bloom.

Let's examine each behavior, describe the predominant symptoms, explain how that behavior may negatively impact on the dispenser and offer some relief or preventive techniques. We will well examine these behaviors in the order of increasing irritation or potential financial loss to the dispenser.

1. The Complainer

Description: This person greets the dispenser with a mantra of woe. The client may verbally attack you. The earmold is irritating. Everything sounds tinny. Or hollow. Or both at once. It isn't as good as the old aid. The client can't hear his or her budgie say "Pretty boy!" as well when the aid is on as when it is off. The aid is too big, too noticeable, too wide, too long, too heavy, etc., without end.

Potential Negative Impact: Each of these 12 behaviors may result in a cancelled purchase. In short, the dispenser may be in a situation in which a refund must be made and may, as a result, be "stuck" with an aid. With single-unit prices of many instruments running at hundreds of dollars, this can be an expensive problem. Further, an unhappy client will probably tell of this unhappiness to 25 people over the next three years, while a contented client may never tell anyone.

However, of the 12 behavior problems we will examine, this one should be the least upsetting to the professional dispenser. As long as the client continues to express complaints, it is a sign that he or she desires to continue with the prosthesis and simply wants something changed. In my first year of practice I saw one such complainer for two additional earmold re-makes and nine microscopic earmold refinements. Because of my sticking with him and eventually getting a satisfactory mold according to his standards, he not only is a satisfied client but has gone out of his way to direct others to my office.

The potential negative impact of this client is primarily in taking a lot of your time.

Relief Strategy: Active listening to the nature of the complaint is most important. Sometimes this takes a bit of imagination. One such person informed me that "everything sounds like I'm listening through a pickle." I asked a few more questions to get a better understanding of the problem. The client had a high-frequency loss and the tone control on the aid was turned all the way to H. By rotating the control back towards N while I continued to talk to her, the patient suddenly interrupted, "That's it! The pickle's gone!" We then re-checked speech discrimination and found that she did just as well with the lower frequency response setting. If I had given up trying to figure out what she meant by "listening through a pickle," the client would have remained unhappy.

I try never to let legitimate complaints get me down. Many clients will growl at you when they are angry at the device. I try not to take such remarks personally and do try to translate the complaint into a plan of action. Again, as long as the person has a specific complaint, you have an excellent chance to satisfy him or her. It is the person who is unhappy, and who can't, or won't, tell you why, that causes more problems.

2. The Know-It-ALL

Description: This person can be an irritant by drawing the rasp of misinformation across your nerves. It is the person who states as fact the most jarring of errors. These clients "know" that hearing aids cost $35. They "know" they can hear high frequencies because their stereo "goes to 48,000 decibels." They "know" that they don't have a nerve loss because they aren't nervous. They "know" there is a health food that the hearing aid people don't want you to know about that cures deafness.

Potential Negative Impact: The Know-It-All is merely a buzzing fly in a restaurant. While the major negative impact is primarily annoyance, you may have to spend more time with this client to correct misconceptions so he or she will not repeat them to others.

Relief Strategy: Years ago, I would patiently drag out my charts, diagrams and underlined texts and try to correct all the hearing misconceptions a client would demonstrate. That was years ago. Slowly, it dawned on me that not one of those people thanked me for correcting their faulty thinking. In fact, most of them were mildly irritated while I was trying to sort out their scrambled facts and replace them with correct ones. Then it came home to me. They were not asking me to correct their faulty ideas. They were asking me to correct their faulty hearing. And quickly. As soon as I had absorbed this fact, I was ready to start trimming my unsolicited lecture series. Unless the person has a misconception that is directly connected to his or her successful adjustment to a hearing aid, I am unlikely to offer anything more thoughtful than a nonjudgmental "Oh?" For example:

Client: My sister may need one of these things. We have the same kind of bones and the doc says my ear bone can't be helped.

Me: Oh? *(pause . . . point to the aid)* Now here's how the battery fits in the drawer.

Client: Yeah, I see. Is this the new kind I heard about that lasts forever?

Me: There are two types of batteries recommended for this aid. Either mercury or zinc/air cells will do. Let's look here for expected battery life.

(Please note that if the misconception bears on the client's use of or adjustment to an aid . . . out come the charts and the lecture series.)

3. The Shrewd Operator

Description. This behavior is best described with several examples. Typically, it is the client who knowingly withholds some information until the last possible moment. I guess these clients believe that by laying out all the facts in advance, they have emotionally bared themselves and have no psychic protection. So, in an effort to keep some sort of "control," they wait until a point in the testing to dramatically announce something—usually an announcement they apparently feel will put you, the dispenser, at a disadvantage.

"I don't want to pay for this, of course. The Veterans' Administration takes care of all my medical bills."

"I had a test like this at Prestige University. The guy there said I should get Brand X. How come you just told me to get Brand Y?" (It is not a question. It's an accusation.)

"I really was born five years earlier. How much do you take off for senior citizens?"

Occasionally, the client is simply getting further proof for what he or she thought was a previous faulty exam. Many people in the history-taking deny any previous hearing tests but later say some faulty thing like, "I'm not surprised. That's what Dr. Kildare told me and Dr. Zhivago, too." Forgive them, for they know not what they do. Frightened, confused, anxious . . . either these clients fear that the examiner is unprofessional and will somehow take advantage of them if they play their ace too soon, or they are defensive from life habit brought on by being the victim in such exchanges. Either is unfortunate.

Potential Negative Impact: The Shrewd Operators, like the Know-It-Alls, take more time. If I knew in advance that three doctors told a client the same thing that I just said, I wouldn't have given that lecture. Instead, I would have asked him what he doesn't understand about his hearing problem. If I knew that the client really expects the VA to pay his bills, I could have correctly referred him to the VA Hospital some 90 minutes sooner.

Relief Strategy: If the Know-It-Alls are a fly in a restaurant, the Shrewd Operators are three flies in your kitchen. The additional irritation is because you know that they don't trust you . . . and that hurts. And one more thing. If the client lets you know that he thinks everyone is a crook, he may be justifying that it's O.K. for him to be a crook. Ask any psychologist.

Your best relief from those who try last-minute financial games is to have pre-established policies.

Have a policy about senior citizens.

Have a policy about those properly referred to the VA, State Assistance programs, etc.

Have a policy about deferred payments, out-of-town checks, insufficient funds reported for a check and so on.

For those patients who withhold data out of fear, I make myself vulnerable. I put it in writing. My test results, my fees, my recommendations. This, more than anything I can say, shows we mean what we say.

4. The Shopper

Description: The Shopper is an unhappy person looking for someone to agree with him or her. This person has probably seen four professionals and may easily go to four more to find a more agreeable diagnosis. Shoppers feel they have been dealt an unfair hand and, like Job, are crying out, "Why me?"

The usual Shopper I have seen is a parent looking for a more favorable diagnosis or prognosis for his or her child. I am a parent. I understand such feelings and my heart goes out to these people. As you may have noted from the descriptions, some Shoppers are also Shrewd Operators.

Potential Negative Impact: Like the others in the Light-Weight Problem group, the Shopper takes more time. There is also increased expenditure sending reports to everyone else who has seen the client and to everyone else who is yet to see the client. Our office title for this went to a family who wanted copies of a test I did on their child to be sent to an otologist in Boston, two otologists in Baltimore, three otologists in Philadelphia, two otologists in Lancaster, three audiologic clinics and the child's hearing clinician and school nurse, and one for themselves. That's $2.80 on postage and $0.84 on photocopies, plus envelopes and office time. All of this for an impedance test for which we charged $7.00.

Relief Strategy: So that photocopy and mailing expenses don't become monstrous, you may wish to establish a documents fee for anyone other than the family and/or the referring source.

All of the behaviors listed under Light-Weight Problems respond favorably to extra time from you in explanations. I give freely of that time.

5. The Careless

Description: The careless user will have the hearing aid back in your office three or four times for repair under the original warranty. This person will break off the battery drawers, crack the microphones, overturn the volume controls and snap off the switches. It is interesting that this behavior is sharply reduced after the first time the client has to pay for the repair.

Potential Negative Impact: When you have to pack and mail the same aid under warranty three or four times, postage and insurance cut a deep slice from the profit margin. Worse, this person will frequently return your loaner aid broken and you have the additional expense of mailing, insuring and repairing your loaner aids. This person may even lose your loaners.

Relief Strategy: You may wish to initiate a charge for mailing and more handling. I have thought about it several times when faced with the Careless but have not done so at this writing. When you provide a loaner, you may wish to have a contract for its safe, prompt return in good working condition, or the restoration/replacement costs will be assessed to the user.

6. The Hermit

Description: Hermits are the people who live alone and like it. Dependency, in any form, is anathema to them. Think for a moment how these clients will be about faithful wearing of a prosthesis. They expect to plug an aid into their ear and get instant good hearing on demand—like getting light from a bulb or water from a tap.

Potential Negative Impact: Beginning with this sort of user through those behaviors which follow rated as equal or greater problems for the dispenser, there is increasing risk that the user will return the device. Under FDA rules, this is then a used prosthesis, and the dispenser may either keep it for loaner stock or may re-sell it only if it is reconditioned, and clearly marked that it is a reconditioned device. In my practice, I prefer not to offer reconditioned instruments, so I try very hard not to recommend an aid to someone whose expectation level is for instant success.

Relief Strategy: In the initial meeting with the client, make a point to ask what he or she expects from an aid. This can be your cue to educate the person prior to dispensing the device. Ask the client to describe a typical week in his or her life. If it sounds like a religious order under vows of silence, ask why the client wants to get an aid at all. The answers are frequently very telling.

"Well, I don't want it at all. It's actually for my sister. She wants me to get one. So I'll wear it when she visits," he grins.

He may very well do that. But he won't get the aid from my office. Not with that emotional set. If he doesn't respond favorably to a lengthy and impassioned explanation I give about daily wearing and gradual increase of wearing time—actually a short course in aural rehabilitation—I advise him to go home and think about it. If that doesn't go down too well with him, I suggest that he get the instrument elsewhere. One more aid dispensed won't solve all my financial problems for life, but one less aid dispensed that I strongly see as unacceptable to the client can be a blessing, for not only won't I have the aid returned, I also won't have him telling all his hearing impaired friends just how unhappy he was that he was pressured into an aid at my office.

7. The Impatient

Description: Mr. John Doe has arrived for his appointment 10 minutes late. I see from a note attached to his folder that he has tried twice to get an earlier appointment. He had, in all, a three-day wait. As I go out to greet him, his first words to me are, "Will this take long?"

This is significant, for each time he called he was reminded that the appointment was for an hour and a half.

While I'm taking his history, he checks his watch twice. His fingers are making drum rolls on the table, then on the chair.

Nevertheless, he is still an otherwise excellent candidate for amplification, so we go ahead with the hearing aid evaluation and the recommendation of an aid. He accepts the idea and an earmold impression is prepared. When informed that everything, i.e., medical clearance, the earmold and the recommended device, will be ready in about 10 days, he looks stunned and says that he thought he could walk out with one of the aids he tried.

Again, this is significant. He is referring to "one of the aids I tried" when I have been spending the last 20 minutes referring to a specific instrument.

The Impatient are poor listeners and worse in following directions. When we do call him to set up the appointment to get the device, he will probably call a few days later to re-schedule the time because "something came up."

Potential Negative Impact: Frequently personable and well-meaning, this client can cause the dispenser problems because he or she is too busy to take the slow steps needed for successful adaptation to amplification. The risk for a returned aid is proportionately higher with this client. You may need additional counselling time, as the client will not remember much of what you have tried to get across.

Relief Strategy: When I sense that I'm face-to-face with the White Rabbit, the one who cries, "I'm late! I'm late! For a very important date!" my own speech . . . slows . . . down . . . a . . . bit. As speaking softly will effectively tone down a shouting child, slowing down your rate of speech may have a calming effect on this behavior. When the client is as calmed as you can get him or her, explain frankly your concern about the ability to stick to a slow, deliberate adjustment schedule. The client will then probably not disappoint you. A challenge to this person is like oxygen, food and water. This person *needs* challenges. Let your impatient clients show you they are able to do what you have doubted that they could.

8. The Liar

Description: This is not the person who, on re-telling a fish story, makes the fish a little bigger each time.

This is the person who walks in unannounced for an appointment and tries to brass it through by saying, "I know your girl gave me this time." There is no way my "girl" could have done that. My "girl" is my wife, who carefully blocked out the time this woman claims is hers for my dentist appointment six months ago.

This is also the person who, after having been advised weeks ago that payment is due upon receipt of the aid, says, "I'm so embarrassed! I forgot my checkbook. Let me take the aid home right now and I'll be right back with the check," when we had a phone call not 10 minutes before her arrival from her husband, who wanted to know how long this was going to take because the moving van was ready to roll.

Years ago, when I was working at a community agency, a hearing aid dealer asked me why I didn't start up my own office and sell hearing aids. I was quite candid with him and said that my concern was about the professional image (then) of hearing aid dealers and that I wouldn't want to be in a situation in which the public might think I was trying to (bleep) them. He roared with laughter and said, "If you ever do dispense aids, you'll be too busy trying to keep the public from (bleep)ing you." He was referring to the Liars.

A young woman once told us she "forgot" the check her mother filled out for her. "I remember, she filled out the whole amount and left it on the kitchen table just before she left to visit her sister in Baltimore." I apologized for her inconvenience but asked her to bring us the check before we could turn over the aid. She sighed and flounced out of the office after asking us to include an extra pack of batteries. She returned a half hour later. We were quite impressed with the clairvoyance of the mother, who not only "filled out the whole amount" before leaving for Baltimore, but predicted that her daughter would ask for another pack of batteries and correctly included their cost on the check. I admit, this is only circumstantial evidence that the daughter was lying . . . but we were wise to protect ourselves, whatever her reason.

Potential Negative Impact: Liars can impact with financial loss. The least they can do is disrupt your scheduling. If you permit it to happen, Liars can cause you to spend much of your energy in trying to track down who really said what to whom.

Relief Strategy: To prevent payment problems, have a firm policy of payment for the prosthesis upon delivery to the client. Another way would be to accept any of the various bank credit cards for payment. Your payment is thus guaranteed, but for a percentage fee.

For those who attempt to push into a different appointment time, we let them . . . with this exception: those who have valid appointments are seen first. I apologize to the client with the bogus appointment, but he or she waits until I have seen the others. After all, it is at least a possibility that the person heard the wrong time or day. We try to be as charitable as possible, but usually the client tells us enough conflicting data that we see the story for what it is.

Occasionally a client will quote someone as saying or doing something that reflects directly on your practice in a negative manner. Our policy is to ignore it on the first telling, but if we hear the report again from another source, I directly contact the person quoted and say something like, "I heard from a client that you allegedly said this, that and so. How can we work together to prevent this sort of false rumor from starting?"

From all the above, one may get the idea that this behavior problem is a significant part of a dispensing practice. In my case it isn't. I have seen this behavior maybe six times in five years relative to payment, and perhaps a dozen times for appointment changes. However, you tend to remember this person a lot more than the 200 previous grateful and satisfied users.

The middle-weight problems, like the light-weight ones, take dispenser time. However, for the light-weight problems, time (in the form of prolonged explanations) is often the prevention or the cure. For middle-weight problems you need time, but you also need office policies and preventive techniques.

9. The Pressured

Description: At first glance, the pressured client seems like the Impatient, but with this important difference. Impatient people put their burden on themselves. As soon as a project is finished, they rush into another task of their choosing. For the Pressured, events beyond their control place additional tasks upon already overburdened humans. A breakdown is only a short distance away.

This is your Pressured Man. Retired recently and living in a new apartment, he expected to sit at home, watch TV, read and putter in the summer garden plot the landlord provides for the tenants. Instead, his wife has a myocardial infarction. He is poorly prepared to take over the home, cook, clean, visit his wife twice a day in the or hospital and cope with his feeling of dread. His transmission is acting up on his seven-year-old car. A daughter, recently divorced, offers to "come home to help," but they end up with daily fights concerning her lifestyle. Her boyfriend, whom her father can't stand, has been laid off and asks to move in with her. When Mr. Pressured says "No!" the daughter threatens to leave. His pastor tells him to forgive his daughter. His former son-in-law gets drunk a few times each week and makes late-night phone calls—calls the daughter won't accept—so Mr. Pressured accepts the call, out of loyalty to his grandchild, who stayed with his father, and then listens to a drunken litany from his former son-in-law.

Meanwhile, his arthritis is flaring up with all the emotional tension he is under, and the pain is robbing him of needed sleep each on night. Then word comes from the hospital. His wife is not responding as well as they had hoped. His visits are to be limited to five minutes, once a day. When he sees her in her weakened, drugged condition, he can barely hear her. One evening, at home, he opens his mail and learns that the apartment is going condominium. When he visits his wife the next day, he decides not to tell her the news about the condo. Again he can barely hear her. On his way home, he impulsively stops by my office and takes the first open time for a hearing aid evaluation. This is a very Pressured Man.

Potential Negative Impact: The drive of the Pressured Patient is their downfall. They simply try to do more than is humanly possible. They are like tragic figures in a Greek classic, mere mortals locked in combat with overwhelming events. They don't mean to cause you any problems. But as their world disintegrates, the hearing aid purchased in good faith is the first thing that goes.

In my first year of private practice, I had to make refunds on four hearing aids. All were from Pressured clients. There is a cynical definition of a fanatic. It is a person who, when the cause is hopeless, redoubles his or her efforts. This is what happens with the Pressured. They will beg you to get the aid. But it takes a low-pressure or no-pressure existence to adjust to amplified living most of the time.

Relief Strategy: The best way to avoid the returned aid of the Pressured client is to resist the pleas that he or she must have one "right away." I beg this person to wait until life is more tranquil. If the person insists, then I provide a loaner device until we know for certain whether he or she can use one.

10. The I'll-Show-You'er

Description: The daughter shoots a meaningful glance to me as her mother misunderstands my question. I repeat the question with different phrasing and the mother answers in a flat, detached voice. When the mother is in the booth, the daughter spills out the story. They haven't been particularly close. Mother is getting to be even more of a cross to bear since everyone must shout at her and repeat things. The mother recently had to move in with the daughter, which increased the tension. The daughter feels guilty about their relationship and wants to buy off the guilt by purchasing a hearing aid for her mother. When they return for the recommended instrument, the daughter says, "Mother, I just know you're going to love this aid."

Mother slowly turns to me. Her eyes narrow. A thin, tight smile creases her mouth while her head bobs slowly up and down. She is no doubt thinking, "I'll show you!" On the 29th day of our purchase-option agreement, the daughter brings back the aid for a refund.

Here is another. Jean makes an appointment for Ralph. He drags himself to our office, but it is Jean who interrupts him with all the answers to my questions. When I ask Ralph how he feels about the possible use of an aid, he shrugs. In a while, we have made a specific recommendation. Jean is ecstatic.

Ralph is non-committal. I bluntly ask him if he would just like to think about it. Before he can answer, Jean is off and running a mile a minute to say that she knows that Ralph will just love it. Ralph turns to look at Jean with a totally bland expression. He is very skilled at hiding his true feelings from her. Jean's final statement is, "Aw, honey, just try it." Ralph shrugs. Two days later, Ralph walks into my office and lays the aid on the counter. "Well," he smirks, "I tried."

Potential Negative Impact: The vengeful are not out to get you. They are out to blast their daughters and their Jeans. If the force of their explosion should wound a few innocent bystanders, well, that's kismet as far as they are concerned. To dispense an unwanted aid is very risky. I have quite enough loaners, thank you, and I don't wish to perjure myself with the FDA by trying to pass the instrument back to the manufacturer as unused.

Relief Strategy: To keep this sort of shrapnel out of your office, only accept the word of the potential user in those situations. If the mother is indifferent, don't provide the aid but encourage her to think about it. Believe me, the daughter will provide sufficient pressure. When Ralph couldn't care less, we simply tell him what his options are and close the file unless we hear from him again. For minors, however, follow the parental direction.

11. The Thief

Description: None, I suspect. Thieves have no telltale behavior clues that are a dead giveaway, but successful Liars may easily become Thieves. Within my first four months of practice, we were hit by a successful Liar who conned me out of an audiometric examination, a hearing aid evaluation, an earmold and a hearing aid. She was, to my naive first impression, the perfect client. She praised the testing. "Wasn't it wonderful. Wasn't it marvelous? My, you must have to study so hard." She artfully stroked every ego need of mine. The aid, to hear her rave about it, was a gift from God. It was perfect. On and on she went. She would have my name in her prayers every night. How lucky she was to have found me, etc., etc.

Then she left the fitting room and stopped at the front desk to make the payment. She rummaged around in her cavernous handbag for nearly five minutes. With eyes misting and her lower lip aquiver, she said that she'd left her checkbook in her other purse. I discreetly nodded to Sandy, who told her that it was O.K., she could bring it in later or mail it to us.

"Oh, God bless you, folks! Oh, you are so good to me!"

It was the last time we ever heard directly from her. We did get some indirect contact several months later, when our collection service caught up with her. She had moved twice since our last contact, and the collection service wanted us to know that she had been located and advised of her debt. And, reported the collection service, "You'll be interested to know that she's telling everyone you sold her the aid against her will, and further, the instrument is defective." When the collection service tried to contact her again, she had once again skipped with no forwarding address.

This was our only major hit by a Thief. I do not count two bad checks, as in both cases full restitution was made. We have had a few minor events. This usually involves testing only and, in every case the client either skipped or gave a bogus address initially.

Potential Negative Impact: Theft, as described above, is financial loss for the dispenser.

Relief Strategy: We have not had this as a major problem. It may be a function of geography. I don't know if this is a major problem in other parts of the country. Since the time we were initially taken for the cost of an aid, we insist, politely, on payment at time of delivery. I don't know how to cope with the occasional client who ducks a testing fee without initiating police state preventive procedures that may be offensive to the vast majority of honest people. As with heavy-weight problems, while they are quite infrequent, you tend to remember them with disproportionate passion.

12. The Disturbed

Description: Various mental health associations tell us that 1 of 10 people will need counselling at some point in life. You may then wonder if a hundred of your first thousand clients may not cause you concern because of their emotional state. It is certainly hoped that no one ever has that experience.

In five years, there were two clients who I felt had disturbed personalities . . . that is, disturbed in a manner that had a direct bearing on their adjustment to amplification. I freely admit that my area of expertise is not psychology, so my terminology "disturbed personalities" may be open to question if not attack. For that reason the descriptions are heavily disguised.

My first Disturbed client was a middle-aged male whose testing, fitting and purchase of a hearing aid was most unremarkable. However, in his third month of use, he made an appointment for a recheck, stating that the device was no longer of benefit. All the retesting produced identical results to those when we recommended the aid. The device checked out on the acoustic analyzer. Client aided discrimination was 88%, while unaided was 52%. He was counselled and discharged. Three days later he was back again. Very carefully, I listened to his description of what he felt the problem was.

In brief, he said that the aid wasn't working. Once again we demonstrated to him that he had improved speech comprehension while wearing the device. Then I got my first inkling that something was disturbed in his personality. He looked at me for nearly a half minute in silence when I concluded my counsel and at last he said, "You have tricked me with your machine." Without another word he left. He did stop at the front desk and offered sympathy to Sandy that she must work "for such a trickster." Then he left. I thought that was the end of it. I was wrong.

For the next 15 months, I was periodically bothered to write detailed, documented, notarized accounts of his testing, subsequent purchase and all related events to several professional societies that were investigating his complaint, and to respond to an inquiry from the hearing aid manufacturer. I was seething! And I could have avoided it all. I had been briefly in touch with this client one more time by phone, and I asked him what he expected me to do. His answer was simple. "Give me all my money back."

Twenty-seven generations of Scottish blood in my veins turned to granite. Never! The aid was quite suitable. He already had it for seven months! Never!

And so we sparred around and around. How much easier it would have been to write the check and go on with life. I had made a bad move, but I am educable and the next time it happened, I was better prepared. Again, initial testing and purchase were unremarkable, but I felt something was peculiar without being able to say what it was. Slowly a pattern developed. Little things would "act up" on the aid worn by the client, a middle-thirtyish computer operator. More significantly, everything she described didn't make acoustic sense. With low frequencies emphasized, she said it sounded hollow and rumbled. The ear-mold was described as getting "tighter and tighter" while I was buffing more surface from it each time, until feedback appeared and we had to make a new mold. Not once did I detect any sign of irritation on her pinna or canal.

During each appointment, she would keep trying to report about her sex life with a variety of lovers and I told her repeatedly that I was not trained to offer advice in that matter. Then I would re-direct her comments to the aid and her hearing. At that point, her observations would defy reason.

"I could hear [a boyfriend] just fine until we get into an argument, then I could never understand another word he ever said from that moment on." She insisted that she couldn't hear anyone at work "but as soon as I leave the office, it turned back on, y'know?" A week later, her story was that it only worked for her in the office, but it shut off when she was out of the office.

Meanwhile, the device continued to check out within specifications on the acoustic analyzer, and her aided speech discrimination in field continued to be 100%. In the fourth month of looking for a solution, she popped into my office without an appointment and asked, "Whatcha gonna do?"

I looked at her for a moment and said that I wasn't smart enough to know what to do to help. How would she like all of her money back? She grinned for the first time in months, pulled the aid from her ear and placed it on my desk. As soon as I handed the check to her, she was out the door like an Olympic sprinter.

Potential Negative Impact: Take your pick. We have loss of time and money. We have frustration, anger, rage and worry. If you believe that you're innocent in the U.S. until proven guilty, it means you haven't had to address the frivolous charges of a Disturbed client who pushes a consumer alert button.

Relief Strategy: When I get that little hunch that tells me something is very strange with the client, I take twice the time I normally spend to find out why the person wants an aid and what he or she expects from it. Try to read the person's mood. In retrospect, both of those clients struck me like poor actors on a stage. I was conscious that they were "acting" during the testing, but since I felt that the audiogram was valid, I attached no significance to that fact.

For protection, we document every procedure in this office and keep careful records on everything. One more thing . . . I am much quicker to refuse "strange" cases and much quicker to cancel the contract and offer the refund.

*   *   *

This list of 12 behaviors may threaten someone who is considering a private dispensing practice. Don't let it get to you. While the list increases in the amount of problem to the dispenser, the frequency of occurrence decreases for each increase in the degree of aggravation.

Of the clients seen in my dispensing practice, less than 6% are "problems," and of that number, the majority are complainers—the first of the light-weights.

This was an attempt to describe the behaviors that bring problems to a dispensing practice. At this writing, I am unaware of another intra-professional source of this information. As some career decisions may be made on the basis of this information, I hope this may mark the start of the profession's acknowledgment of these behavior problems and the sharing of techniques to cope with them.

H. F. M.

Index